Cognitive Behavioral Therapy

Guest Editor

BUNMI O. OLATUNJI, PhD

PSYCHIATRIC CLINICS OF NORTH AMERICA

www.psych.theclinics.com

September 2010 • Volume 33 • Number 3

SAUNDERS an imprint of ELSEVIER, Inc.

W.B. SAUNDERS COMPANY
A Division of Elsevier Inc.

1600 John F. Kennedy Boulevard ● Suite 1800 ● Philadelphia, PA 19103-2899

http://www.theclinics.com

PSYCHIATRIC CLINICS OF NORTH AMERICA Volume 33, Number 3
September 2010 ISSN 0193-953X, ISBN-13: 978-1-4377-2491-2

Editor: Sarah E. Barth

Psychiatric Clinics of North America (ISSN 0193-953X) is published quarterly by Elsevier Inc., 360 Park Avenue South, New York, NY 10010-1710. Months of issue are March, June, September, and December. Business and Editorial Offices: 1600 John F. Kennedy Blvd., Suite 1800, Philadelphia, PA 19103-2899. Periodicals postage paid at New York, NY and additional mailing offices. Subscription prices are $248.00 per year (US individuals), $430.00 per year (US institutions), $125.00 per year (US students/residents), $297.00 per year (Canadian individuals), $535.00 per year (Canadian Institutions), $369.00 per year (foreign individuals), $535.00 per year (foreign institutions), and $185.00 per year (international & Canadian students/residents). Foreign air speed delivery is included in all *Clinics'* subscription prices. All prices are subject to change without notice. **POSTMASTER:** Send address changes to *Psychiatric Clinics of North America*, Elsevier Health Sciences Division, Subscription Customer Service, 3251 Riverport Lane, Maryland Heights, MO 63043. Customer Service: 1-800-654-2452 (US). From outside the United States, call 1-314-447-8871. Fax: 1-314-447-8029. E-mail: journalscustomerservice-usa@elsevier.com (for print support) and journalsonlinesupport-usa@elsevier.com (for online support).

Reprints. For copies of 100 or more, of articles in this publication, please contact the Commercial Reprints Department, Elsevier Inc., 360 Park Avenue South, New York, New York 10010-1710. Tel.: (212) 633-3813, Fax: (212) 462-1935, E-mail: reprints@elsevier.com.

Psychiatric Clinics of North America is covered in *MEDLINE/PubMed (Index Medicus)*, *Current Contents/Social and Behavioral Sciences, Social Science Citation Index, Embase/Excerpta Medica,* and PsycINFO.

Printed and bound by CPI Group (UK) Ltd, Croydon, CR0 4YY

Transferred to Digital Print 2012

Contributors

GUEST EDITOR

BUNMI O. OLATUNJI, PhD
Assistant Professor, Department of Psychology, Vanderbilt University,
Nashville, Tennessee

AUTHORS

LESLEY A. ALLEN, PhD
Associate Professor, Department of Psychiatry, Robert Wood Johnson Medical School,
University of Medicine and Dentistry of New Jersey, Piscataway, New Jersey

KIMBERLY A. BABSON, MA
Department of Psychology, University of Arkansas, Fayetteville, Arkansas

CHRISTAL L. BADOUR, BA
Department of Psychology, University of Arkansas, Fayetteville, Arkansas

ANNIE N. BANDUCCI, BA
Center for Addictions, Personality, and Emotion Research; Department of Psychology,
University of Maryland, College Park, Maryland

DANIELLE A. BLACK, PhD
The Family Institute at Northwestern University, Evanston, Illinois

STEPHANIE BOTH, PhD
Outpatient Clinic for Psychosomatic Gynecology and Sexology (VRSP), Leiden University
Medical Center, Poortgebouw-Zuid, Leiden, The Netherlands

JOSH M. CISLER, MA
Predoctoral Fellow, Department of Psychiatry and Behavioral Sciences, National Crime
Victims Research and Treatment Center, Medical University of South Carolina,
Charleston, South Carolina

ZAFRA COOPER, DPhil, DipPsych
Department of Psychiatry, Warneford Hospital, Oxford University, Oxford,
United Kingdom

BRETT J. DEACON, PhD
Assistant Professor, Department of Psychology, University of Wyoming,
Laramie, Wyoming

ELLEN DRIESSEN, MSc
Faculty of Psychology and Education, Department of Clinical Psychology,
VU University Amsterdam, Amsterdam, The Netherlands

CHRISTOPHER G. FAIRBURN, DM, FMedSci, FRCPsych
Department of Psychiatry, Warneford Hospital, Oxford University, Oxford, United Kingdom

ANGELA FANG, BA
Department of Psychology, Boston University, Boston, Massachusetts

MATTHEW T. FELDNER, PhD
Department of Psychology, University of Arkansas, Fayetteville, Arkansas

CHRISTOPH FLÜCKIGER, PhD
Department of Clinical Psychology and Psychotherapy, The University of Bern, Bern, Switzerland

SHANA A. FRANKLIN, BA
Psychology Department, The University of Wisconsin-Milwaukee, Milwaukee, Wisconsin

K.A. GANASEN, MBChB
Department of Psychiatry, University of Cape Town, Cape Town, South Africa

BRIDGET A. HEARON, MA
Graduate Research Assistant, Department of Psychology, Boston University, Boston, Massachusetts

STEFAN G. HOFMANN, PhD
Department of Psychology, Boston University, Boston, Massachusetts

STEVEN D. HOLLON, PhD
Professor, Department of Psychology and Psychiatry, Vanderbilt University, Nashville, Tennessee

CHRISTOPHER J. HOPWOOD, PhD
Assistant Professor of Psychology, Department of Psychology, Michigan State University, East Lansing, Michigan

J.C. IPSER, MA
Department of Psychiatry, University of Cape Town, Cape Town, South Africa

DAVID KINGDON, MD, FRCPsych
Professor of Mental Health Care Delivery, Department of Psychiatry, University of Southampton, Royal South Hants Hospital, Southampton, Hampshire, United Kingdom

LAURA E. KNOUSE, PhD
Clinical Fellow in Psychology, Behavioral Medicine Service, Department of Psychiatry, Massachusetts General Hospital and Harvard Medical School, Boston, Massachusetts

C.W. LEJUEZ, PhD
Director, Center for Addictions, Personality and Emotion Research; Professor of Psychology, Department of Psychology, University of Maryland, College Park, Maryland

NEHJLA M. MASHAL, MA
Department of Psychology, Northwestern University, Evanston, Illinois

ALEXIS K. MATUSIEWICZ, BA
Center for Addictions, Personality and Emotion Research; Department of Psychology, University of Maryland, College Park, Maryland

R. KATHRYN MCHUGH, MA
Graduate Research Assistant, Department of Psychology, Boston University, Boston, Massachusetts

REBECCA MURPHY, DClinPsych
Department of Psychiatry, Warneford Hospital, Oxford University, Oxford, United Kingdom

BUNMI O. OLATUNJI, PhD
Assistant Professor, Department of Psychology, Vanderbilt University, Nashville, Tennessee

MICHAEL W. OTTO, PhD
Professor, Department of Psychology, Boston University, Boston, Massachusetts

PETER PHIRI, BSc
Researcher, Royal South Hants Hospital, Southampton, Hampshire, United Kingdom

SHANAYA RATHOD, MD, MRCPsych
Consultant Psychiatrist and Associate Medical Director, Hampshire Partnership NHS Foundation Trust, Winchester, Hampshire, United Kingdom

STEVEN A. SAFREN, PhD
Associate Professor, Harvard Medical School; Director, Behavioral Medicine, Department of Psychiatry, Massachusetts General Hospital, Boston, Massachusetts

ALICE T. SAWYER, MA
Department of Psychology, Boston University, Boston, Massachusetts

D.J. STEIN, MD, PhD
Department of Psychiatry, University of Cape Town, Cape Town, South Africa

SUZANNE STRAEBLER, APRN - Psychiatry, MSN
Department of Psychiatry, Warneford Hospital, Oxford University, Oxford, United Kingdom

MONIEK M. TER KUILE, PhD
Outpatient Clinic for Psychosomatic Gynecology and Sexology (VRSP), Leiden University Medical Center, Poortgebouw-Zuid, Leiden, The Netherlands

JACQUES J.D.M. VAN LANKVELD, PhD
Faculty of Psychology and Neuroscience, Department of Clinical Psychological Science, Maastricht University, Maastricht, The Netherlands

MICHAEL R. WALTHER, MS
Psychology Department, The University of Wisconsin-Milwaukee, Milwaukee, Wisconsin

DOUGLAS W. WOODS, PhD
Psychology Department, The University of Wisconsin-Milwaukee, Milwaukee, Wisconsin

ROBERT L. WOOLFOLK, PhD
Professor, Department of Psychology, Rutgers University; Visiting Professor, Department of Psychology, Princeton University, Princeton, New Jersey

RICHARD E. ZINBARG, PhD
Department of Psychology, Northwestern University; The Family Institute at Northwestern University, Evanston, Illinois

Contents

> Attention-deficit/hyperactivity disorder (ADHD) is a valid and impairing psychological disorder that persists into adulthood in a majority of cases and is associated with chronic functional impairment and increased rates of comorbidity. Cognitive behavioral therapy (CBT) approaches for this disorder have emerged recently, and available evidence from open and randomized controlled trials suggests that these approaches are promising in producing significant symptom reduction. A conceptual model of how CBT may work for ADHD is reviewed along with existing efficacy studies. A preliminary comparison of effect sizes across intervention packages suggests that targeted learning and practice of specific behavioral compensatory strategies may be a critical active ingredient in CBT for adult ADHD. The article concludes with a discussion of future directions and critical questions that must be addressed in this area of clinical research.

> Cognitive behavioral therapy (CBT) for substance use disorders has shown efficacy as a monotherapy and as part of combination treatment strategies. This article provides a review of the evidence supporting the use of CBT, clinical elements of its application, novel treatment strategies for improving treatment response, and dissemination efforts. Although CBT for substance abuse is characterized by heterogeneous treatment elements such as operant learning strategies, cognitive and motivational elements, and skills-building interventions, across protocols several core elements emerge that focus on overcoming the powerfully reinforcing effects of psychoactive substances. These elements, and support for their efficacy, are discussed.

> Cognitive behavioral therapy (CBT) complements medication management and evidence has shown its effectiveness in managing positive and negative symptoms, promoting treatment resistance, and improving insight, compliance, and aggression in schizophrenia. There is emerging evidence in early intervention, comorbid substance misuse, and reducing relapse and hospitalization. CBT is now recommended by most clinical guidelines for schizophrenia. Treatment is based on engaging the patient in a therapeutic

relationship, developing an agreed formulation, and then the use of a range of techniques for hallucinations, delusions, and negative symptoms. This article gives an overview of the current status of CBT for schizophrenia.

Cognitive behavioral therapy (CBT) is efficacious in the acute treatment of depression and may provide a viable alternative to antidepressant medication (ADM) for even more severely depressed unipolar patients when implemented in a competent fashion. CBT also may be of use as an adjunct to medication treatment of bipolar patients, although there have been few studies and they are not wholly consistent. CBT does seem to have an enduring effect that protects against subsequent relapse and recurrence following the end of active treatment, which is not the case for medications. Single studies that require replication suggest that patients who are married or unemployed or who have more antecedent life events may do better in CBT than in ADM, as might patients who are free from comorbid Axis II disorders, whereas patients with comorbid Axis II disorders seem to do better in ADM than in CBT. There also are indications that CBT may work through processes specified by theory to produce change in cognition that in turn mediate subsequent change in depression and freedom from relapse following treatment termination, although evidence in that regard is not yet conclusive.

Numerous clinical trials have supported the efficacy of cognitive behavioral therapy (CBT) for the treatment of anxiety disorders. Accordingly, CBT has been formally recognized as an empirically supported treatment for anxiety-related conditions. This article reviews the evidence supporting the efficacy of CBT for anxiety disorders. Specifically, contemporary meta-analytic studies on the treatment of anxiety disorders are reviewed and the efficacy of CBT is examined. Although the specific components of CBT differ depending on the study design and the anxiety disorder treated, meta-analyses suggest that CBT procedures (particularly exposure-based approaches) are highly efficacious. CBT generally outperforms wait-list and placebo controls. Thus, CBT provides incremental efficacy above and beyond nonspecific factors. For some anxiety disorders, CBT also tends to outperform other psychosocial treatment modalities. The implications of available meta-analytic findings in further delineating the efficacy and dissemination of CBT for anxiety disorders are discussed.

Patients presenting with somatoform disorders often incur excessive health care charges and fail to respond to standard treatment. The purpose of this article is to provide an overview of the diagnostic criteria and demographic and clinical characteristics of each somatoform disorder and to examine the research assessing the efficacy of cognitive behavioral therapy (CBT) for each disorder. The review shows that CBT has received some empirical support for somatization, hypochondriasis, and body dysmorphic disorder. However, there are few data on the impact of treatment on health care use, especially when the cost of CBT is factored into the equation. Too few methodologically sound studies have been published on the treatment of conversion disorder or of pain disorder to make any conclusions.

Sexual dysfunctions in women are classified into disorders of desire, arousal, orgasm, and pain (including dyspareunia and vaginismus). As the cognitive behavioral treatment (CBT) procedures differ among these sexual disorders, the treatments for each disorder are reviewed separately. The efficacy of CBT differs depending on the specific sexual dysfunction to be treated. It is concluded that only a few CBT treatments for women's sexual dysfunction have yet been empirically investigated in a methodologically sound way and little is known about which of the treatment components are most effective.

Cognitive behavioral therapy (CBT) is the leading evidence-based treatment for bulimia nervosa. A new "enhanced" version of the treatment appears to be more potent and has the added advantage of being suitable for all eating disorders, including anorexia nervosa and eating disorder not otherwise specified. This article reviews the evidence supporting CBT in the treatment of eating disorders and provides an account of the "transdiagnostic" theory that underpins the enhanced form of the treatment. It ends with an outline of the treatment's main strategies and procedures.

More than 70 million people in the United States experience primary insomnia (PI) at some point in their life, resulting in an estimated $65 billion in health care costs and lost productivity. PI is therefore one of the most common health care problems in the United States. To mollify the negative effects of PI, scholars have sought to evaluate and improve treatments of this costly health care problem. A breadth of research has demonstrated that cognitive behavioral therapy (CBT) is an effective intervention for PI. The goal of this article is to provide an overview of CBT for PI, including evidence regarding treatment efficacy, effectiveness, and practitioner considerations.

A variety of treatment approaches have been used to manage tic symptoms in Tourette syndrome and other tic disorders. Pharmacological interventions remain the most common approach, but in the past 3 decades, various nonpharmacological treatment options have emerged including: (1) massed practice, (2) relaxation training, (3) self-monitoring, (4) function-based/contingency management procedures, (5) habit reversal training, (6) exposure and response prevention, and (7) cognitive behavior therapy. Each of these procedures is described along with the evidence reflecting its efficacy and usefulness. A synthesis of the findings and implications is provided, including directions and recommendations for future treatment and research.

This article provides a comprehensive review of cognitive behavioral therapy (CBT) treatments for personality disorders (PDs), including a description of the available treatments and empirical support, drawing on research published between 1980 and 2009. Research generally supports the conclusion that CBT is an effective treatment modality for reducing symptoms and enhancing functional outcomes among patients with PDs, thereby making it a useful framework for clinicians working with patients with PD symptomatology. There is a clear need, however, to develop and evaluate CBT in order to provide specific and more unambiguous treatment recommendations with particular relevance for understudied PDs.

There has long been interest in combining pharmacotherapy with psychotherapy, including cognitive behavioral therapy (CBT). More recently, basic research on fear extinction has led to interest in augmentation of CBT with the N-methyl Daspartate (NMDA) glutamate receptor partial agonist D-cycloserine (DCS) for anxiety disorders. In this article, the literature on clinical trials that have combined pharmacotherapy and CBT is briefly reviewed, focusing particularly on the anxiety disorders. The literature on CBT and DCS is then systematically reviewed. A series of randomized placebo-controlled trials on panic disorder, obsessive-compulsive disorder, social anxiety disorder, and specific phobia suggest that low dose DCS before therapy sessions may be more effective compared with CBT alone in certain anxiety disorders. The strong translational foundation of this work is compelling, and the positive preliminary data gathered so far encourage further work. Issues for future research include delineating optimal dosing, and demonstrating effectiveness in real-world settings.

This article reviews the current state of empirical research on the purported "new wave" of cognitive behavioral therapy (CBT). A particular emphasis is given to mindfulness-based treatments and acceptance and commitment therapy (ACT). Mindfulness-based approaches and ACT are evaluated with regard to their efficacy and comparison with traditional CBT. Deviations from CBT are explained within the context of theory, specifically in terms of the role of cognitions. These differences, however, are not irreconcilable in requiring a separate classification of "new wave" treatments. While subtle and important differences on the theoretical and procedural level might exist, available data do not favor one treatment over another, and do not suggest differential mechanisms of action that warrant a dramatic separation from the CBT family of approaches. Instead, the "new wave" treatments are consistent with the CBT approach, which refers to a family of interventions rather than a single treatment. Thus, the term "new wave" is potentially misleading because it is not an accurate reflection of the contemporary literature.

The Academy for Psychological Clinical Science and the independent accrediting entity it created, the Psychological Clinical Science Accreditation system, have recently launched a movement aimed at reforming all of clinical psychology. If this movement is successful, it will result in a greater emphasis on empirical science in the practice of clinical psychology. As cognitive behavioral therapy (CBT) is the approach that currently has the greatest number of controlled scientific studies supporting it, this should be an impetus for CBT to grow. The very same scientific evidence that supports the efficacy of CBT, however, also shows that CBT is far from fully efficacious. Several recent trends that hold great promise to enhance the effectiveness of CBT are discussed, such as greater integration of CBT with biological approaches, cognitive science, systemic approaches, motivational interviewing, and strengths-based approaches.

THE CLINICS ARE NOW AVAILABLE ONLINE!

Access your subscription at:
www.theclinics.com

Preface: The Current Status of Cognitive Behavioral Therapy for Psychiatric Disorders

Bunmi O. Olatunji, PhD[a], Steven D. Hollon, PhD[b]

KEYWORDS

- Cognitive behavioral therapy • Psychological disorders
- Efficacy • Dissemination

Cognitive behavioral therapy (CBT) is one of the most extensively researched psychotherapies and is increasingly being recognized as the gold standard for many psychological disorders.[1] CBT is now regarded as the psychological treatment of choice by many as managed care organizations are necessarily interested in ensuring that clinicians provide the most effective and least extensive, intensive, intrusive, and costly interventions. Although early implementations of CBT were largely indicated for anxiety and mood disorders,[2] more recent clinical and research efforts have begun to develop CBT for an increasingly wider range of problems. The diverse range of disorders covered in this special issue reflects the significant advances that have been made over the years in the application of CBT. Indeed, disorders traditionally considered resistant to psychotherapy (eg, hypochondriasis) are now conceptualized within a cognitive (ie, dysfunctional beliefs) and behavioral (ie, safety-seeking) framework and the CBT treatment derived from this model has produced encouraging results.[3] Although the empirical evidence supporting the efficacy of CBT is very promising,[4] there remains a noticeable gap between the evidence and clinical use of CBT among practitioners.

BROADLY DEFINING THE PRACTICE OF CBT

CBT generally refers to interventions that use behavioral and cognitive techniques and are derived from scientifically supported theoretical models.[5] Although the actual

[a] Department of Psychology, Vanderbilt University, 301 Wilson Hall, 111 21st Avenue South, Nashville, TN 37203, USA
[b] Department of Psychology and Psychiatry, Vanderbilt University, 301 Wilson Hall, 111 21st Avenue South, Nashville, TN 37203, USA
E-mail addresses: olubunmi.o.olatunji@vanderbilt.edu (B.O. Olatunji); steven.d.hollon@vanderbilt.edu (S.D. Hollon).

Psychiatr Clin N Am 33 (2010) xiii–xix
doi:10.1016/j.psc.2010.04.015

mechanism underlying the effectiveness of CBT for a broad range of disorders is not well understood, CBT operates under the assumption that psychological disorders are mediated by distorted cognitions and maladaptive behaviors. Thus, symptoms of various disorders can be improved by modifying the cognitions and behaviors that led to their development. The practice of CBT is collaborative, structured, and goal oriented[1] and current forms of CBT target core components of a given disorder. For example, CBT interventions for panic disorder target catastrophic misinterpretations of somatic sensations of panic and their perceived consequences, and exposure procedures focus directly on the fear of somatic sensations. CBT is typically delivered over the course of 12 to 20 sessions. Treatment begins with a thorough evaluation of the presenting problem and this initial evaluation consists of a detailed functional analysis of symptoms. Although the assessment may require some consideration of past events, such information is generally gathered only if it is directly relevant to the solution of here-and-now problems.

A key feature of CBT is the establishment of a strong, collaborative working relationship with the patient. This is often initiated in the context of educating the patient about the nature of the disorder, explaining the CBT model of the etiology and maintenance of the disorder and the intervention derived from the model. Psychoeducation that includes information on the course of treatment may also enhance patient motivation for change as well as the determination of clear treatment goals. To gather information on the patient's symptoms, patients are taught how to monitor their symptoms. Self-monitoring helps patients become aware of the timing and occurrence of target symptoms, providing additional information on potential opportunities for intervention. CBT also places emphasis on systematic monitoring of symptom change. This may take the form of having a patient's complete objective symptoms measured throughout the course of treatment. This provides an objective assessment of symptoms relative to established norms, which symptoms have improved, and which symptoms require more attention. Monitoring outcome can also help guide the clinician with regard to case formulation or consideration of alternative CBT interventions if expected treatment goals are not achieved.

At the beginning of each treatment session, an agenda is set with input from the patient. Particular attention is given to events that occurred since the previous session that are relevant to the patient's goals for treatment. Part of the agenda for the treatment sessions should focus on anticipating difficulties that may occur before the next treatment session. These difficulties should then be discussed in the context of problem solving and the implementation of necessary cognitive and behavioral skills. Although the specific interventions used during CBT may vary, the decision on which interventions to use should be informed by cognitive and learning theories that view disorders within a framework of reciprocally connected behaviors, thoughts, and emotions that are activated and influenced by environmental and interpersonal events. CBT is also a very active treatment with an emphasis on homework, which should follow naturally from the problem-solving process in the treatment session. The use of homework in CBT draws from the understanding of therapy as a process in which the patient learns to master new skills. At the end of each CBT treatment session, patients should be provided with an opportunity to summarize lessons learned during the session.

THE STATUS OF CBT

CBT originated from behavior therapy, which translated Pavlovian and other behavior methods into interventions for excessive fear and anxiety, and the later addition of cognitive principles resulted in a broader treatment approach that is now the first-line psychological treatment for many disorders.[6] Although the theoretical foundation of CBT has made it quite amenable to empirical investigation, much remains unknown with regard to its theoretical and procedural boundaries (what is CBT?) as well as the mechanism of change (what makes CBT effective?) for various psychological disorders.

Is CBT Coming in Waves?

The operational definition of CBT can be complicated by philosophical differences in areas of emphasis. This issue is best reflected in the emergence of a so-called "*The Third Wave*" of CBT.[7] Chronologically, the first wave of treatments emphasized empiricism and linked behavioral principles to clinical change. The second wave of CBT was largely influenced by the information-processing model of cognition followed by the extension of such models to clinical phenomena. The third wave of CBT treatments are characterized by a focus on contextual change and the construction of flexible/effective skills. Although emphasis on cognitions and emotions is common in most contemporary CBT interventions, third-wave CBT treatments are theorized to primarily target the function of cognitions and emotions rather than their form, frequency, or situational sensitivity.

Acceptance and commitment therapy (ACT)[8] is perhaps the most heavily touted third-wave treatment. ACT is proposed to be based on the philosophical tradition of functional contextualism, which involves the prediction and influence of psychological events, such as thoughts, feelings, and behaviors, by focusing on variables that may be manipulated in their context. ACT uses acceptance and mindfulness strategies, together with commitment and behavior change strategies, to increase psychological flexibility. Although this treatment is increasingly being applied to a wide range of psychological problems,[9] there is concern that the promotion and dissemination of ACT and other third-wave CBT interventions may be getting ahead of the data.[10,11] Given the relative lack of studies rigorously evaluating the incremental efficacy (ie, more effective than standard CBT) of ACT (and other third-wave treatments), it remains unclear if the third-wave interventions are functionally distinct from contemporary CBT and if they are suited to carry the CBT tradition into the next century.[7]

Which CBT Components Matter?

Component-controlled randomized controlled trials hold substantial promise in delineating the mechanism of action in CBT. Constructing the appropriate combination of CBT components relative to nonspecific control conditions would allow for multiple component comparisons. Such comparisons allow for strong experimental tests of key components of CBT that would facilitate the identification of the underlying principles of CBT that serve as the mechanisms of change. Component-controlled studies may reveal that cognitive and behavioral components of CBT produce equivalent outcomes. However, equivalent outcomes would be predicted to be mediated by distinct theoretical mechanisms of action. Despite the substantial knowledge to be gained from component-controlled treatment outcome studies, few such investigations exist. The lack of component-controlled CBT evaluations in the empirical literature precludes definitive conclusions about the specific mechanism of change. The inability to consistently identify the active ingredient of CBT is partially attributable to inconsistencies in defining the specific treatment components of CBT. For example, "cognitive" components (running behavioral experiments to test beliefs) of CBT for some disorders (obsessive-compulsive disorder) often overlap with "behavioral" components (exposure). This cross contamination in techniques complicates efforts to determine which components (cognitive or behavioral) account for treatment gains. Studies that have been able to operationalize distinct CBT components have produced robust effects for behavioral interventions. For example, Dimidjian and colleagues[12] found that behavioral activation was comparable to antidepressant medication, and both significantly outperformed cognitive therapy for severely depressed patients. More recent research has shown that behavioral activation is nearly as enduring as cognitive therapy in the treatment of depression.[13]

Is CBT Better Than Other Treatments?

Strong inferences regarding the efficacy of CBT require direct comparisons with other treatments.[14] This line of inquiry has direct relevance for the claims about the general equivalence of all forms of psychotherapy. Often referred to as the Dodo bird verdict, it has been posited that there is no convincing evidence that different treatments are differentially effective and, furthermore, that most evidence demonstrates the equivalence of all psychosocial treatments.[15] Although the Dodo bird verdict has been welcomed by many and accepted, perhaps reluctantly, by many others,[16] the demonstrated outcomes for CBT relative to other psychosocial treatments present a significant challenge to the Dodo bird verdict. For example, there is now clear evidence that CBT is more efficacious than credible control treatments for anxiety disorders, that various forms of CBT differ in their efficacy depending on the anxiety disorder being treated, and that CBT is disorder specific, such that changes are primarily observed in anxiety symptoms relative to depressive symptoms among patients with an anxiety disorder.[17]

Although CBT may be more efficacious than credible control treatments for some disorders, definite claims regarding the incremental efficacy of CBT may be limited by the observation that credible control treatments are often not "bona fide" treatments. That is, they are not typically intended to be therapeutic. Future treatment outcome research comparing CBT to truly "bona fide" treatments will provide an even stronger empirical basis for claims about the incremental efficacy of CBT. It should be noted that such concerns about the efficacy of CBT are not limited to its comparison with other "bona fide" treatments. Indeed, researchers continue to pursue important questions about the efficacy of CBT compared with pharmacotherapy. The comparative and combined effect of CBT and pharmacotherapy has been most heavily investigated in the mood and anxiety disorders.[18] A general theme that emerges from these findings is that CBT is at least equally as effective as pharmacotherapy, more enduring than pharmacotherapy, and cheaper than pharmacotherapy; however, research on the combination of CBT and pharmacotherapy continues to yield complex findings. Combined treatment may have beneficial effects for those with chronic depression and in cases to prevent the return of depression. In the anxiety disorders, there are some benefits in the short term, but combined treatment may limit the maintenance of treatment gains offered by CBT alone.

Is CBT Being Used?

Although CBT is regarded as the gold standard of psychosocial treatments by many, its dissemination has been less than adequate. Indeed, only a minority of individuals with various psychological disorders receive CBT. For example, one study found that complementary and alternative medicine treatments accounted for 31.3% of all mental health visits.[19] There is also evidence that when CBT is being delivered, it is done so suboptimally.[20] A recent review of the literature suggests that 2 obstacles prevent effective dissemination of CBT[21]: (1) commonly held beliefs among clinicians, and (2) gaps in knowledge about CBT, including its delivery and training modes. Although there is substantial evidence to the contrary,[22] one belief that prevents effective dissemination is that research trials supporting the efficacy of CBT have limited generalizability to clinical practice because patients in these trials are perceived to be less severe than patients in the real world. Many clinicians also lack knowledge about how to effectively convey CBT skills, what the principles of change in CBT are, and the minimum dose of CBT that patients require.

Lack of CBT knowledge may be the biggest obstacle to the dissemination of CBT. Recent attempts to address this issue have focused on condensing and simplifying CBT. In fact, simplified variations of CBT that can be implemented over the phone or on the computer are becoming increasingly more popular. Although this approach maximizes external validity, it remains unclear if this is the best solution for inadequate CBT dissemination. Disseminating CBT in this manner may result in insufficient application of important CBT principles. This alone may largely account for concerns that CBT effects sizes tend to be more robust in research trials than what is observed in the community. Optimal dissemination of CBT will be contingent on translating basic and applied research that directly informs our understanding of how and why CBT is effective. This approach may ultimately lead to a movement away from applying different CBT packages that are often complex and target different disorders to a "unified" treatment approach that focuses on distilling common empirically supported treatment principles.[23] Mastery of separate CBT protocols for different disorders requires a significant amount of training, which is a major obstacle to dissemination. Research identifying empirically supported treatment principles may ultimately remove this obstacle. Shafran and colleagues[21] also recommend the following to facilitate the dissemination of CBT:

- Treatment developers should state how the existing trials address comorbidity and produce treatment guidelines and manuals; such manuals should be easily accessible and available at a reasonable cost.
- Clinicians should have easy access to training in diagnostic assessments and routine outcome measures. They should be encouraged to use outcome measures at regular intervals during treatment to monitor progress.
- Effectiveness studies should provide adequate training and supervision for therapists when studying how well treatments work in routine clinical populations.
- CBT trials and effectiveness studies should be analyzed for therapist effects and should establish the effects of levels of training on clinician competence and patient outcomes.
- The skill level that is required for a therapist to obtain good outcomes should be identified; this requires reliable assessment measures of competence.
- There is a need for more research on efficient ways of disseminating treatment procedures.
- The mechanisms of action of efficacious treatments should be studied.
- Methods to establish which patients would benefit from lower intensity interventions and which require more face-to-face contact are required.

Is CBT for Everyone?

Approximately 50% to 80% of patients undergoing CBT for affective disorders respond to treatment, which suggests that many patients achieve less than optimal response or do not respond at all.[24] More research is clearly needed to delineate who will benefit from CBT. That is, what are the robust and consistent predictors of CBT outcome? There are 2 distinct ways in which pretreatment factors can predict outcome. A *prognostic* variable is one that predicts outcome irrespective of the treatment, whereas a *prescriptive* variable predicts a different pattern of outcomes between treatment modalities.[1] Prognostic variables can indicate which kinds of patients are especially refractory to treatment irrespective of the type of intervention. Thus, they may indicate which patients require a more intensive course of treatment or a different modality of treatment. On the other hand, when 2 treatments are found not to differ in outcome, pretreatment markers may identify a group of patients who fare considerably better in one treatment than the other. For example, a recent study on the treatment of depression found that the prognostic variables of chronic depression, older age, and lower intelligence each predicted poor response to either cognitive therapy or antidepressant medication.[25] The study also found that 3 prescriptive variables—marriage, unemployment, and having experienced a greater number of recent life events—each predicted superior response to cognitive therapy relative to antidepressant medication. Future research identifying similar markers could be used prescriptively and would clearly have significant clinical utility, as they would allow individual patients to receive the treatment that is the most likely to lead to a rapid reduction in symptoms.

THE SPECIAL ISSUE ON CBT

Although CBT has taken its rightful place as the gold standard of psychosocial treatments for various psychological disorders, many questions remain unanswered. The questions highlighted here represent only the tip of the iceberg. In addition to taking stock in what we do know about CBT and its efficacy across various disorders, there is a need to begin to formulate an empirical agenda for how CBT can be advanced in future research. This agenda should include novel methods for enhancing the efficacy of CBT for different disorders as well as novel approaches to the dissemination of the core principles of CBT. These, among other reasons, makes this special issue on CBT a timely one. Several colleagues were invited to review the latest evidence on the efficacy of CBT for various disorders, including attention-deficit hyperactivity disorder, substance use disorders, schizophrenia, mood disorders, anxiety disorders, somatoform disorders, sexual dysfunction, eating disorders, sleep disorders, tic disorders, and personality disorders. The range of disorders covered here will make this special issue a valuable resource for researchers and practitioners. This special issue may also prove useful in CBT training across various disciplines. In addition to reviewing the available research on the efficacy of CBT for various disorders, the series of articles assembled here attempts to address many of the questions posed in this introduction in varying degrees. Articles are included that address the issue of augmenting CBT pharmacotherapy and the empirical status of the "new wave" of CBT. The special issue then concludes with a commentary on the future of CBT, which by all accounts is a very promising one.

REFERENCES

1. Hollon SD, Beck AT. Cognitive and cognitive-behavioral therapies. In: Lambert MJ, editor. Bergin and Garfield's handbook of psychotherapy and behavior change. 5th edition. New York: Wiley; 2004.
2. Brewin CR. Theoretical foundations of cognitive-behavior therapy for anxiety and depression. Annu Rev Psychol 1996;47:33–57.
3. Olatunji BO, Deacon BJ, Abramowitz JS. Is hypochondriasis an anxiety disorder? Br J Psychiatry 2009;194:481–2.
4. Butler AC, Chapman JE, Forman EM, et al. The empirical status of cognitive-behavioral therapy: a review of meta-analyses. Clin Psychol Rev 2006;26:17–31.
5. Deacon BJ, Abramowitz JS. Cognitive and behavioral treatments for anxiety disorders: a review of meta-analytic findings. J Clin Psychol 2004;60:429–41.

6. Rachman S. Psychological treatment of anxiety: the evolution of behavior therapy and cognitive behavior therapy. Annu Rev Clin Psychol 2009;5:97–119.
7. Hayes SC. Acceptance and commitment therapy, relational frame theory, and the third wave of behavior therapy. Behav Ther 2004;35:639–65.
8. Hayes SC, Strosahl K, Wilson KG. Acceptance and commitment therapy: an experiential approach to behavior change. New York: Guilford Press; 1999.
9. Hayes SC, Luoma J, Bond F, et al. Acceptance and commitment therapy: model, processes, and outcomes. Behav Res Ther 2006;44:1–25.
10. Corrigan P. Getting ahead of the data: a threat to some behavior therapies. The Behavior Therapist 2001;24:189–93.
11. Scheel KR. The empirical bases of dialectical behavior therapy: summary, critique, and implications. Clin Psychol Sci Pract 2000;7:68–86.
12. Dimidjian S, Hollon SD, Dobson KS, et al. Randomized trial of behavioral activation, cognitive therapy, and antidepressant medication in the acute treatment of adults with major depression. J Consult Clin Psychol 2006;74:658–70.
13. Dobson KS, Hollon SD, Dimidjian S, et al. Randomized trial of behavioral activation, cognitive therapy, and antidepressant medication in the prevention of relapse and recurrence in major depression. J Consult Clin Psychol 2008;76: 468–77.
14. Borkovec TD, Castonguay LG. What is the scientific meaning of empirically supported therapy? J Consult Clin Psychol 1998;66:136–42.
15. Wampold BE, Mondin GW, Moody M, et al. A meta-analysis of outcome studies comparing bona fide psychotherapies: empirically, "All must have prizes." Psychol Bull 1997;122:203–15.
16. Hunsley JY, Di Giulio G. Dodo bird, phoenix, or urban legend? The question of psychotherapy equivalence. The Scientific Review of Mental Health Practice 2002;1:11–22.
17. Hofmann SG, Smits JA. Cognitive-behavioral therapy for adult anxiety disorders: a meta-analysis of randomized placebo-controlled trials. J Clin Psychiatry 2008; 69:621–32.
18. Otto MW, Smits JAJ, Reese HE. Combined psychotherapy and pharmacotherapy for mood and anxiety disorders in adults: review and analysis. Clin Psychol Sci Pract 2005;12:72–86.
19. Wang PS, Lane M, Olfson M, et al. Twelve month use of mental health services in the USA. Results from the National Comorbidity Survey Replication. Arch Gen Psychiatry 2005;62:629–40.
20. Kessler RC, Merikangas KR, Wang PS. Prevalence, comorbidity and service utilization of mood disorders in the United States at the beginning of the twenty-first century. Annu Rev Clin Psychol 2007;3:137–58.
21. Shafran R, Clark DM, Fairburn CG, et al. Mind the gap: improving the dissemination and implementation of CBT. Behav Res Ther 2009;47:902–9.
22. Weisz JR, Weersing VR, Henggleler SW. Jousting with straw men: comment on Westen, Novotny and Thompson-Brenner (2004). Psychol Bull 2005;131:418–26 [discussion: 427–3].
23. Moses EB, Barlow DH. A new unified treatment approach for emotional disorders based on emotion science. Curr Dir Psychol Sci 2006;15:146–50.
24. Barlow D. Anxiety and its disorders: the nature and treatment of anxiety and panic. 2nd edition. New York: Guilford Press; 2002.
25. Fournier JC, DeRubeis RJ, Shelton RC, et al. Prediction of response to medication and cognitive therapy in the treatment of moderate to severe depression. J Consult Clin Psychol 2009;77:775–87.

Current Status of Cognitive Behavioral Therapy for Adult Attention-Deficit Hyperactivity Disorder

Laura E. Knouse, PhD*, Steven A. Safren, PhD

KEYWORDS

- Attention-deficit/hyperactivity disorder
- Psychosocial treatment • Cognitive behavioral therapy
- Adults • Treatment outcome

Attention-deficit/hyperactivity disorder (ADHD) is a valid psychiatric disorder characterized by severe and impairing levels of inattention, hyperactivity, and impulsivity.[1] As a developmental disorder, it appears in childhood and is associated with lags in the development of sustained attention and behavioral inhibition relative to same-aged peers, contributing to functional impairment across academic, behavioral, and social domains.[2,3] Once believed to be a childhood-limited disorder, longitudinal and cross-sectional data demonstrate that the disorder persists into adulthood in a majority of cases, causing disruption in multiple areas of adult functioning, including employment, intimate relationships, and motor vehicle driving.[4,5] In addition, adults with ADHD are at a significantly elevated risk for comorbid disorders, including depression, anxiety, substance use, and personality disorders.[6,7] Recent prevalence studies suggest that 4.4% of American adults may suffer from ADHD[8] and cross-national prevalence estimates are reasonably comparable (3.4%).[9]

Because ADHD has only been well characterized and widely recognized, diagnosed, and treated within approximately the past 20 years, many adults with ADHD present for diagnosis and treatment after having suffered with the disorder, untreated,

Some of the investigator time for preparation of this paper was supported by NIH Grant 5R01MH69812 to Steven A. Safren and by the Kaplen Fellowship on Depression from Harvard Medical School to Laura E. Knouse.
Behavioral Medicine Service, MGH Department of Psychiatry, One Bowdoin Square, 7th Floor, Boston, MA 02114, USA
* Corresponding author.
E-mail address: lknouse@partners.org

Psychiatr Clin N Am 33 (2010) 497–509
doi:10.1016/j.psc.2010.04.001
0193-953X/10/$ – see front matter © 2010 Elsevier Inc. All rights reserved.

for the majority of their lives. In addition, adults with ADHD continue to be faced with skepticism from those around them, fueled by persistent and scientifically uninformed perceptions that ADHD is not a real disorder with real consequences and costs. On the contrary, the available data overwhelmingly support the validity of this condition and the chronic, multi-domain impairments that it confers upon its sufferers.[4,10]

Fortunately, researchers interested in ADHD in adults have been able to begin to develop and test effective treatments for this condition. This article addresses the current status of evidence for cognitive behavioral therapy (CBT) interventions for adults with ADHD. Although stimulant medications are considered first-line treatments for ADHD, many adults with ADHD cannot or will not take medication and, of those that do, many continue to experience significant residual symptoms.[11] Depending upon baseline symptom severity, even those considered responders by the standards of most medication trials (ie, 30% or more reduction in symptoms[12]) may continue to experience significant and impairing symptoms. Thus, there has been an increasing demand for psychosocial approaches targeting ADHD-related behavioral deficits, though the supply of empirically-based strategies appears to be accumulating more slowly than that of recommendations based only upon clinical experience.

First, a conceptual rationale for the use of CBT for adults with this neurobiologically based disorder is presented followed by a review of existing empirical evidence for these approaches. Integrating the reviewed studies, preliminary comparisons are then made across treatment packages and possible active ingredients common to the most effective CBT approaches are discussed. Finally, challenges in psychosocial treatment research with this population awaiting resolution are highlighted.

COGNITIVE BEHAVIORAL THERAPY FOR ADULT ATTENTION-DEFICIT/HYPERACTIVITY DISORDER: CONCEPTUAL BASIS

Given that prior research supports a strong neurobiological basis for ADHD, what is the conceptual basis for applying CBT to the disorder in adults? Consistent with current theories of ADHD, the treatment model proposed by Safren and colleagues[13] (**Fig. 1**) begins with the premise that neuropsychological impairments are at the core of the disorder. Deficits in sustained attention, inhibitory control, working memory, and motivation underlie the cardinal symptoms of ADHD: inattention, hyperactivity, and impulsivity.[3,14] These deficits contribute to functional impairment and produce disruption in adaptive behavior, including use of higher-level organization and planning strategies that might ameliorate symptom-related difficulties. Thus, these underlying neuropsychological impairments hinder individuals with ADHD from acquiring and using the compensatory strategies that might support their areas of need, which results in symptom maintenance and exacerbation and further contributions to functional impairment.

As a result of these chronic functional impairments persisting since childhood, many adults with ADHD have had multiple failure experiences and chronic underachievement. In addition, many adults have likely received ongoing negative social feedback from parents, teachers, and peers. Such experiences can lead to the development of maladaptive negative cognitions and beliefs that decrease motivation and increase avoidance behavior and mood disturbance, reinforcing this cycle and further decreasing the likelihood that an adult with ADHD will consistently engage in the difficult work of acquiring and using compensatory strategies.

This conceptual model[13] and emerging empirical data described later, support using behavioral skills training to target the acquisition and especially the maintenance

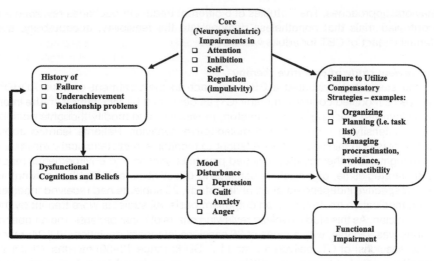

Fig. 1. Illustration of cognitive behavioral model of ADHD. *From* Safren S, Sprich S, Chulvick S, et al. Psychosocial treatments for adults with ADHD. Psychiatr Clin North Am 2004;27:349.

of compensatory skills, in addition to medication treatment targeting core symptoms as key components of optimal treatment of ADHD in adults. Critical to this model is the *consistent* performance of concrete, overlearned compensatory skills because, as Barkley[14] points out, ADHD is characterized not as a disorder of knowledge but of performance. These compensatory behavioral strategies can lead to decreases in associated functional impairments. Finally, cognitive interventions may target dysfunctional patterns of thought and associated emotions that contribute to avoidance, procrastination, and attentional shifts. Though the primary symptoms of ADHD are most certainly neurobiological in nature, cognitive behavioral interventions can play an integral role in breaking the link between core symptoms and continued failure and underachievement.

COGNITIVE BEHAVIORAL THERAPY FOR ADULT ATTENTION-DEFICIT/HYPERACTIVITY DISORDER: EMPIRICAL BASIS

As the authors have discussed elsewhere,[15] the current evidence for the use of psychosocial approaches in treating adults with ADHD can best be described as emerging and lags behind the evidence base for medication treatment of adult ADHD[11] and cognitive behavioral treatment for other adults disorders (eg, mood and anxiety disorders). Bearing these limitations in mind, the preliminary evidence base for cognitive behavioral approaches applied to this population are promising.

Uncontrolled Studies

The first preliminary examination of psychotherapy outcomes in adults with ADHD collected information on treatment history from 60 adults with ADHD presenting to an outpatient practice and engaging in traditional, insight-oriented psychotherapy.[16] Accordingly, traditional, insight-oriented psychotherapy was unsuccessful, pointing to the need for structured, skills-based interventions. Subsequent published evaluations of psychosocial treatments for ADHD in adults all involve some form of skills training in behavioral or cognitive strategies and thus are reviewed here as cognitive behavioral approaches. The 7 studies of 6 different treatment packages reviewed are uncontrolled trials that nonetheless demonstrate the feasibility, acceptability, and potential impact of CBT for adults with ADHD.

Chart review study of cognitive therapy

The first study that evaluated a CBT approach to the treatment of adult ADHD[17] employed a modified cognitive therapy (CT) as described by McDermott.[18] The intervention involved teaching patients to stop, reevaluate, and modify thoughts contributing to intensifying emotions and maladaptive behavior. Patients learned about negative biases in thinking and were taught to monitor and systematically reevaluate their thoughts. The therapy also included psychoeducation and environmental modification strategies (ie, organization, scheduling of activities, and problem solving). In this retrospective independent chart review study, 26 subjects had received modified CT and medication treatment on an outpatient basis. All subjects were treated by the same clinician. As this study involved reviewing charts of clinic patients, the number of sessions was variable, with a mean of 36 sessions (standard deviation [SD] 24; range 10–103 sessions) of CT, delivered over 11.7 (SD 8; range 13–30) months. Clinician-rated Clinical Global Impression (CGI) scores were assigned for ADHD symptoms, anxiety symptoms, and depression symptoms at baseline, at medication stabilization, and at post-CT treatment.

All CGI scores decreased significantly from baseline to the time of medication stabilization, and from medication stabilization to the endpoint of CT, providing preliminary evidence for the impact of CT above and beyond medication treatment. Sixty nine percent of subjects were classified as "much improved" or "very much improved." Prospective baseline and endpoint self-report measures were also available for 12 individuals. On the self-report measures, participants showed significant improvement in core ADHD symptoms (33% reduction) and associated anxiety and depressive symptoms. Limitations included challenges to internal validity and a variable and generally long course of treatment. However, the study also provided promising evidence that the combination of medication and structured, skills-based treatment could have a significant impact for adults with ADHD.

Dialectical behavioral therapy

A group of investigators in Germany have adapted Linehan's[19] dialectical behavior therapy (DBT) skills training group treatment for the treatment of ADHD in adults and have studied its efficacy in a small, nonrandomized controlled trial (N = 15)[20] and in a larger, multisite open trial (N = 72).[21] DBT is a cognitive behavioral approach developed for the treatment of borderline personality disorder that blends traditional change-oriented CBT skills with acceptance-based and mindfulness-based skills. The investigators adapted DBT skills training based on the premise that ADHD and borderline personality disorder share overlapping features, including problems with affect regulation, impulse control, self-esteem, and interpersonal relationships. The modified DBT treatment for ADHD was delivered in 13 group-formatted sessions with educational and discussion topics including psychoeducation about ADHD; neurobiology and mindfulness training (2 sessions); "chaos and control,"[20] which is a discussion of disorganized behavior followed by concrete advice about how to plan and organize aspects of participants' lives; dysfunctional behavior/behavior analysis (2 sessions); emotion regulation; psychoeducation about depression; psychoeducation about impulse control; psychoeducation about stress; psychoeducation about substance dependency; discussion of relationships and self-respect; and a summary discussion and next steps.

In the first trial of this intervention,[20] 8 subjects were assigned to the group treatment and 7 subjects acted as a waitlist control group without random assignment. Based on pre-to-post analyses, participants in the DBT skills group showed significant improvements in self-reports on measures of depression, a checklist of ADHD symptoms, and other measures of psychopathology and impairment. The control group did not achieve any significant differences, although 4 of these 7 subjects were lost to follow-up.

In the larger, multisite open trial (N = 72),[21] 66 participants completed the study and showed significant reductions from pretreatment to posttreatment in self-reported ADHD symptoms on 2 measures with medium and small effect sizes. Self-reported depressive symptoms decreased significantly with a medium effect size. Participants reported that they felt better educated and able to cope with their ADHD symptoms. The investigators report that they are currently undertaking a large, multisite, randomized controlled trial comparing medication to group skills training with the combination of these treatment modalities.

Group metacognitive therapy

Solanto and colleagues[22] developed a group treatment for adults with ADHD targeting problems in time management, organization, and planning. They described metacognitive therapy as a cognitive behavioral intervention intended to "enhance the development of an overarching set of executive self-management skills," emphasizing repeated practice of skills to make them more habitual and automatic.[22] Skill modules included time management, behavioral activation, procrastination, organization, and planning. During each weekly 2-hour session, groups of 5 to 8 participants first discussed at-home application of skills, received feedback from group members, and were given new skill information and homework assignments from group leaders. Thirty adults diagnosed with ADHD participated in either an 8-session or 12-session version of the treatment. Seventy percent of participants were receiving ongoing medication treatment for their ADHD symptoms. At posttreatment assessment, participants showed significant reductions in inattentive symptoms as measured by the Conners' Adult ADHD Rating Scale (CAARS) and the Brown ADD Scales. A total of 47% of the sample fell below the clinical cutoff for inattentive symptoms on the CAARS posttreatment and participants reported significant improvements in targeted skills. Solanto and colleagues[23] then conducted a randomized controlled trial (RCT) of metacognitive therapy, the initial results of which are summarized in a later section that reviews the existing RCTs.

Combined medication and cognitive behavioral therapy

In an open study of 43 adults diagnosed with ADHD, Rostain and Ramsay[24] examined the effects of 6 months of combined medication and CBT. Participants received 16 50-minute individual CBT sessions and Adderall titrated to the participants' optimal dosage, up to 20 mg twice a day. CBT focused on teaching individualized coping strategies and identifying and modifying maladaptive patterns of thinking that could interfere with effective coping. Content included psychoeducation about ADHD, helping the client to conceptualize their difficulties from a CBT perspective, training coping strategies, working on treatment-interfering behavior both behaviorally and cognitively, and building on strengths. At posttreatment, adults receiving combined medication treatment and CBT showed significant reductions in clinician-rated ADHD symptoms with a large effect size and in Clinical Global Impression of ADHD (reduced from 5.28 to 3.40). Significant reductions in comorbid anxiety and depression symptoms were also observed. Because of the use of a combined treatment approach, it is unclear the extent to which improvements were differentially associated with medication versus CBT. However, the results demonstrate the potential efficacy of a combined treatment package.

Cognitive behaviorally oriented group rehabilitation

In Finland, Virta and colleagues[25] tested their group intervention, described as cognitive behaviorally oriented group rehabilitation. A total of 29 adults with ADHD completed weekly group sessions covering a range of topics including a substantial psychoeducation and social support component. Topics for the 10 to 11 sessions included 2 psychoeducation sessions, motivation and initiation, organization, attention, emotion regulation, memory, communication, impulsivity and comorbidity, self-esteem, and conclusion. Skills relevant to each area were discussed and assigned for homework. Participants were assessed at 2 time points before group participation with no significant differences in study measures between the 2 pretreatment time periods. At posttreatment, 31% of the group members showed at least 20% improvement on a self-report adult ADHD rating scale; however, there were no changes in observed symptom ratings made by the subjects' significant others. Follow-up data were later reported[26] for 25 of the 29 participants at 3 and 6 months posttreatment. The 11 group members who had showed at least 20% reduction in self-reported symptoms maintained their reductions in ADHD symptoms at 3 and 6 months. The 14 remaining participants showed no effect on their ADHD symptoms at any time during the trial.

Mindfulness meditation training

CBT approaches have, in recent years, been successfully incorporating mindfulness-based skills to address mood and anxiety symptoms. Zylowska and colleagues[27] conducted an open trial of modified mindfulness meditation training with 24 adults and 8 adolescents with ADHD. Their hypothesis was that the attention control cultivated during mindfulness exercises would improve sustained attention and emotion regulation for patients with ADHD. Eight weekly sessions provided education about and practice of mindfulness skills, including weekly out-of-session practice assignments. As a group, treatment completers self-reported significant decreases in inattentive and hyperactive-impulsive symptoms, with 30% of participants showing a treatment response of 30% symptom reduction or more. Completers also showed pre-to-post improvements on neuropsychological attention conflict and set shifting. It is unclear to what extent improvements in performance on these tests correspond to improved performance in real-life situations that place demands on executive functions[28] and practice effects must be ruled out in subsequent investigations. This approach is unique compared with the other interventions described here, in that it proposes to change cognitive processing directly rather than to train skills that compensate for symptom-related deficits.

Randomized Controlled Trials

There are 3 published randomized trials of psychosocial interventions for adult ADHD and 1 recently completed trial.

Cognitive remediation program

An Australian research group examined a therapist-delivered[29] and self-directed[30] psychosocial treatment for adults with ADHD. Their cognitive remediation program (CRP) consisted of 8 2-hour group sessions led by a clinical psychologist, the provision of a support person or coach, and a participant workbook for use in completing homework assignments. The researchers' 3-pronged approach involved retraining cognitive functions, helping participants develop internal and external coping strategies, and work on restructuring the environment to support success for adults with

ADHD. Individual sessions targeted motivation, concentration, listening, impulsivity, organization, anger management, and self-esteem. Each session involved review of prior skills and homework assignments, introduction of a new skill, and assignment of new homework. The support person, either someone known to the participant or an assigned coach, worked with the participant to remind them of sessions, take notes in session, and have at least weekly supportive telephone contacts with the participant between sessions.

A total of 22 individuals were randomly assigned to the treatment group and 21 to the waiting-list control.[29] Some of the subjects were on medications (stabilized) and others were not. Self-report assessments occurred pretreatment and posttreatment for both groups. Participants in the cognitive remediation program also completed measures at 2-month and 1-year follow-ups. At posttreatment, individuals assigned to the treatment condition reported reduced ADHD symptoms, better organizational skills, and reduced anger problems than individuals assigned to the control group. Compared to their baseline reports, adults in the cognitive remediation program maintained lower ADHD symptoms and better organization at both follow-up assessments. However, data were not available to compare these treatment effects to those in the control condition. Although the conclusions that can be drawn from this study were perhaps limited by the use of self-report measures as the only outcome measures, this randomized controlled trial provided evidence of symptom reduction associated with psychosocial treatment while beginning to control for threats to validity, such as regression to the mean.

The more self-directed version[30] used a self-help book that included the following topics: (1) education about ADHD, (2) how to overcome attention and motivational difficulties, (3) listening skills, (4) organizational skills, (5) impulse-control techniques, (6) cognitive strategies for anger management, and (7) cognitive strategies for self-esteem. Three therapist-led sessions (beginning, middle, and end of treatment) were included, which were geared toward review and monitoring of progress. Support people (in this study, trained undergraduate and graduate students) were again assigned to aid participants.

There were 17 individuals (stable on medications or unmedicated) assigned to the treatment group and 18 assigned to the control group. Statistically significant differences emerged between the 2 groups' self-report outcome measures of ADHD symptoms, organizational skills, and self-esteem at posttreatment. Compared to baseline, CRP participants also had improved ratings at the 2-month follow-up. These findings further strengthen the evidence for the effects of skills-based, psychosocial intervention for adults with ADHD. In addition, the study illustrates a novel, potentially cost-effective method of combining self-help with the use of a nonprofessional supportive person to promote change.

Cognitive behavioral therapy for attention-deficit/hyperactivity disorder in medication-treated adults with residual symptoms

Our clinical research group completed a randomized controlled trial of cognitive behavioral therapy for adults with ADHD already receiving medication treatment but experiencing significant residual symptoms.[31] The 3 core modules of the treatment were (1) organizing and planning, (2) reducing distractibility, and (3) cognitive restructuring (adaptive thinking). There were 12 to 15 individual sessions that each began by therapist and patient setting an agenda. Symptom severity and medication adherence from the previous week were reviewed via a rating scale and discussed. During each session, skills-based homework was assigned to be completed over the course of the week and the next session included review of the homework and all previously learned skills. Initial sessions began with psychoeducation, the conceptual model of ADHD and rationale for compensatory skill use, and motivational exercises. Major foundational skills established and reinforced during the first module—organization and planning skills—included use of a simple calendar and task-list system, prioritization strategies, breaking down overwhelming tasks into manageable pieces, and training of problem-solving skills. Skills in the distractibility module included increasing awareness of attention span, breaking down tasks to fit within this span, use of visual and auditory reminders to cue assessment of on-task behavior, and reducing distractions in the physical environment. The last core module (focusing on adaptive thinking) included cognitive restructuring skills from those outlined by Beck,[32] including use of thought records, identification of cognitive errors, and formulation of rational responses, adapted for adults with ADHD.

Three additional modules were optional depending on participants' needs and preferences, including (1) application of skills to procrastination, (2) anger and frustration management, and (3) communication skills. However, as we delivered the treatment, we found that the core modules alone involve a great deal of behavioral change and that adding these additional modules became overwhelming for patients. Hence, in the revised treatment,[33] we dropped the modules on communication skills and anger/frustration management because these were not observed to be relevant for most patients, but retained the procrastination module because many participants found it helpful.

A randomized controlled trial (N = 31) found the cognitive behavioral treatment previously described to be superior to continued medications alone.[31] Participants completed a battery of self-report measures and an independent evaluation with an assessor who was blind to treatment assignment. At the outcome assessment, those randomized to CBT (n = 16) had lower independent assessor-rated ADHD symptoms and global severity and self-reported ADHD symptoms than those randomized to continued psychopharmacology alone (n = 15). Those in the CBT group also had lower independent-assessor rated and self-reported anxiety, lower independent assessor-rated depression, and a trend toward lower self-reported depression. We also examined the number of treatment responders in each condition, using a conservative outcome of a CGI score reduction in 2 points or more. Following this method, there were significantly more treatment responders among subjects who received CBT (56%) compared with those who did not (13%). Our group has recently completed a larger-scale, randomized controlled trial of CBT versus applied relaxation training for adults receiving medication treatment for ADHD, for which final data analyses are pending.

Group metacognitive therapy

Solanto and colleagues[23] recently completed a randomized controlled trial comparing metacognitive therapy (described earlier) to group supportive psychotherapy. Participants completing group metacognitive therapy (n = 45) had significantly greater reductions in inattentive ADHD symptoms than those completing group supportive therapy (n = 43) as measured by self-report and ratings by a clinician blinded to group status. Significant others' ratings of inattentive symptoms also showed significantly greater change for the metacognitive therapy group and a greater number were considered treatment responders as defined by at least 30% change on clinician ratings of inattentive symptoms. This randomized controlled trial, comparing a cognitive behavioral intervention to active supportive treatment, shows positive results in the context of the most methodologically rigorous test of a psychosocial treatment for adult ADHD to date.

COMPARISON OF COGNITIVE BEHAVIORAL THERAPY–ORIENTED APPROACHES

The available data on CBT for adult ADHD suggest that these interventions, as a group, show promise as efficacious interventions; however, more studies of the same treatment and more methodologically rigorous trials are needed. Despite the small overall number of trials, a range of distinct but related approaches have emerged. Can any preliminary conclusions be drawn from existing data regarding the most effective approaches at this stage? If so, common features might suggest promising directions for further treatment development and support for specific clinical recommendations. Caution must be exercised in comparing treatments to one another at this early stage because (1) most programs have only been tested in a single study, (2) a host of factors could account for differences in effect sizes across studies besides features of the treatment itself, and (3) measures used vary widely across studies. However, this necessary caution does not preclude, at this stage, some well-placed critical thinking about what may work best for adults with ADHD.

To generate hypotheses about the most effective emerging psychosocial treatments, effect sizes (standardized mean differences; Cohen's *d*) were calculated for ADHD symptom measures from pretreatment to posttreatment as reported in 8 of the published treatment trials described earlier representing 7 distinct treatment packages (**Table 1**). All were structured, skills-based programs where statistics necessary to calculate effect sizes were reported. Outcome measures varied considerably across studies and thus the most comparable measures are reported: self-report or investigator-report of ADHD total or inattentive symptoms using either *Diagnostic and Statistical Manual of Mental Disorders (DSM)*-based or other established rating. Because uncontrolled trials using pre-to-post data may overestimate the effect of the intervention compared with controlled trials, only pre-to-post effect sizes from the active treatment group of controlled trials are reported.[20,29,31] Effect sizes and descriptors for each study are displayed in **Table 1** and rank is ordered by magnitude of effect size on total symptoms.

From this preliminary examination, nearly all treatment packages (with the exception of Virta and colleagues[25]) resulted in large effect sizes (0.8+)[34] on total ADHD symptoms and results were similar for studies that reported inattentive ADHD symptoms. Overall, these data provide support for these skills-based, psychosocial approaches in the treatment of adult ADHD, with a mean effect size for total symptoms of 1.12 and for inattentive symptoms of 0.99. However, as discussed earlier, this conclusion is based on uncontrolled pre-to-post findings from intervention groups, which may overestimate efficacy. In comparing treatment packages, note that neither number of treatment sessions nor format of intervention (group vs individual) appeared to be associated with treatment effects. The program by Virta and colleagues,[25] which showed small effect sizes on self-reported symptoms, covered a broad range of topics with a new topic or broad skill area introduced each session. It appears that less emphasis was placed on the acquisition, repeated practice, and reinforcement of specific compensatory skills directly targeting core symptom-related deficits (ie, 5 of the 11–12 sessions). In contrast, the group intervention developed by Solanto and colleagues,[22] showed a much larger effect size and focused each session upon compensatory skills and their repetition. The investigators state their belief that, "...development of new, more adaptive habits and functional routines in adults with ADHD demands a certain degree of unambiguous emphasis and repetition so that desired behaviors (eg, checking a planner every day) ultimately become automatic and no longer dependent on the individual's active executive or decision-making functions."[22] This type of repetition of adaptive skills to become habits is also at the core of

Table 1
Effect sizes and study characteristics for published trials of psychosocial treatments of adult ADHD arranged by magnitude of effects on total ADHD symptom scores

Treatment	Format	Sessions	n^a	Measure	ES Total ADHD	ES ADHD inatt
CBT-oriented rehabilitation[25]	Group	10–11	29	BADDS total	0.38	—
				BADDS attention	—	0.33
Mindfulness meditation training[27]	Group	8	23	ADHD-RS total	0.80	—
				ADHD-RS inattention	—	0.97
Adapted DBT for adult ADHD[20,21]	Group	13	74	ADHD checklist	0.91	—
Combined medication and CBT[24]	Individual	16	38	BADDS-I total	1.02	—
				BADDS-I attention	—	1.25
Metacognitive therapy[22]	Group	10	30	BADDS total	1.57	—
				BADDS attention	—	1.09
				CAARS inattention	—	1.22
Cognitive remediation program[29]	Group	8	22	ADHD checklist[b]	1.65	—
CBT for medication-treated adults with residual symptoms[31]	Individual	12–15	16	ADHD CSS	1.74	—
				ADHD checklist-I	1.97	—
	—	Total	232	Mean pooled ES	1.12	0.99

Effect sizes are presented for pre- to post-treatment measurement of current self-reported or investigator-rated ADHD symptoms on established checklists. Separate effects are calculated for overall and inattentive ADHD symptoms when available.

Abbreviations: ADHD checklist-I, ADHD checklist-independent assessor; ADHD-CSS, ADHD current symptoms scale self-report; ADHD-RS, ADHD rating scale self-report; BADDS, Brown Attention-Deficits Disorder Scales self-report; BADDS-I, BADDS investigator report; CAARS, Conners' Adult ADHD Rating Scale self-report; ES, effect size (Cohen's *d*).

[a] Sample sizes reflect those used to calculate a pre-to-post effect size for active treatment groups. Thus, for trials with control groups[20,29,31] only the findings from the active treatment group are included to enable appropriate comparisons across studies.

[b] This ADHD self-report checklist was based on symptoms from *DSM-III-R*. All other ADHD checklists based on symptoms from *DSM-IV*.

the authors' approach,[33] which also has a similar effect size to the Solanto intervention. These preliminary findings raise the hypothesis that the active ingredient in successful CBT for adult ADHD is the introduction and, most importantly, repetition and reinforcement of compensatory skills that target core symptoms versus covering a broad range of topics in a treatment at the sacrifice of enough repetition and practice of newly acquired core skills. After a more solid base of efficacy trials to attain a designation of CBT as an empirically supported treatment for ADHD, comparative effectiveness studies may be able to more definitively test this hypothesis in the future.

Examination of elements common to the most effective treatments also reveals some important themes. Based on total ADHD symptoms, 3 treatments showed effect sizes more than half of one standard deviation above the others (see **Table 1**) and a closer examination indicates common features that may contribute to treatment effectiveness. These features involve teaching of specific skills and strategies and emphasis on practice of those skills outside of session. These are highly structured programs, elements of which include (1) short-term work, averaging about 10 sessions; (2) manualized content and; (3) inclusion of client handouts or a workbook to guide work outside of the session. With respect to the content, the 3 treatments with the largest effect sizes (1) focus mostly on learning of compensatory skills to ameliorate ADHD-related difficulties, (2) focus on organization and planning skills, and (3) consider skills to deal with difficulties in motivation. To varying degrees, all 3 programs also target the role of internal processes (thoughts, feelings) in increasing or decreasing the likelihood of appropriate skill use. For example, metacognitive therapy[22] teaches positive and negative visualization of long-term consequences, whereas the program by Safren and colleagues[33] includes a module on adaptive thinking skills. Overall, these programs can be described as primarily behavioral, incorporating cognitive elements to the degree that these processes block adaptive behavior and skill use. These preliminary findings suggest that psychoeducation alone, even when it covers the range of topics that might be relevant to adults with ADHD, is not sufficient to have a significant impact on ADHD symptoms and that it is critical to learn and practice specific skills.

SUMMARY AND FUTURE DIRECTIONS

The conceptual and empirical basis for CBT approaches in adult ADHD is growing and suggests that targeted, skills-based interventions have a role in effectively treating this disorder. At this stage of development, however, subsequent studies must progress in methodological rigor. Additional randomized controlled trials with active control groups are needed and intervention packages must be tested across multiple trials by more than 1 research group. Importantly, nearly all published trials to date have only examined acute outcomes and we have virtually no data on the longer-term impact of these interventions on symptoms and functioning. The measurement of treatment outcomes is another topic that requires additional study and perhaps additional discussion and debate among researchers. Should the primary outcome measure in studies of CBT for adult ADHD be symptoms, skill use, or functioning? In medication trials, when participants report needing compensatory strategies to manage symptoms, this is sometimes considered evidence of a lack of treatment effect. However, for CBT, these reports may instead be indicative of treatment success.

The role of medication, CBT, and the combination of these treatments is another topic that requires further study. Although some have speculated that adequate psychopharmacological control of core symptoms is necessary for effective CBT,[13] results from existing trials including medicated and unmedicated participants have not, thus far, supported this idea.[21,22,27,29] Future studies examining this question must take into account other possible correlates, including baseline constellation and severity of symptoms and comorbidity. As discussed previously in this article, preliminary data suggest possible differential treatment effects with regard to a treatments' focus on repeated practice of compensatory skills versus a more broad-based psychoeducational model. This hypothesis will require additional study as more rigorous randomized controlled trials emerge. However, it does not seem too early in this stage of the field's development to begin to define what works in CBT for adults with ADHD. Finally, as CBT treatments targeting ADHD symptoms emerge and become more refined, future approaches must begin to address the needs of adults with ADHD who suffer from comorbid disorders. The optimal combination, integration, and timing of known efficacious CBT interventions for mood, anxiety, and substance-use disorders with treatment of ADHD is an untouched area of clinical research relevant for the majority of adults with this disorder.

REFERENCES

1. American Psychiatric Association. Diagnostic and statistical manual of mental disorder-text revision. 4th edition. Washington, DC: American Psychiatric Association; 2000.
2. Barkley RA. Attention-deficit hyperactivity disorder: a handbook for diagnosis and treatment. 3rd edition. New York: Guilford Press; 2006.
3. Nigg JT. What causes ADHD? New York: Guilford Press; 2006.
4. Barkley RA, Murphy KR, Fischer M. ADHD in adults: what the science says. New York: Guilford Press; 2008.
5. Biederman J, Faraone SV, Spencer T, et al. Patterns of psychiatric comorbidity, cognitive, and psychosocial functioning in adults with attention-deficit hyperactivity disorder. Am J Psychiatry 1993;150:1792.
6. McGough JJ, Smalley SL, McCracken JT, et al. Psychiatric comorbidity in adult attention deficit hyperactivity disorder: findings from multiplex families. Am J Psychiatry 2005;162:1621.
7. Miller TW, Nigg JT, Faraone SV. Axis I and II comorbidity in adults with ADHD. J Abnorm Psychol 2007;116:519.
8. Kessler RC, Adler L, Barkley RA, et al. The prevalence and correlates of adult ADHD in the United States: results from the National Comorbidity Survey Replication. Am J Psychiatry 2006;163:716.
9. Fayyad J, de Graaf R, Kessler R, et al. Cross-national prevalence and correlates of adult attention-deficit hyperactivity disorder. Br J Psychiatry 2007;190:402.
10. Barkley RA, Cook EH, Dulcan M, et al. Consensus statement on ADHD. Eur Child Adolesc Psychiatry 2002;11:96.
11. Prince J, Wilens T, Spencer T, et al. Pharmacotherapy of ADHD in adults. In: Barkley RA, editor. Attention-deficit hyperactivity disorder: a handbook for diagnosis and treatment. 3rd edition. New York: Guilford; 2006. p. 704.
12. Steele M, Jensen PS, Quinn DMP. Remission versus response as the goal of therapy in ADHD: a new standard for the field? Clin Ther 1892;28:2006.
13. Safren S, Sprich S, Chulvick S, et al. Psychosocial treatments for adults with ADHD. Psychiatr Clin North Am 2004;27:349.
14. Barkley RA. Behavioral inhibition, sustained attention, and executive functions: constructing a unifying theory of ADHD. Psychol Bull 1997;121:65.

15. Knouse LE, Cooper-Vince C, Sprich S, et al. Recent developments in the psychosocial treatment of adult ADHD. Expert Rev Neurother 2008;8:1537.
16. Ratey JJ, Greenberg MS, Bemporad JR, et al. Unrecognized attention-deficit hyperactivity disorder in adults presenting for outpatient psychotherapy. J Child Adolesc Psychopharmacol 1992;2:582.
17. Wilens TE, McDermott SP, Biederman J, et al. Cognitive therapy in the treatment of adults with ADHD: a systematic chart review of 26 cases. J Cognitive Psychother Int Quarterly 1999;13:215.
18. McDermott SP. Cognitive therapy for adults with attention-deficit/hyperactivity disorder. In: Brown TE, editor. Attention-deficit disorders and comorbidities in children, adolescents, and adults. Washington, DC: American Psychiatric Press; 2000. p. 569.
19. Linehan MM. Skills training manual for treating borderline personality disorder. New York: Guilford; 1993.
20. Hesslinger B, Tebartz van Elst L, Nyberg E, et al. Psychotherapy of attention deficit hyperactivity disorder in adults: a pilot study using a structured skills training program. Eur Arch Psychiatry Clin Neurosci 2002;252:177.
21. Philipsen A, Richter H, Peters J, et al. Structured group psychotherapy in adults with attention deficit hyperactivity disorder: results of an open multicentre study. J Nerv Ment Dis 2007;195:1013.
22. Solanto MV, Marks DJ, Mitchell KJ, et al. Development of a new psychosocial treatment for adult ADHD. J Atten Disord 2008;11:728.
23. Solanto MV, Marks DJ, Wasserstein J, et al. Efficacy of meta-cognitive therapy (MCT) for adult ADHD. Am J Psychiatry, in press.
24. Rostain AL, Ramsay JR. A combined treatment approach for adults with ADHD–results of an open study of 43 patients. J Atten Disord 2006;10:150.
25. Virta M, Vedenpää A, Gronroos N, et al. Adults with ADHD benefit from cognitive-behaviorally oriented group rehabilitation: a study of 29 participants. J Atten Disord 2008;12:218.
26. Salakari A, Virta M, Gronroos N, et al. Cognitive-behaviorally-oriented group rehabilitation of adults with ADHD: results of a 6-month follow-up study. J Atten Disord 2010;13:516–23.
27. Zylowska L, Ackerman DL, Yang MH, et al. Mindfulness meditation training in adults and adolescents with ADHD: a feasibility study. J Atten Disord 2008; 11:737.
28. Burgess PW. Theory and methodology in executive function research. In: Rabbitt P, editor. Methodology of frontal and executive function. Hove (UK): Psychology Press; 1997. p. 81.
29. Stevenson CS, Whitmont S, Bornholt L, et al. A cognitive remediation programme for adults with attention deficit hyperactivity disorder. Aust N Z J Psychiatry 2002; 36:610.
30. Stevenson CS, Stevenson RJ, Whitmont S. A self-directed psychosocial intervention with minimal therapist contact for adults with attention deficit hyperactivity disorder. Clin Psychol Psychother 2003;10:93.
31. Safren SA, Otto MW, Sprich S, et al. Cognitive-behavioral therapy for ADHD in medication-treated adults with continued symptoms. Behav Res Ther 2005;43:831.
32. Beck JS. Cognitive therapy: basics and beyond. New York: Guilford Press; 1995.
33. Safren SA, Perlman CA, Sprich S, et al. Mastering your adult ADHD: a cognitive-behavioral therapy approach. New York: Oxford University Press; 2005.
34. Cohen J. Power analysis for the behavioral sciences. 2nd edition. Hillsdale (NJ): Lawrence Erlbaum; 1988.

Cognitive Behavioral Therapy for Substance Use Disorders

R. Kathryn McHugh, MA*, Bridget A. Hearon, MA,
Michael W. Otto, PhD

KEYWORDS

- Substance use disorders • Cognitive behavioral therapy
- Contingency management • Relapse prevention
- Motivational interviewing

Substance use disorders (SUDs) are heterogeneous conditions characterized by recurrent maladaptive use of a psychoactive substance associated with significant distress and disability. These disorders are common, with lifetime rates of substance abuse or dependence estimated at more than 30% for alcohol and more than 10% for other drugs, and past year point prevalence rates of 8.5% for alcohol and 2% for other drugs.[1,2] As understanding of the nature of substance use patterns has improved, a greater specificity of psychosocial and pharmacologic treatments has followed, with evidence for the efficacy and cost-effectiveness of these approaches. This article provides an overview of the evidence for, and clinical application of, cognitive behavioral therapy (CBT) for SUDs. In this article, CBT refers to both behavioral and cognitive behavioral interventions. Given the scope of the literature, this review focuses on the treatment of alcohol and drug use disorders, not including nicotine. For review of the literature on CBT for smoking cessation see Ref.[3]

To clarify key terms used in this manuscript, the term substance use is defined as consuming alcohol or any illicit psychoactive substance or improper use of any prescribed or over-the-counter medication. SUD as used here refers to a diagnosis of substance abuse and substance dependence. Symptoms of substance abuse reflect the external consequences of problematic use, such as failure to fulfill role obligations, legal problems, physically hazardous use, and interpersonal difficulty resulting from use. Symptoms of substance dependence reflect more internal consequences of use, such as physical withdrawal upon discontinuation of a substance and difficulty with cutting down or controlling the use of a substance.

This work was supported in part by NIDA award DA017904 to Dr Otto.
Disclosures: Dr Otto has served as a consultant and receives research support from Organon (Schering-Plough). Ms McHugh and Ms Hearon have no disclosures to report.
Department of Psychology, Boston University, 648 Beacon Street, 6th Floor, Boston, MA 02215, USA
* Corresponding author.
E-mail address: rkmchugh@bu.edu

Psychiatr Clin N Am 33 (2010) 511–525
doi:10.1016/j.psc.2010.04.012
0193-953X/10/$ – see front matter © 2010 Elsevier Inc. All rights reserved.

psych.theclinics.com

EFFICACY OF CBT FOR SUDS

Evidence from numerous large-scale trials and quantitative reviews supports the efficacy of CBT for alcohol and drug use disorders.[4,5] Our group conducted a meta-analytic review of CBT for drug abuse and dependence including 34 randomized controlled trials (with 2340 patients treated) and found an overall effect size in the moderate range (d = 0.45), with effect sizes ranging from small (d = 0.24) to large (d = 0.81) depending on the substance targeted. Larger treatment effect sizes were found for treatment of cannabis, followed by treatments for cocaine, opioids, and, with the smallest effect sizes, polysubstance dependence. Of individual treatment types, there was some evidence for greater effect sizes for contingency management (CM) approaches (see later discussion) relative to relapse prevention (RP) or other cognitive behavioral treatments. In all cases, these advantages were computed relative to control conditions, most frequently general drug counseling or treatment as usual. Similar results for alcohol and illicit drugs were reported in a meta-analytic review of CBT trials by Magill and Ray.[5] Evidence also supports the durability of treatment effects over time.[6] In a study of psychosocial treatment of cocaine dependence, Rawson and colleagues[7] reported that 60% of patients in the CBT condition provided clean toxicology screens at 52-week follow-up.

CBT for SUDs includes several distinct interventions, combined or used in isolation, many of which can be administered in individual and group formats. Specific behavioral and cognitive behavioral interventions administered to individuals are reviewed later in this article, followed by a review of family-based treatments. The evaluation of CBT for SUDs in special populations such as those diagnosed with other Axis I disorders (ie, dual diagnosis), pregnant women, and incarcerated individuals is beyond the scope of the current review, so this article focuses on SUD treatment specifically.

Individual and Group Treatments

CBT for SUDs encompasses a variety of interventions that emphasize different targets. This section reviews individual and group treatments including motivational interventions, CM strategies, and RP and related interventions that a focus on functional analysis.

Motivational interventions

At the outset of considering treatment, motivation for treatment and the likelihood of treatment adherence needs to be considered. To address motivational barriers to change, motivational enhancement techniques have been created and tested. Motivational interviewing (MI)[8] is an approach based on targeting ambivalence toward behavior change relative to drug and alcohol use, with subsequent application to motivation and adherence to a wide variety of other disorders and behaviors, including increasing adherence to CBT for anxiety disorders.[9–11] Treatments based on the MI model are used as stand-alone interventions and in combination with other treatment strategies for SUDs. A meta-analytic review of interventions based on MI found effect sizes across studies in the small to moderate range for alcohol and the moderate range for drug use compared with a placebo or no-treatment control group, and similar efficacy to active treatment comparisons.[12] MI is typically offered in an individual format (although group formats are also used) often consisting of a brief treatment episode. Greater efficacy may be achieved when a higher dose of treatment is used.[12]

Contingency management

As treatment is initiated, a primary challenge is countering the robust reinforcing effects of the drug. CM approaches are grounded in operant learning theory and involve the administration of a nondrug reinforcer (eg, vouchers for goods) following demonstration of abstinence from substances. Many clinical trials have supported the efficacy of CM for various substances such as alcohol,[13] cocaine,[14] and opioids.[15] Meta-analytic reviews indicate that effect sizes for the efficacy of CM across studies are moderate, with greater efficacy for some substances (opioids, cocaine) relative to others (tobacco, polydrug use).[4,16] To allow for greater cost-efficacy of CM approaches, researchers have investigated the role of lottery-type strategies for distribution of reinforcers. For example, the punchbowl method rewards negative screens for drug use with the opportunity to draw a prize from a punchbowl. Most prizes have low monetary value (eg, $1), but the inclusion of rarer large prizes (eg, $50) saves money while offering a successful inducement for abstinence.[17] CM procedures may use stable or escalating reinforcement schedules, in which reinforcer value increases as duration of abstinence increases.[18] In addition to contingencies linked to negative drug screens (eg, from swab or urine toxicology screens), adaptive behaviors ranging from attendance at prenatal visits to medication adherence have been successfully modified with CM approaches.[19,20]

A limitation of CM is the availability of funds for providing the reinforcers in clinical settings. The establishment of job-based reinforcements have been introduced as alternatives to aid the clinical adoption of these methods.[21,22] CM strategies have also been incorporated into couples' interactions (using the reinforcers available to the couples) to aid the reduction of drug use (see later discussion).

Relapse prevention and other treatments

Another well-researched cognitive behavioral approach to drug abuse has emphasized a functional analysis of cues for drug use and the systematic training of alternative responses to these cues. The RP approach focuses on the identification and prevention of high-risk situations (eg, favorite bars, friends who also use) in which a patient may be more likely to engage in substance use.[23] Techniques of RP include challenging the patient's expectation of perceived positive effects of use and providing psychoeducation to help the patient make a more informed choice in the threatening situation. A meta-analysis reviewing the efficacy of RP across 26 studies examining alcohol and drug use disorders as well as smoking found a small effect ($r = 0.14$) for RP reducing substance use, but a large effect ($r = 0.48$) for improvement in overall psychosocial adjustment.[24]

Similar CBT strategies have also been developed that, in addition to attending to the functional cues for drug use, may include a broader range of psychoeducation, cognitive reappraisal, skills training, and other behavioral strategies. Individual CBT packages vary in the degree to which each of these components is used. For example, a cognitive behavioral intervention for cocaine dependence developed by Carroll[25] includes components of functional analysis, behavioral strategies to avoid triggers, and building problem-solving, drug refusal and coping skills. Evidence for the efficacy of CBT for SUDs is supported in meta-analytic reviews, with effect size estimations in the low moderate range using heterogeneous comparison conditions[4] and large effect sizes compared with no-treatment control groups.[5]

Couples and Family Treatments

Although substance abuse treatment often occurs in an individual or group format, the disorder itself has strong ties to the patient's social environment. Accordingly, several promising treatments have been developed that use the support of the partner, family, and community to aid the patient in achieving abstinence. The community reinforcement approach (CRA),[26] similar to CM, focuses on altering contingencies within the environment (eg, inclusion of favorable non–alcohol-related activities in the patient's daily schedule) to make sober behavior more rewarding than substance use. The efficacy of the CRA approach for alcohol dependence has been supported through several meta-analyses,[27–29] with usefulness also shown in drug-dependent populations, such as patients who are dependent on cocaine[30] and opioids.[31]

Another treatment that uses the support of a significant other is behavioral couples therapy (BCT). In this treatment it is assumed that there is a reciprocal relationship between relationship functioning and substance abuse, whereby substance use can have a detrimental effect on the relationship, and that this relationship distress can lead to increased substance use.[32] Therefore, the focus of this treatment involves improving a partner's coping with substance-related situations as well as improving overall relationship functioning. Interventions commonly include psychoeducation, training in withdrawal of relationship contact contingent on drug use, and the application of reinforcement (eg, enhanced recognition of positive qualities and behaviors) contingent on drug-free days, and including the scheduling of mutually pleasurable nondrug activities to decrease opportunities for drug use and to reward abstinence.[33]

A recent meta-analysis has shown considerable support for the use of BCT rather than individually based counseling treatments (not including CBT) in alcohol use disorders[34] such that those in the BCT condition showed reduced frequency of use and consequences of use, as well as greater relationship satisfaction at follow-up. In addition, a meta-analysis conducted by Stanton and Shadish[35] found that BCT was associated with strong treatment retention, perhaps because of successful incorporation of the patient's home environment and desired support system in the treatment.

Combination Treatment Strategies

There has been the hope that combination treatment strategies (eg, CBT plus pharmacotherapy) will lead to especially enhanced drug treatment outcomes. However, like the results for mood and anxiety disorders,[36] this approach has frequently met with equivocal outcomes. Some studies have supported the combination of naltrexone and CBT for alcohol dependence.[37–39] In contrast, the COMBINE study evaluated combinations of naltrexone, acamprosote, and behavioral interventions for alcohol dependence in 1383 patients and found that naltrexone, behavioral interventions, and their combination resulted in the best drinking outcomes; however, combination treatment did not exhibit additive efficacy relative to monotherapy.[40] The addition of behavioral strategies such as CM has been shown to enhance the efficacy of opioid agonist therapies, such as methadone.[7] Other strategies have been successful, such as the addition of disulfiram to CBT[41] and citalopram to CBT or CM for cocaine dependence.[42]

The combination of psychosocial approaches has also yielded mixed results. For example, the combination of CBT and CM yielded the highest effect sizes (in the large range) relative to other interventions alone in a meta-analysis of treatments for drug dependence, but only 2 studies contributed to these effect sizes, undermining confidence in this approach.[4] In contrast, several studies have not shown additive effects with the combination of behavioral therapies, such as cue exposure and CBT,[43] and CM and CBT.[7] More studies of the combination of efficacious monotherapies are needed to determine the strongest treatment strategies for alcohol and drug use disorders.

Relative Efficacy Across Treatments

Studies evaluating the relative efficacy of different cognitive behavioral approaches for SUDs have yielded equivocal results regarding the relative benefits of these approaches for drug use outcomes. In a comparison of BCT with individual CBT for alcohol dependence, similar efficacy was noted with some cost advantages of individual CBT relative to BCT.[44] In a study comparing CM with CBT for stimulant dependence, CM showed better acute efficacy; however, at follow-up, efficacy was similar for both treatments.[45] Similar results have been found comparing CM with CBT for opioid-dependent patients in methadone maintenance treatment.[7] In the Project MATCH trial of the treatment of alcohol dependence, 3 evidence-based psychosocial treatment strategies (including CBT and an MI-based treatment) found similar overall outcomes across treatment conditions immediately after treatment[46] and at 3-year follow-up.[47] Attempts to match patients to treatments based on baseline characteristics has yet to yield a clear sense of the front-line treatments based on the individual.[46] However, results of effect size analysis across treatment trials provide support for the most robust treatment effects for CM for drug use[4] and combined psychosocial treatments (eg, CBT + cue exposure) for alcohol use.[5]

EFFECTIVENESS OF CBT FOR SUDS

Although empirical support for these interventions is promising, it is most often garnered through efficacy studies in which the treatment is performed in optimal conditions. However, most SUD treatments occur in service provision settings in conditions that are not optimal. A limited body of effectiveness research has been conducted examining these treatments without the stringent controls afforded by efficacy trials.

Several studies examined the effectiveness of CM as a supplement to traditional drug counseling. The studies initially provided large rewards (as much as $1000) for sustained abstinence from substance use,[48–50] but effectiveness studies have recently focused on providing low-cost CM as a more feasible addition to traditional counseling programs. Petry and Martin[15] examined the addition of CM to standard community-based treatment (methadone maintenance and monthly individual counseling) for patients dependent on cocaine and opioids. CM in this study was delivered through a raffle format using a fixed ratio schedule in which drug-free urine samples afforded patients the opportunity to draw from a fish bowl for prizes valued between $1 and $100; patients in the CM condition achieved longer durations of abstinence through a 6-month follow-up period relative to those who did not receive CM.

The study of the effectiveness of motivational enhancement strategies has yielded mixed results. In a large effectiveness trial of motivational enhancement therapy for Spanish-speaking patients seeking treatment of substance use, Carroll and colleagues[51] found small advantages for this treatment relative to TAU only among those in the sample seeking treatment of alcohol problems. This finding of an advantage for motivational enhancement in alcohol- and not drug-using samples was consistent with prior investigations.[52] Similarly, a study conducted by Gray and colleagues[53] examined the effects of single-session MI delivered by youth workers for alcohol, nicotine, and cannabis use among young people. At 3-month follow-up, those who received MI reported significantly fewer days of alcohol use than those who did not receive MI; however, significant differences were not found for cigarette or cannabis use, indicating that the extent of benefit of MI is more modest than that identified by efficacy research studies. Results for the improvement of retention with motivational enhancement in effectiveness studies have been more promising.[54] There is a clear need for more effectiveness research to better understand the application of CBT outside controlled research settings.

CLINICAL ELEMENTS OF CBT FOR SUDS

As implied earlier, CBT for SUDs varies according to the particular protocol used and, given the variability in the nature and effects of different psychoactive substances, the substance targeted. However, across protocols, several core elements emerge. Consistent across interventions is the use of learning-based approaches to target maladaptive behavioral patterns, motivational and cognitive barriers to change, and skills deficits.

One of the core principles underlying CBT for SUDs is that substances of abuse serve as powerful reinforcers of behavior. In time, these positive (eg, enhancing social experiences) and negative (eg, reducing negative affect) reinforcing effects become associated with a wide variety of internal and external stimuli. The core elements of CBT are intended to mitigate the strongly reinforcing effects of substances of abuse by increasing the contingency associated with nonuse (eg, vouchers for abstinence) or by building skills to facilitate reduction of use and maintenance of abstinence, and facilitating opportunities for rewarding nondrug activities.

Despite these commonalities, as the aforementioned studies show, length of treatment can vary greatly even within the rubric of CBT for SUDs (eg, single-session MI, 12-session BCT). Research on duration and intensity of treatment is mixed, with some correlational studies indicating a positive relationship between longer duration and positive outcome, and others indicating no differential effects of treatment duration.[46,55,56]

Case Conceptualization and Functional Analysis

During assessment and early treatment sessions, case conceptualization requires consideration of the heterogeneity of SUDs. For example, the relative contribution of affective and social/environmental factors can vary widely across patients. A patient with co-occurring panic disorder and alcohol dependence may be experiencing cycles of withdrawal, alcohol use, and panic symptoms that serve as a barrier to reduction of alcohol consumption and amelioration of panic symptoms.[57] Alternatively, patients without co-occurring psychological disorders may face different barriers and skills deficits, such as difficulty refusing offers for substances or a perceived need for substances in social situations. Therefore, all of these factors must be considered before embarking on treatment.

Consistent with general CBT models, treatment of SUDs benefits from the use of a regular structure, including agenda setting, identification of goals, and the assignment and review of homework. This structure is particularly important for subgroups for whom cognitive deficits, difficulty concentrating, or organizational and problem-solving skills deficits are present, because it can help such patients to more easily remember and apply treatment techniques outside the treatment session. Functional analysis is an important component of treatment from the earliest stages. The identification of antecedents or triggers for use is critical to determining the appropriate situations and behaviors to target. For example, identifying high-risk situations for use, such as liquor stores or areas where drugs are commonly sold, and encouraging the patient to avoid such situations (particularly in the early stages of recovery) can be used in this stage. Such stimulus-control strategies may serve as an important precursor to building skills for resilience in these settings because it facilitates initial achievement of abstinence. These analyses will also help clarify for the clinician whether drugs are used as part of social repertoires, used to enhance positive activities, or used to cope with difficult situations or emotions. Independent assessment of drug use motives can also aid this aspect of the functional analysis. For example, the

Revised Drinking Motives Questionnaire[58] may provide important information about the nature of drinking motives and its association with particular triggers, such as mood disturbance.[59]

Cognitive and Motivational Strategies

Once high-risk situations and events are identified (including people and places, as well as internal cues such as changes in affect), CBT can be directed to altering the likelihood that these events are encountered (providing alternative nondrug activities, or activities with sober individuals) as well as rehearsing nondrug alternatives to these cues. Motivational and cognitive interventions can be provided to enhance motivation for these alternative activities, while also working to decrease cognitions that enhance the likelihood of drug use. In addition to the elements of MI (ie, assessment, dispassionate presentation of information, and elucidation and discussion of ambivalence about drug abstinence), broader cognitive strategies can target the cognitive distortions specific to substance abuse, including rationalizing use (eg, "I will just use this once," "One drink won't hurt me," "It has been a bad day; I deserve to use") and giving up (eg, "Why even try," "I will always be an addict"). In such circumstances, eliciting evidence from the patient regarding the accuracy of these thoughts can help to identify alternative appraisals that may be more adaptive and better reflect the patient's experience. Similarly, providing psychoeducation on the nature of such thoughts and the role that they may play in recovery can help the patient to gain awareness about how such thinking patterns contribute to the maintenance of the disorder. As with other disorders, rehearsal of cognitive restructuring in the context of drug cues may enhance the availability of these skills outside the treatment setting.[60]

As part of cognitive restructuring, expectancies, or beliefs about the consequences of use, are another important target for intervention. It is common to find that patients maintain a belief that use of a particular substance will help some problematic aspect of their life or given situations. For example, a patient may believe that a family holiday would not be enjoyable without alcohol use. Similar to cognitive restructuring techniques, evaluating evidence for expectancies and designing behavioral experiments can be used to target this issue. In this instance, the patient would be encouraged to refrain from drinking at the holiday party and assess the degree to which the event was enjoyable. In addition, the patient could evaluate evidence from past holidays to compare the consequences and benefits of alcohol use in these settings.

Shifting Contingencies

As noted earlier, a variety of CM procedures have shown success in helping patients reduce drug use. The cognitive behavioral therapist needs to consider how abstinence is to be rewarded as part of treatment. In addition to consideration of traditional CM rewards (monetary prizes, vouchers for goods, or treatment privileges such as take-home doses of methadone) the arrangement of social contingencies, such as is evident in BCT approaches, should be considered. In treatment, the question is how contingencies can be arranged to encourage initial experiences of abstinence and entry into nondrug activities. When this goal is achieved, treatment becomes concerned with identification of more naturally occurring rewards for abstinence (eg, greater employment, relationship, and social success). Problem-solving strategies and programming and rehearsal of steps to broader goal attainment may need to be provided, depending on the skills available to the patient.

Several approaches to the treatment of drug use patterns have emphasized exposure to the cues for drug use. Research has shown moderate success for exposure to external cues for use such as drug paraphernalia or the drugs themselves.[61,62] Accordingly, attention has also shifted to exposure to internal cues for drug use. Pilot studies in illicit drug use[63,64] and smoking cessation[65,66] have provided early support for this approach. For these approaches in smoking cessation, attention has been on reduction of fears of anxiety sensations that may amplify the aversiveness of withdrawal and affective consequences of nicotine cessation. By pre-exposing individuals to some of these sensations in interoceptive exposure procedures, the aversiveness of these sensations can be reduced, with resulting reduction in smoking behavior.[65,66]

Skills Training

Skills training can be broadly conceptualized as targeting interpersonal, emotion regulation, and organizational/problem-solving deficits. Clinical trials examining the addition of coping and communication skills training have shown positive outcomes and are common components of CBT for substance abuse.[61,62] The use of strategies should be based on case conceptualization, building from patient reports and behavioral observation of such deficits. Interpersonal skills-building exercises may target repairing relationship difficulties, increasing the ability to use social support, and effective communication. For patients with strong support from a family member or significant other, the use of this social support in treatment may benefit goals for abstinence and relationship functioning. In addition, the ability to reject offers for substances can be a limitation and constitutes a challenge to recovery. Rehearsal of socially acceptable responses to offers for alcohol or drugs provides the patient with a stronger skill set for applying these refusals outside of the session. If relevant, this rehearsal can be supplemented by imaginal exposure or emotional induction to increase the degree to which the rehearsal is similar to the patient's high-risk situations for drug use.

Emotion regulation skills can include distress tolerance and coping skills. Through the use of problem-solving exercises and the development of a repertoire for emotion regulation, the patient can begin to determine and use nondrug alternatives to distress. Strategies for coping with negative affect, such as using social supports, engaging in pleasurable activities, and exercise can be introduced and rehearsed in the session. The development of pleasurable sober activities is of particular importance given the amount of time and energy that is often taken for substance use activities (ie, obtaining, using, and feeling the effects of substances). When reducing substance use, patients can be left with a sense of absence where time was dedicated to use, which can serve as an impediment to abstinence. Thus, concurrently increasing pleasant and goal-directed activities while reducing use can be crucial for facilitating initial and maintained abstinence.

Goal-setting deficits can be targeted within the session as part of the treatment. Guiding patients in setting treatment goals can serve as a first practice of this skill. Assisting patients in setting smaller goals in the service of longer-term goals is also an important exercise. The inability to delay long-term pleasure for short-term pleasure is a characteristic feature of SUDs, and thus the ability to set long-term goals may be compromised.[67] Particularly for patients with more severe substance dependence, skills building may require shifting the patient's relevant skills and goals from those of an illicit lifestyle to those of a more normative lifestyle. Thus, the skills that may have been adaptive while actively using (interpersonal skills needed to obtain drugs and to connect with other substance users, the ability to manipulate those around you, to do things without being caught) may translate poorly to reconnecting with family and sober friends, obtaining and maintaining a job, and building healthy life activities.

Clinical Challenges

There are many challenges that may arise in the treatment of SUDs and that can serve as barriers to successful treatment. These include acute or chronic cognitive deficits, medical problems, social stressors, and lack of social resources. In addition, certain populations, such as pregnant women and incarcerated patients, may present particular challenges. In each of these circumstances, the use of functional analysis to arrive at strong case conceptualization and the flexible use of treatment components is important. For example, among individuals with low levels of literacy, the use of written homework forms may need to be replaced by alternative means of monitoring home practice (eg, using simplified forms or having the patient call to leave a phone message regarding completion of an assignment).

The shift in the social and environmental contexts associated with use relative to nonuse lifestyles can be a particular challenge. For example, among individuals who have long histories of substance misuse, there are often significant life consequences, such as unemployment, family difficulties, and reduced social networks. In such groups, their fit to society is within the context of others with similar misuse problems. The illicit drug use culture, characterized at times by other illicit behaviors (eg, drug dealing, theft, prostitution) and the valuation of particular skills (eg, the ability to make a drug deal at 2:00 AM), varies dramatically from a more mainstream culture. Thus, in treatment, the patient not only is being asked to transition to a culture in which he or she may have few skills and resources but also to relinquish the parts of his or her life in which there is a sense of effectiveness and belonging. The sense of belonging to the substance use culture can increase ambivalence for change, particularly when measurable life changes occur at a slow pace. In such cases, it is critical to establish alternatives for achieving a sense of belonging, including social connection and effectiveness. Depending on the resources available to the patient, this may include joining some type of social group (eg, a sports club), volunteer work, or other activity-based social opportunities.

NOVEL TREATMENT STRATEGIES

Despite the success of the strategies described earlier, much work remains to be done to improve rates of treatment response. In addition to the treatment techniques previously described, several novel approaches are being studied to enhance behavioral treatments for SUDs. One new approach is the use of computer-assisted delivery of treatment. A recent study conduced by Carroll and colleagues[68] compared the addition of biweekly computer-based CBT to a standard drug counseling treatment. Results indicate that those who received the computer-based treatment had significantly higher numbers of drug-free urine tests and longer periods of abstinence, with benefits continuing through a 6-month follow-up.[69]

Another novel approach is the use of a medication, D-cycloserine (DCS), to augment exposure-based treatments. DCS works as a partial agonist targeting N-methyl-D-aspartate (NMDA) receptors, which enhance glutamate neurotransmission, thereby facilitating extinction.[70] DCS has been applied successful in augmenting exposure-based treatments for anxiety disorders.[71] Several animal studies have shown that administration of DCS coupled with an extinction paradigm has deterred reacquisition of cocaine- and alcohol-seeking behavior[72,73] and facilitated extinction of withdrawal-associated place aversion in morphine-dependent rats.[74] Such promising findings in the animal literature suggest that further application with human populations is warranted. Our group is currently evaluating the addition of DCS to an exposure-based CBT protocol from treatment-resistant opioid dependence. In this treatment, DCS, when administered before exposure sessions, is hypothesized to facilitate extinction learning to achieve more rapid and more robust treatment response.

DISSEMINATION OF CBT FOR SUDS

Many effective behavioral techniques for the treatment of substance use have been identified; however, use of such techniques is often scarce or nonexistent in service provision settings. Several reasons have been cited for this limitation in technology transfer, including a commonly held belief that addiction is a moral failing rather than a brain disease, thus preventing the adoption of a medical model, availability of resources to implement new treatments, and the resistance to change shown by many organizations and individual clinicians.[75] In response to the lack of effective diffusion of evidence-based treatments, there has recently been an increase in resource allocation for targeting dissemination and implementation efforts. For example, the National Institute on Drug Abuse (NIDA) in conjunction with the Addiction Technology Transfer Center (ATTC) and Substance Abuse and Mental Health Services Administration (SAMHSA) instituted a blending initiative in 2001 to help combine the knowledge and skill of researchers, clinicians, policymakers, and dissemination programs to help develop and implement evidence-based treatments that could be used in community settings.

One outcome of the blending initiative was the inception of the Clinical Trials Network (CTN), a 17-site regional research and training center that collaborates with many community treatment programs to study the effectiveness of specific interventions in diverse community settings and patient populations. Other efforts to increase access to CBT and other evidence-based treatments for SUDs are also underway.[76–78] Future research focusing on methods to bridge the gap between theory and practice in a way that supports clinicians so that systemic change can truly be effective is of particular importance.

SUMMARY

CBT for SUDs includes a broad range of behavioral treatments including those targeting operant learning processes, motivational barriers to improvement, and the traditional variety of other cognitive behavioral interventions. Overall, these interventions have shown efficacy in controlled trials and may be combined with each other or with pharmacotherapy to provide more robust outcomes. Despite this heterogeneity, core elements emerge based in a conceptual model of SUDs as disorders characterized by learning processes and driven by the strongly reinforcing effects of substances of abuse. Particular challenges to the field include the determination of the most effective combination treatment strategies and improving the dissemination of CBT to service provision settings. Novel treatment strategies including more scalable modalities (such as computer-based programs) and combination strategies to improve rates or speed of treatment response (such as DCS) may aid in the transportability of treatments outside research settings.

REFERENCES

1. Compton WM, Thomas YF, Stinson FS, et al. Prevalence, correlates, disability, and comorbidity of DSM-IV drug abuse and dependence in the United States: results from the national epidemiologic survey on alcohol and related conditions. Arch Gen Psychiatry 2007;64:566–76.

2. Hasin DS, Stinson FS, Ogburn E, et al. Prevalence, correlates, disability, and co-morbidity of DSM-IV alcohol abuse and dependence in the United States: results from the national epidemiologic survey on alcohol and related conditions. Arch Gen Psychiatry 2007;64:830–42.
3. Vidrine JI, Cofta-Woerpel L, Daza P, et al. Smoking cessation 2: behavioral treatments. Behav Med 2006;32:99–109.
4. Dutra L, Stathopoulou G, Basden SL, et al. A meta-analytic review of psychosocial interventions for substance use disorders. Am J Psychiatry 2008;165:179–87.
5. Magill M, Ray LA. Cognitive-behavioral treatment with adult alcohol and illicit drug users: a meta-analysis of randomized controlled trials. J Stud Alcohol Drugs 2009;70:516–27.
6. Carroll KM, Rounsaville BJ, Nich C, et al. One-year follow-up of psychotherapy and pharmacotherapy for cocaine dependence. Delayed emergence of psychotherapy effects. Arch Gen Psychiatry 1994;51:989–97.
7. Rawson RA, Huber A, McCann M, et al. A comparison of contingency management and cognitive-behavioral approaches during methadone maintenance treatment for cocaine dependence. Arch Gen Psychiatry 2002;59:817–24.
8. Miller WR, Rollnick S. Motivational interviewing: preparing people for change. 2nd edition. New York: Guilford Press; 2002.
9. Merlo LJ, Storch EA, Lehmkuhl HD, et al. Cognitive behavioral therapy plus motivational interviewing improves outcome for pediatric obsessive-compulsive disorder: a preliminary study. Cogn Behav Ther 2009;1:24–7.
10. Simpson HB, Zuckoff A, Page JR, et al. Adding motivational interviewing to exposure and ritual prevention for obsessive-compulsive disorder: an open pilot trial. Cogn Behav Ther 2008;37:38–49.
11. Westra HA, Arkowitz H, Dozois DJ. Adding a motivational interviewing pretreatment to cognitive behavioral therapy for generalized anxiety disorder: a preliminary randomized controlled trial. J Anxiety Disord 2009;23:1106–17.
12. Burke BL, Arkowitz H, Menchola M. The efficacy of motivational interviewing: a meta-analysis of controlled clinical trials. J Consult Clin Psychol 2003;71: 843–61.
13. Petry NM, Martin B, Cooney JL, et al. Give them prizes, and they will come: contingency management for treatment of alcohol dependence. J Consult Clin Psychol 2000;68:250–7.
14. Higgins ST, Wong CJ, Badger GJ, et al. Contingent reinforcement increases cocaine abstinence during outpatient treatment and 1 year of follow-up. J Consult Clin Psychol 2000;68:64–72.
15. Petry NM, Martin B. Low-cost contingency management for treating cocaine- and opioid-abusing methadone patients. J Consult Clin Psychol 2002;70:398–405.
16. Prendergast M, Podus D, Finney J, et al. Contingency management for treatment of substance use disorders: a meta-analysis. Addiction 2006;101:1546–60.
17. Sindelar J, Elbel B, Petry NM. What do we get for our money? Cost-effectiveness of adding contingency management. Addiction 2007;102:309–16.
18. Stitzer M, Petry N. Contingency management for treatment of substance abuse. Annu Rev Clin Psychol 2006;2:411–34.
19. Carroll KM, Ball SA, Nich C, et al. Targeting behavioral therapies to enhance naltrexone treatment of opioid dependence: efficacy of contingency management and significant other involvement. Arch Gen Psychiatry 2001;58:755–61.
20. Elk R, Mangus L, Rhoades H, et al. Cessation of cocaine use during pregnancy: effects of contingency management interventions on maintaining abstinence and complying with prenatal care. Addict Behav 1998;23:57–64.

21. DeFulio A, Donlin WD, Wong CJ, et al. Employment-based abstinence reinforcement as a maintenance intervention for the treatment of cocaine dependence: a randomized controlled trial. Addiction 2009;104:1530–8.

22. Silverman K, Wong CJ, Needham M, et al. A randomized trial of employment-based reinforcement of cocaine abstinence in injection drug users. J Appl Behav Anal 2007;40:387–410.

23. Marlatt GA, Gordon JR, editors. Relapse prevention: maintenance strategies in the treatment of addictive behaviors. New York: Guilford Press; 1985.

24. Irvin JE, Bowers CA, Dunn ME, et al. Efficacy and relapse prevention: a meta-analytic review. J Consult Clin Psychol 1999;67:563–70.

25. Carroll KM. A cognitive-behavioral approach: treating cocaine addiction. Rockville (MD): National Institute on Drug Abuse; 1998.

26. Hunt GM, Azrin NH. A community reinforcement approach to alcoholism. Behav Res Ther 1973;11:91–104.

27. Finney JW, Monahan SC. The cost-effectiveness of treatment for alcoholism: a second approximation. J Stud Alcohol 1996;57:229–43.

28. Holder H, Longabaugh R, Miller WR, et al. The cost effectiveness of treatment for alcoholism: a first approximation. J Stud Alcohol 1991;52:517–40.

29. Miller WR, Brown JM, Simpson TL, et al. What works? A methodological analysis of the alcohol treatment outcome literature. In: Hester RK, Miller WR, editors. Handbook of alcoholism treatment approaches: effective alternatives. Needham (MA): Allyn & Bacon; 1995. p. 12–44.

30. Higgins ST, Budney AJ, Bickel WK, et al. Outpatient behavioral treatment for cocaine dependence one-year outcome. Exp Clin Psychopharmacol 1995;3:205–12.

31. Abbott PJ, Weller SB, Delaney HD, et al. Community reinforcement approach in the treatment of opiate addicts. Am J Drug Alcohol Abuse 1998;24:17–30.

32. Epstein EE, McCrady BS. Behavioral couples treatment of alcohol and drug use disorders: current status and innovations. Clin Psychol Rev 1998;18:689–711.

33. O'Farrell TJ, Fals-Stewart W. Behavioral couples therapy for alcoholism and drug abuse. New York: Guilford Press; 2006.

34. Powers MB, Vedel E, Emmelkamp MG. Behavioral couples therapy (BCT) for alcohol and drug use disorders: a meta-analysis. Clin Psychol Rev 2008;28:952–62.

35. Stanton DM, Shadish WR. Outcome, attrition, and family-couples treatment for drug abuse: a meta-analysis and review of the controlled, comparative studies. Psychol Bull 1997;122:170–91.

36. Otto MW, Smits JAJ, Reese HE. Combined psychotherapy and pharmacotherapy for mood and anxiety disorders in adults: review and analysis. Clin Psychol Sci Pract 2005;12:72–86.

37. Anton RF, Moak DH, Latham P, et al. Naltrexone combined with either cognitive behavioral or motivational enhancement therapy for alcohol dependence. J Clin Psychopharmacol 2005;25:349–57.

38. Feeney GF, Connor JP, Young RM, et al. Combined acamprosate and naltrexone, with cognitive behavioural therapy is superior to either medication alone for alcohol abstinence: a single centres' experience with pharmacotherapy. Alcohol Alcohol 2006;41:321–7.

39. Walters D, Connor JP, Feeney GF, et al. The cost effectiveness of naltrexone added to cognitive-behavioral therapy in the treatment of alcohol dependence. J Addict Dis 2009;28:137–44.

40. Anton RF, O'Malley SS, Ciraulo DA, et al. Combined pharmacotherapies and behavioral interventions for alcohol dependence: the combine study: a randomized controlled trial. JAMA 2006;295:2003–17.

41. Carroll KM, Fenton LR, Ball SA, et al. Efficacy of disulfiram and cognitive behavioral therapy in cocaine-dependent outpatients; a randomized placebo-controlled trial. Arch Gen Psychiatry 2004;61:264–72.
42. Moeller FG, Schmitz JM, Steinberg JL, et al. Citalopram combined with behavioral therapy reduces cocaine use: a double-blind, placebo-controlled trial. Am J Drug Alcohol Abuse 2007;33:367–78.
43. Kavanagh DJ, Sitharthan G, Young RM, et al. Addition of cue exposure to cognitive-behaviour therapy for alcohol misuse: a randomized trial with dysphoric drinkers. Addiction 2006;101:1106–16.
44. Vedel E, Emmelkamp PM, Schippers GM. Individual cognitive-behavioral therapy and behavioral couples therapy in alcohol use disorder: a comparative evaluation in community-based addiction treatment centers. Psychother Psychosom 2008; 77:280–8.
45. Rawson RA, McCann MJ, Flammino F, et al. A comparison of contingency management and cognitive-behavioral approaches for stimulant-dependent individuals. Addiction 2006;101:267–74.
46. Project MATCH Research Group. Matching alcoholism treatments to client heterogeneity: Project MATCH posttreatment drinking outcomes. J Stud Alcohol 1997;58:7–29.
47. Project MATCH Research Group. Matching alcoholism treatments to client heterogeneity: Project MATCH three-year drinking outcomes. Alcohol Clin Exp Res 1998;22:1300–11.
48. Higgins ST, Budney AJ, Bickel WK, et al. Incentives improve outcomes in outpatient behavioral treatment of cocaine-dependence. Arch Gen Psychiatry 1994;51: 568–76.
49. Silverman K, Wong CJ, Higgins ST, et al. Increasing opiate abstinence through voucher-based reinforcement therapy. Drug Alcohol Depend 1996;41:157–65.
50. Silverman K, Wong CJ, Umbricht-Schneiter A, et al. Broad beneficial effects of cocaine abstinence reinforcement among methadone patients. J Consult Clin Psychol 1998;66:811–24.
51. Carroll KM, Martino S, Ball SA, et al. A multisite randomized effectiveness trial of motivational enhancement therapy for Spanish-speaking substance users. J Consult Clin Psychol 2009;77:993–9.
52. Ball SA, Martino S, Nich C, et al. Site matters: multisite randomized trial of motivational enhancement therapy in community drug abuse clinics. J Consult Clin Psychol 2007;75:556–67.
53. Gray E, McCambridge J, Strang J. The effectiveness of motivational interviewing delivered by youth workers in reducing drinking, cigarette, and cannabis smoking among young people: quasi-experimental pilot study. Alcohol Alcohol 2005;40:535–9.
54. Carroll KM, Ball SA, Nich C, et al. Motivational interviewing to improve treatment engagement and outcome in individuals seeking treatment for substance abuse: a multisite effectiveness study. Drug Alcohol Depend 2006;81:301–12.
55. McCrady BS, Ziedonis D. American Psychiatric Association practice guideline for substance use disorders. Behav Med 2001;32:309–36.
56. Miller WR, Hester R. Inpatient alcoholism treatment: who benefits? Am Psychol 1986;41:794–805.
57. Cosci F, Schruers KR, Abrams K, et al. Alcohol use disorders and panic disorder: a review of the evidence of a direct relationship. J Clin Psychiatry 2007;68:874–80.
58. Cooper ML. Motivations for alcohol use among adolescents: development and validation of a four-factor model. Psychol Assess 1994;6:117–28.

59. Grant VV, Stewart SH, Mohr CD. Coping-anxiety and coping-depression motives predict different daily mood-drinking relationships. Psychol Addict Behav 2009; 23:226–37.

60. Otto MW, O' Cleirigh CM, Pollack MH. Attending to emotional cues for drug abuse: bridging the gap between clinic and home behaviors. Sci Pract Perspect 2007;3:48–56.

61. Monti PM, Rohsenow DJ, Swift RM, et al. Naltrexone and cue exposure with coping and communication skills training for alcoholics: treatment process and 1-year outcomes. Alcohol Clin Exp Res 2001;25:1634–47.

62. Rohsenow DJ, Monti PM, Rubonis AV, et al. Cue exposure with coping skills training and communication skills training for alcohol dependence: 6- and 12-month outcomes. Addiction 2001;96:1161–74.

63. Otto MW, Safren SA, Pollack MH. Internal cue exposure and the treatment of substance use disorders: lessons from the treatment of panic disorder. J Anxiety Disord 2004;18:69–87.

64. Pollack MH, Penava SA, Bolton E, et al. A novel cognitive-behavioral approach for treatment-resistant drug dependence. J Subst Abuse Treat 2002;23:335–42.

65. Zvolensky MJ, Lejuez CW, Kahler CW, et al. Integrating an interoceptive exposure-based smoking cessation program into the cognitive-behavioral treatment of panic disorder: theoretical relevance and case demonstration. Cogn Behav Pract 2003;10:347–57.

66. Zvolensky MJ, Yartz AR, Gregor K, et al. Interoceptive exposure-based cessation intervention for smokers high in anxiety sensitivity: a case series. J Cogn Psychother 2008;22:347–66.

67. Reynolds B. A review of delay-discounting research with humans: relations to drug use and gambling. Behav Pharmacol 2006;17:651–67.

68. Carroll KM, Ball SA, Martino S, et al. Computer-assisted delivery of cognitive-behavioral therapy for addiction: a randomized trial of CBT4CBT. Am J Psychiatry 2008;165:881–8.

69. Carroll KM, Ball SA, Martino S, et al. Enduring effects of a computer-assisted training program for cognitive behavioral therapy: a 6-month follow-up of CBT4CBT. Drug Alcohol Depend 2009;100:178–81.

70. Hood WF, Compton RP, Monahan JB. D-Cycloserine: a ligand for the N-methyl-D-aspartate coupled glycine receptor has partial agonist characteristics. Neurosci Lett 1989;98:91–5.

71. Otto MW, Basden SL, Leyro TM, et al. Clinical perspectives on the combination of D-cycloserine and cognitive-behavioral therapy for the treatment of anxiety disorders. CNS Spectr 2007;12:51–6, 59–61.

72. Dhonnchadha BAN, Szalay JJ, Achat-Mendes C, et al. D-Cycloserine deters reacquisition of cocaine self-administration by augmenting extinction learning. Neuropsychopharmacology 2009;2:357–67.

73. Groblewski PA, Lattal KM, Cunningham CL. Effects of D-cycloserine on extinction and reconditioning of ethanol-seeking behavior in mice. Alcohol Clin Exp Res 2009;33:772–82.

74. Myers KM, Carlezon WA. D-Cycloserine facilitates extinction of naloxone-induced place aversion in morphine-dependent rats. Biol Psychiatry 2010;67:85–7.

75. Condon TP, Miner LL, Balmer CW, et al. Blending addiction and research and practice: strategies for technology transfer. J Subst Abuse Treat 2008;35:156–60.

76. Cook JM, Walser RD, Kane V, et al. Dissemination and feasibility of a cognitive-behavioral treatment for substance use disorders and posttraumatic stress disorder in the veterans administration. J Psychoactive Drugs 2006;38:89–92.

77. McHugo GJ, Drake RE, Whitley R, et al. Fidelity outcomes in the National Implementing Evidence-based Practices Project. Psychiatr Serv 2007;58:1279–84.
78. Squires DD, Gumbley SJ, Storti SA. Training substance abuse treatment organizations to adopt evidence-based practices: the Addiction Technology Transfer Center of New England Science to Service Laboratory. J Subst Abuse Treat 2008;34:293–301.

Cognitive Behavioral Therapy for Schizophrenia

Shanaya Rathod, MD, MRCPsych[a],*, Peter Phiri, BSc[b],
David Kingdon, MD, FRCPsych[c]

KEYWORDS

- Schizophrenia • Cognitive behavioral therapy
- Psychosis • CBT

Although pharmacotherapy remains the main treatment of schizophrenia, up to 75% of patients are dissatisfied and discontinue their initially prescribed medication (typical or atypical) in an 18-month period[1] by stopping or changing to another drug. Treatment resistance is another problem. Even when patients with schizophrenia adhere to prescribed medication regimes, up to 50% will have ongoing positive or negative symptoms, with 20% to 30% of people with such persistent symptoms of schizophrenia demonstrating very little symptomatic response to adequate trials of conventional antipsychotic medications.[2] A recent cost-effectiveness analysis evaluating total population-level costs and effectiveness (measured in disability-adjusted life years averted) concluded that the most cost-effective interventions in schizophrenia were those using older antipsychotic drugs combined with psychosocial treatment, delivered via a community-based service model.[3]

Cognitive behavioral therapy (CBT) is an evidence-based adjunct to medication in the treatment of schizophrenia. The treatment is acceptable to patients. It is regarded as an essential treatment in clinical treatment guidelines in the United States (eg, American Psychiatric Association Steering Committee on Practice Guidelines,[4,5] Patient Outcome Research Team[6]) and the United Kingdom and Europe (eg, National Institute of Clinical Excellence[7,8]). Evidence has developed from case studies, randomized controlled trials, and meta-analyses[9,10] confirming its effectiveness in persistent positive and negative symptoms of schizophrenia.

[a] Hampshire Partnership NHS Foundation Trust, Melbury Lodge, Winchester, Hampshire SO22 5DG, UK
[b] Royal South Hants Hospital, Southampton, Hampshire SO14 0YG, UK
[c] Department of Psychiatry, University of Southampton, Royal South Hants Hospital, Southampton, Hampshire SO14 0YG, UK
* Corresponding author.
E-mail address: shanaya.rathod@hantspt-mid.nhs.uk

Psychiatr Clin N Am 33 (2010) 527–536
doi:10.1016/j.psc.2010.04.009
0193-953X/10/$ – see front matter © 2010 Elsevier Inc. All rights reserved.

DEVELOPMENT AND TECHNIQUES

Cognitive behavioral techniques in psychosis were first used in 1952 by Beck[11] in a patient who was paranoid about the Federal Bureau of Investigation. The patient was encouraged to trace the antecedents of the delusion and behavioral techniques such as reality testing were used. The patient was eventually able to recognize that all his alleged persecutors were normal people going about their daily business. Subsequently, Hole and colleagues[12] described 8 patients with chronic delusions, half of whom appeared to improve when cognitive and behavioral techniques were used.

CBT for schizophrenia has developed against a backdrop of intense skepticism because of past failures of other individual psychotherapies. However, unlike therapies for schizophrenia evaluated in the 1970s and 1980s, CBT is based on the general principles of cognitive therapy developed by Beck for depression. These techniques are more structured and collaborative. They involve discussion of thoughts, feelings, and actions to understand symptoms better. Therapy draws on the patient's beliefs and experiences. CBT for schizophrenia differs from other psychosocial interventions because it is based on the stress vulnerability model developed by Zubin and Spring[13] and further elaborated by Nuechterlein and colleagues.[14] This model emphasizes the interaction between life events, circumstances, and individual genetic, physiological, psychological, and social predispositions that lead to variation in vulnerability to psychotic breakdown.

In CBT there is a strong focus on engagement of the patient. Agendas are less explicit, feelings are elicited with great care, and homework is used. Assessment is based on clinical practice. Emphasis is placed on understanding the first episode in detail because it often holds the key to current beliefs and perceptions. For example, hallucinations may have first emerged with a drug-related experience or paranoia following a traumatic event. Information on current beliefs and how they were arrived at is assembled into a formulation that draws together predisposing, precipitating, perpetuating, and protective factors with current and underlying concerns with the interactions between thoughts, feelings, and behaviors. A rationale based on a vulnerability-stress model is explored with the patient using normalizing of symptoms where appropriate and forming part of the continuum between normal and distressing or disturbing experiences. Methods to draw up and debate or explore key beliefs in other disorders are applied such as Socratic questioning and guided discovery.[15,16]

Specific work with hallucinations, delusions, and negative symptoms can assist in reattribution of the experiences and beliefs to the self rather than others or external sources. Ways of coping with persistent hallucinations and strong beliefs allow behavioral change including socialization to occur. This in turn can help break the cycle of isolation and distress that frequently fuels the dysfunctional beliefs. Negative symptoms are conceptualized in terms of their positive value to the individual (eg, reduction of anxiety or protection against increase in voices or paranoia), and then alternative ways for the individual to control and manage these symptoms are found. This may initially involve improving understanding of the positive symptoms (eg, paranoia, voices, and anxiety) better and then, through long-term goals-setting (instilling hope) and short-term graded collaborative task assignment, begin a process of developing behavioral activation (**Fig. 1**).

The affective and nonaffective psychoses are varied in presentation and psychosocial interventions are becoming increasingly tailored to these differences. These relatively distinct approaches are detailed in **Fig. 1**.[15] In summary, when drug misuse is a precipitating factor, approaches using a combination of motivational interviewing,

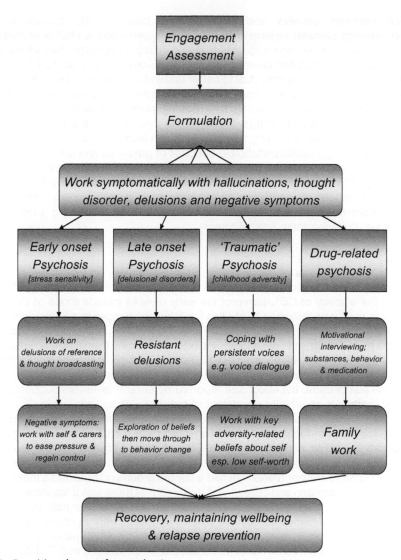

Fig. 1. Cognitive therapy for psychosis.

CBT, and family work are showing promise.[17] Experience of severe childhood adversity has been an issue for a group of patients with schizophrenia who also meet criteria for borderline personality disorder. Management of both the psychotic and emotional symptoms is necessary. Onset of psychosis may also be an important factor to consider in management[18] with the early onset group presenting major issues in relation to socialization; later onset often presents with systematized delusions requiring specific psychological work.

Relapse prevention is a key aspect of working to prevent reemergence and exacerbation of psychosis using CBT. Two general methods have been used in cognitive therapy to promote collaboration with pharmacotherapy regimens. The first is specific discussion of medication and associated beliefs with psychoeducation regarding the balance between benefits and side effects. Involving the patient in the decision-making process regarding treatment (eg, providing a choice of possible medications to consider and negotiation about dosage) improves their chances of compliance. The second and complementary approach is a more gradual one aimed at broadly working with the individual to better understand their problems (eg, voices), their development (eg, through early traumatic events or drug misuse), normalizing symptoms appropriately, enhancing their coping skills, and discussing what part medication might have in assisting with such coping. As part of this broader approach, cognitive therapy involves helping the patients to develop alternative explanations for their symptoms (eg, misinterpretation in the case of paranoia) and the understanding that these symptoms could be triggered by stressful events while they were vulnerable, biologically or psychosocially. Patients may then be more likely to recognize the potential benefit of medication in reducing their distressing experiences (eg, through improved sleep or reduced stimulation) and by improving their coping capacity (eg, buffering them against stress).

EVIDENCE

More than 30 randomized controlled trials and meta-analyses have been published reporting the efficacy of CBT. Some of the early reviews include those of Bouchard and colleagues[19] who reviewed 15 studies focusing on changes in positive symptoms as the main outcome measure and Rector and Beck[20] who examined 7 randomized controlled trials. Pilling and colleagues[21] included the results from 8 randomized trials; a review published by NICE[7] included 13 randomized clinical trials (including the review by Pilling and colleagues[21]) with data from 1297 patients.

Over the last decade, the effect size reported by several reviewers suggested that cognitive therapy is an effective treatment of patients with schizophrenia. Gould and colleagues[22] calculated effect sizes for 7 studies involving 340 subjects and reported mean effect size for reduction of psychotic symptoms as 0.65. Follow-up analyses in 4 studies indicated that patients receiving CBT continued to make gains over time (effect size 0.93). Tarrier and Wykes[23] reviewed 20 trials of CBT, mainly of treatment-resistant schizophrenia that had a control group and reported a mean effect size of 0.37. Zimmermann and colleagues[9] reported that there was a significant reduction in positive symptoms and there was a higher benefit of CBT for patients suffering an acute psychotic episode versus the chronic condition with an effect size of 0.57 versus 0.27 following a review of 14 studies including 1484 patients published between 1990 and 2004. Pfammatter and colleagues[24] concluded that CBT for persistent positive symptoms emerges as an effective adjunct to pharmacotherapy with an effect size of 0.47. Wykes and colleagues[10] published a meta-analysis of 34 trials of CBT for psychosis and reported overall beneficial effects for the target symptom with effect size of 0.40, as well as significant effects for positive symptoms, negative symptoms, functioning, mood, and social anxiety with effects ranging from 0.35 to 0.44. They did not find an effect on hopelessness. The meta-analysis concluded that improvements in one domain were correlated with improvements in others and noted that effect sizes were related to the strength of the control condition and the methodological rigor of the trial.

Besides benefits in persistent positive and negative symptoms of schizophrenia, CBT-based techniques have demonstrated an improvement in medication adherence.[25] CBT-based brief interventions[26] have led to a statistically significant improvement in overall insight, symptoms of psychosis, and depression at posttherapy assessment. CBT has been shown to affect time to hospitalization[27] with the effect maintained at 24-months follow-up, although in this study occupational recovery did not improve.[28] Although there are reported benefits in relapse,[29] in studies in which hospitalization was excluded as a proxy for relapse, Lynch and colleagues[30] did not find CBT to have a significant effect.

There is emerging evidence that CBT in psychosis is superior to treatment-as-usual (TAU) in reducing the incidence of aggression during treatment and in the follow-up period.[31] CBT is also proving beneficial in comorbid conditions (eg, anxiety associated with psychosis).[32] There are some positive reports for broader CBT-based psychosocial interventions for psychosis and substance misuse[17] and early intervention in psychosis[33] although there are methodological difficulties with some of these trials and further research with larger sample sizes is progressing.

Gaps remain, in particular, in mediation analyses that clarify exactly how CBT for psychosis produces its effects. Few studies have provided much information and so this is becoming a focus of future work. Although CBT for psychosis is based on Beckian models and methods of intervention, it has been supplemented in a range of ways and these have differed at least in emphasis from study to study. For example, some studies have focused on delusions and hallucination, whereas others have emphasized the importance of also working with negative symptoms.

Although most of the research on CBT for schizophrenia has been conducted in the United Kingdom, several studies are being conducted in Europe, the United States, and Canada.[34] Rector and colleagues[35] reported significant clinical effects for positive, negative, and overall symptom severity for patients treated in the CBT arm, although there were no statistically significant differences between the treatment groups after treatment.

NEUROBIOLOGICAL EVIDENCE

There is emerging evidence that gray matter volume of the frontal, temporal, parietal, and cerebellar areas that are known to be involved in the coordination of mental activity, cognitive flexibility, and verbal learning and memory predict responsiveness to CBT in patients with psychosis.[36] In this study, improvement in positive symptoms was associated with greater right cerebellum gray matter volume and with the left precentral gyrus and right inferior parietal lobule gray matter volumes in negative symptoms. Improvement in general psychopathology was associated with greater right superior temporal gyrus, cuneus, and cerebellum (Crus I) gray matter volumes. However, gray matter volume in these brain areas did not correlate with the severity of baseline symptoms. In another functional study, CBT plus TAU patients showed significant improvement in relation to the TAU-alone group at follow-up. This correlated with stronger dorsolateral prefrontal cortex activity (although within the normal range) and connectivity with the cerebellum, which predicted responsiveness to CBT in schizophrenia.[37]

PREDICTORS OF OUTCOME

Being female,[38,39] a shorter duration of untreated illness, a shorter duration of illness,[39] higher levels of insight, higher levels of admissions,[40] and patients with low level of convictions in their delusions[38] have been associated with better outcome with CBT. Despite its potential to improve insight,[26] CBT has been less successful with patients with very low levels of insight[40,41] and severe primary negative symptoms[42] including affective blunting and alogia[43] although modification of techniques and longer treatment periods (20 sessions) in some studies has been more successful with these patients.[44]

For certain types of psychotic symptoms (eg, command hallucinations linked to trauma, or systematized or grandiose delusions), distressing affects can emerge as the psychotic symptom is worked with but can also be successfully managed.[45] Brief CBT is often not indicated for such presentations and 20 to 50 sessions with a CBT expert can be indicated.[46]

CULTURAL ADAPTATIONS OF CBT

Cultural adaptations and understanding of ethnic, cultural, and religious interpretations is an area that currently remains underdeveloped.[47,48] In the Insight study, the African Caribbean group at 3 months and the Black African group at 1 year follow-up analysis showed higher dropout rates and significantly poorer change in insight compared with the White group.[49] Literature from other cultural groups recommends the adaptation of CBT for use with ethnic minority populations as necessary and possible.[50] The evidence base includes very few adequately powered randomized trials of CBT in which specific ethnic groups are included in adequate numbers to assess treatment efficacy and effectiveness. Qualitative work has indicated a range of appropriate adaptations[51] that are now being evaluated.

LIMITATIONS

Criticisms of CBT research have been made[30]; specifically that studies did not shown effects better than those of nonspecific intervention or effects on relapse. These criticisms have been refuted as, for example, studies dismissed as negative showed enduring effects present at 18 months and 5 years and in general, the assertions of noneffect may be attributed to the limited selection of studies. Relapse prevention has been more difficult to demonstrate and a large new study has produced negative findings in this area. Again, however, the exclusion of studies using hospitalization as a proxy for relapse led to a substantial underestimate of effect.[52]

Nevertheless investigator allegiance is an issue in that control interventions; for example, supportive therapy and befriending have not been delivered by experts in that particular therapy modality.[53] In this way, the nonspecific factors were well controlled for but the quality of the control intervention could be improved further. Engagement of patients in therapy has also been expressed as a concern[54] but specific approaches to this[15] can allow for common goals and agendas to be developed that make productive work possible. Further research in understanding the relative efficacy of CBT in schizophrenia compared with expert delivery of, for example, interpersonal therapy, or supplementing by using, for example, mindfulness, would nonetheless be of value.

Although there is strong evidence supporting the implementation of CBT for patients with psychosis, the potential mechanisms of action remain unclear as stated earlier. There are a variety of approaches to the delivery and conceptual underpinnings within different research groups, and the degree of consensus or disagreements regarding what are the intrinsic components have not been explored. Morrison and Barratt's[55] study uses the Delphi method to try to establish what a group of experts in CBT for psychosis view as important. Experts were invited to participate in 3 rounds of producing and rating statements that addressed areas such as principles, assessment, models, formulation, change strategies, homework, and therapists' assumptions to consolidate consensus of opinion. Seventy-seven items were endorsed as important or essential for CBT for psychosis by more than 80% of the panel. These recommendations should ensure greater fidelity in clinical practice, allow greater evaluation of adherence within clinical trials, facilitate the development of competency frameworks, and be of value in relation to training and dissemination of CBT for psychosis.

SUMMARY

CBT should be considered as a component of a comprehensive treatment package with social interventions and antipsychotic medication. In the United Kingdom, and even more elsewhere, there remain limitations in service delivery because of inadequate numbers of trained providers. There also needs to be more research into the active ingredients of CBT, predictors of outcome, role in comorbidities and benefits of cultural adaptations.

CBT for schizophrenia continues to be more widely practiced in the United Kingdom than in the United States.[56,57] In contrast, in the mid-twentieth century psychotherapies for schizophrenia were much more widely available in the United States than in the United Kingdom. Lack of evidence for these has contributed to the adoption of a biological model that may have, albeit inadvertently, led to dismissal of any psychological approach as likely to be beneficial. The reemergence of biopsychosocial-vulnerability-stress models and evidence of the effectiveness of CBT in clinical practice may assist in establishing a more balanced position. The presence of universal health care with sector-based responsibility for services with mental health parity in the United Kingdom may also have contributed to the differences in approach to health care delivery in the United States and elsewhere.

REFERENCES

1. Lieberman JA, Stroup TS, McEvoy JP, et al. Effectiveness of antipsychotic drugs in patients with chronic schizophrenia. N Engl J Med 2005;353:1209–23.
2. Conley RR, Buchanan RW. Evaluation of treatment-resistant schizophrenia. Schizophr Bull 1997;23(4):663–74.
3. Chisholm D, Gureje O, Saldivia S, et al. Schizophrenia treatment in the developing world: an interregional and multinational cost-effectiveness analysis. Bull World Health Organ 2008;86:542–51.
4. American Psychiatric Association Steering Committee on Practice Guidelines 2000. American Psychiatric Association practice guidelines for the treatment of psychiatric disorders: compendium 2000. Washington, DC: American Psychiatric Association; 2000.
5. American Psychiatric Association. Practice guideline for the treatment of patients with schizophrenia, second edition. Am J Psychiatry 2004;161:1–56.
6. Kreyenbuhl J, Buchanan RW, Dickerson FB. The Schizophrenia Patient Outcomes Research Team (PORT): updated treatment recommendations 2009. Schizophr Bull 2010;36(1):94–103.
7. National Institute for Clinical Excellence. Clinical guideline 1: schizophrenia. Core interventions in the treatment and management of schizophrenia in primary and secondary care. Available at: London: NICE; 2002 http://www.nice.org.uk. Accessed April 19, 2010.
8. National Institute for Clinical Excellence. Clinical guideline: schizophrenia (CG1). London: Department of Health; 2009.
9. Zimmermann G, Favrod J, Trieu VH, et al. The effect of cognitive behavioral treatment on the positive symptoms of schizophrenia spectrum disorders: a meta-analysis. Schizophr Res 2005;77(1):1–9.

10. Wykes T, Steel C, Everitt B, et al. Cognitive behaviour therapy for schizophrenia: effect sizes, clinical models, and methodological rigor. Schizophr Bull 2008;34: 523–37.

11. Beck AT. Successful outpatient psychotherapy of a chronic schizophrenic with a delusion based on borrowed guilt. Psychiatry 1952;15:305–12.

12. Hole RW, Rush AJ, Beck AT. A cognitive investigation of schizophrenic delusions. Psychiatry 1979;42:312–9.

13. Zubin J, Spring B. Vulnerability—a new view on schizophrenia. J Abnorm Psychol 1977;86:103–26.

14. Nuechterlein KH, Dawson ME, Ventura J, et al. The vulnerability-stress model of schizophrenic relapse: a longitudinal study. Acta Psychiatr Scand Suppl 1994; 382:58–64.

15. Kingdon D, Turkington D. Cognitive therapy of schizophrenia. New York: Guilford Press; 2005.

16. Wright J, Turkington D, Kingdon D, et al. Cognitive-behavior therapy for severe mental illness. An illustrated guide. Arlington (VA): American Psychiatric Publishing; 2009.

17. Haddock G, Barrowclough C, Tarrier N, et al. Cognitive-behavioural therapy and motivational intervention for schizophrenia and substance misuse: 18-month outcomes of a randomised controlled trial. Br J Psychiatry 2003;183(5): 418–26.

18. Howard R, Rabins PV, Seeman MV, et al. Late-onset schizophrenia and very-late-onset schizophrenia-like psychosis: an international consensus. The International Late-Onset Schizophrenia Group. Am J Psychiatry 2000;157(2): 172–8.

19. Bouchard S, Vallieres A, Roy M, et al. Cognitive restructuring in the treatment of psychotic symptoms of schizophrenia: a critical analysis. Behav Ther 1996;27: 257–77.

20. Rector N, Beck A. Cognitive behavioural therapy for schizophrenia: an empirical review. J Nerv Ment Dis 2001;189:278–87.

21. Pilling S, Bebbington P, Kuipers E, et al. Psychological treatments in schizophrenia: I. Meta-analysis of family intervention and cognitive behaviour therapy. Psychol Med 2002;32:763–82.

22. Gould RA, Mueser KT, Bolton E, et al. Cognitive therapy for psychosis in schizophrenia: an effect size analysis. Schizophr Res 2001;48:335–42.

23. Tarrier N, Wykes T. Is there evidence that cognitive behaviour therapy is an effective treatment for schizophrenia? A cautious or cautionary tale? Behav Res Ther 2004;2(12):1377–401.

24. Pfammatter M, Junghan UM, Brenner HD. Efficacy of psychological therapy in schizophrenia: conclusions from meta-analyses. Schizophr Bull 2006;32(Suppl 1): S64–80.

25. Kemp R, Hayward P, Applewhaite G, et al. Compliance therapy in psychotic patients: a randomised controlled trial. Br Med J 1996;312:345–9.

26. Turkington D, Kingdon D, Turner T. The effectiveness of a brief cognitive behavioural intervention in schizophrenia. Br J Psychiatry 2002;180(6):523–7.

27. Turkington D, Kingdon D, Rathod S, et al. Outcomes of an effectiveness trial of cognitive-behavioural intervention by mental health nurses in schizophrenia. Br J Psychiatry 2006;189:36–40.

28. Malik N, Kingdon D, Pelton J, et al. Effectiveness of brief cognitive-behavioral therapy for schizophrenia delivered by mental health nurses: relapse and recovery at 24 months. J Clin Psychiatry 2009;70(2):201–7.

29. Gumley A, O'Grady M, Mcnay L, et al. Early intervention for relapse in schizophrenia: results of a 12-month randomized controlled trial of cognitive behavioural therapy. Psychol Med 2003;33(3):419–31.
30. Lynch D, Laws KR, McKenna PJ. Cognitive behavioural therapy for major psychiatric disorder: does it really work? A meta-analytical review of well-controlled trials. Psychol Med 2010;40:9–24.
31. Haddock G, Barrowclough C, Shaw JJ, et al. Cognitive-behavioural therapy v. social activity therapy for people with psychosis and a history of violence: randomised controlled trial. Br J Psychiatry 2009;194(2):152–7.
32. Naeem F, Kingdon D, Turkington D. Cognitive behaviour therapy for schizophrenia: relationship between anxiety symptoms and therapy. Psychol Psychother Theor Res Pract 2006;79(Pt 2):1–13.
33. Morrison AP, French P, Walford L, et al. Cognitive therapy for the prevention of psychosis in people at ultra-high risk: randomised controlled trial. Br J Psychiatry 2004;185:291–7.
34. Pinto A, La Pia S, Mennella R, et al. Cognitive-behavioral therapy for clozapine clients with treatment-refractory schizophrenia. Psychiatr Serv 1999;50: 901–4.
35. Rector NA, Seeman MV, Segal ZV. Cognitive therapy of schizophrenia: a preliminary randomized controlled trial. Schizophr Res 2003;63:1–11.
36. Premkumar P, Fannon D, Kuipers E, et al. Structural magnetic resonance imaging predictors of responsiveness to cognitive behaviour therapy in psychosis. Schizophr Res 2009;115(2–3):146–55.
37. Kumari V, Peters ER, Fannon D, et al. Dorsolateral prefrontal cortex activity predicts responsiveness to cognitive-behavioral therapy in schizophrenia. Biol Psychiatry 2009;66(6):594–602.
38. Brabban A, Tai S, Turkington D. Predictors of outcome in brief cognitive behavior therapy for schizophrenia. Schizophr Bull 2009;35(5):859–64.
39. Drury V, Birchwood M, Cochrane R, et al. Cognitive therapy and recovery from acute psychosis: a controlled trial. II. Impact on recovery time. Br J Psychiatry 1996;169:602–7.
40. Garety P, Fowler D, Kuipers E, et al. London-East Anglia randomised controlled trial of cognitive-behavioural therapy for psychosis. II: predictors of outcome. Br J Psychiatry 1997;171:420–6.
41. Naeem F, Kingdon D, Turkington D. Predictors of response to cognitive behaviour therapy in the treatment of schizophrenia: a comparison of brief and standard interventions. Cognit Ther Res 2008;32(5):651–6.
42. Garety PA, Fowler D, Kuipers E. Cognitive-behavioral therapy for medication-resistant symptoms. Schizophr Bull 2000;26(1):73–86.
43. Tarrier N, Yusupoff L, Kinney C, et al. Randomised controlled trial of intensive cognitive behavior therapy for patients with chronic schizophrenia. Br Med J 1998;317:303–7.
44. Sensky T, Turkington D, Kingdon D, et al. A randomized controlled trial of cognitive-behavioral therapy for persistent symptoms in schizophrenia resistant to medication. Arch Gen Psychiatry 2000;57(2):165–72.
45. Birchwood M, Trower P. The future of cognitive–behavioural therapy for psychosis: not a quasi-neuroleptic. Br J Psychiatry 2006;188:107–8.
46. Turkington D, McKenna P. Is cognitive behavioural therapy a worthwhile treatment for psychosis? Br J Psychiatry 2003;182:477–9.
47. Rathod S, Naeem F, Phiri P, et al. Expansion of psychological therapies. Br J Psychiatry 2008;193:256.

48. Rathod S, Kingdon D. Cognitive behaviour therapy across cultures. Psychiatry 2009;8(9):370-1.
49. Rathod S, Kingdon D, Smith P, et al. Insight into schizophrenia: the effects of cognitive behavioural therapy on the components of insight and association with sociodemographics - data on a previously published randomised controlled trial. Schizophr Res 2005;74:2-3, 211-9.
50. Daffenbacher L. Agreement and response to neglected variables in cognitive-behavioural treatments. Couns Psychol 1988;16:314-7.
51. Rathod S, Kingdon D, Phiri P, et al. Developing culturally sensitive cognitive behaviour therapy for psychosis for ethnic minority patients by exploration and incorporation of service users and health professionals views and opinions. Behav Cogn Psychother, in press.
52. Kingdon D. Over-simplification and exclusion of non-conforming studies can demonstrate absence of effect: a lynching party? Psychol Med 2010;40(1):25-7.
53. Paley G, Shapiro D. Lessons from psychotherapy research for psychological interventions for people with schizophrenia. Psychol Psychother Theor Res Pract 2002;75:5-17.
54. Kingdon D, Kirschen H. Who does not get cognitive-behavioral therapy for schizophrenia when therapy is readily available? Psychiatr Serv 2006;57:1792-4.
55. Morrison AP, Barratt S. What are the components of CBT for psychosis? A Delphi study. Schizophr Bull 2010;36:136-42.
56. Christie-Smith D, Gartner C. Highlights of the 2002 Institute on Psychiatric Services. Psychiatr Serv 2003;54(1):12-7.
57. Turkington D, Kingdon D, Weiden P. Cognitive behaviour therapy for schizo-phrenia. Am J Psychiatry 2006;163:365-73.

Cognitive Behavioral Therapy for Mood Disorders: Efficacy, Moderators and Mediators

Ellen Driessen, MSc[a],*, Steven D. Hollon, PhD[b]

KEYWORDS

- Cognitive behavioral therapy • Mood disorder
- Depression • Efficacy • Moderator • Mediator

Clinical depression is one of the most common and debilitating of the psychiatric disorders.[1] Lifetime prevalence has been estimated at 16.2% and rates of comorbidity and risk for suicide are high.[2] Up to one-third of all patients have episodes that last longer than 2 years, and more than three-quarters of all patients who recover from one episode go on to have at least one more.[3] Although there are efficacious treatments for depression, many patients do not receive adequate treatment, and still more are refractory to available interventions.[4]

Depression can be defined as a syndrome and a disorder. As a syndrome it involves episodes of sadness, loss of interest, pessimism, negative beliefs about the self, decreased motivation, behavioral passivity, suicidal thoughts and impulses, and changes in sleep, appetite, and sexual interest. As a disorder it comes in 2 forms. The unipolar type, which affects approximately 10% of men and 20% of women, includes only episodes of depression. Heritability estimates for unipolar depression have ranged from approximately 25% in less severe samples up to 50% in more severe samples.[5] In the bipolar form, which is commonly known as manic depression, patients also (or exclusively) experience episodes of mania or hypomania that are in many ways the opposite of depression. Manic episodes are marked by euphoria or irritability, sleeplessness, grandiosity, recklessness, and uncontrollable impulses that can lead to buying sprees and sexual promiscuity.[6]

Preparation of this manuscript was supported by National Institute of Mental Health Grant MH01697 (K02) to the second author.

[a] Faculty of Psychology and Education, Department of Clinical Psychology, VU University Amsterdam, Van der Boechorststraat 1, 1018 BX Amsterdam, The Netherlands
[b] Department of Psychology, Vanderbilt University, 306 Wilson Hall, Nashville, TN 37240, USA
* Corresponding author.
E-mail address: e.driessen@psy.vu.nl

Cognitive behavioral therapy (CBT) refers to a family of interventions that are among the best-known empirically supported treatments for depression. There are several different specific interventions that vary in their constituent components, with cognitive therapy (CT) being the most widely practiced, but all these interventions are closely related and the terms CBT and CT are used interchangeably in this article. CBT is based on the premise that inaccurate beliefs and maladaptive information processing (forming the bases for repetitive negative thinking) have a causal role in the cause and maintenance of depression. This cognitive model posits that when maladaptive thinking is corrected, acute distress and the risk for subsequent symptom return are reduced.[7] This article focuses on the efficacy of individual CBT in the treatment of acute phase depression and the prevention of subsequent symptom return in adult populations, with an emphasis on the moderation and mediation of response.

THE EFFICACY OF CBT IN THE ACUTE PHASE OF DEPRESSION
Meta-analytic Findings

CBT has a medium effect size ($d = 0.67$) relative to a variety of control conditions ranging from the absence of treatment to nonspecific controls.[8] Translated into numbers needed to treat (NNT), this effect size corresponds to an NNT of 2.75; this means that for just less than every 3 patients treated with CBT, one will get better solely because of having come into therapy. By way of comparison, medication treatment of severe hypertension produces an NNT of 15 and taking aspirin alone for myocardial infarction produces an NNT of 40 relative to no treatment (see NNT readings at http://www.evidence-based-medicine.co.uk). Effect sizes tend to be larger when CBT is compared with wait-list controls ($d = 0.88$) than when CBT is compared with care-as-usual ($d = 0.38$) or nonspecific controls ($d = 0.38$).[8] These findings suggest that CBT is more efficacious than its absence and somewhat more efficacious than the mobilization of hope and therapist contact. Effect sizes tend to be lower in high-quality studies or when corrected for publication bias.[8] It has been reported that the efficacy of CBT when delivered individually did not differ from the efficacy of a group format ($d = 0.15$, nonsignificant [ns]), but the quality of the relevant studies is low, limiting our confidence in this conclusion.[9]

Gloaguen and colleagues[10] found CBT superior to an assortment of other psychotherapies, but this estimate was likely inflated by the inclusion of nonbona fide therapies intended only to control for nonspecific factors.[11] This is in line with Cuijpers and colleagues,[8] who found no significant differences when comparing CBT with other psychotherapies. Gloaguen and colleagues[10] also found CBT moderately superior to antidepressant medication (ADM); however, this estimate was likely to be inflated by the inclusion of early studies that did a questionable job of implementing pharmacotherapy.[12] For example, Rush and colleagues[13] found CBT superior to the ADM imipramine in the treatment of depressed outpatients, but started medication withdrawal 2 weeks before the end of treatment, and Blackburn and colleagues[14] found CBT superior to either amitriptyline or clomipramine in a general practice sample, but had such a poor response to ADM (14%) as to raise questions about the adequacy of the pharmacotherapy as implemented by the general practitioners. Subsequent studies that implemented pharmacotherapy more adequately typically found comparable outcomes between CBT and ADM.[15,16] This result is in line with findings of a more recent meta-analysis by Cuijpers and colleagues[8] that suggests that CBT and ADM are equally efficacious in the treatment of major depression.

Combining CBT with ADM results in higher effect sizes than medication alone ($d = 0.27$, $P<.05$; NNT = 6.58).[8] This finding means that the combination produces a modest increment compared with medication monotherapy; combining CBT with ADM improves acute response for 1 out of nearly every 6 patients. Combined treatment produces only a small nonsignificant effect relative to CBT alone ($d = 0.15$; ns; NNT = 11.9), an effect about half the magnitude of adding CBT to medications.[8] However, these estimates are based on controlled treatment trials that often provide greater training and supervision than is the case in practice. Whether most patients have access to comparably trained CBT therapists is a matter of conjecture. Combining medications with CBT as typically practiced in applied settings may enhance treatment response.

CBT has been found to work better than its absence and may work for specific reasons. CBT seems to be at least as efficacious as other active treatments, including medications. Adding CBT to ADM has resulted in a modest improvement of efficacy. The benefits of adding medication to CBT relative to CBT alone have been less apparent, although these effects might be larger in applied clinical practice than in the controlled setting of a treatment trial.

CBT for Severe Depression

The National Institute of Mental Health Treatment of Depression Collaborative Research Program (TDCRP) was the first major trial comparing CBT with a pill-placebo control and the results were not supportive of CBT. Although there were no differences across the full sample,[17] CBT was no more efficacious than pill-placebo and less efficacious than either the ADM imipramine or interpersonal psychotherapy (IPT) among patients with more severe depressions.[18] The results of the TDRCP had a major effect on the field, because of the size of the sample and the rigor of the design. It led many to conclude that CBT was not efficacious with more severe depressions, and subsequent guidelines strongly suggested that such patients should not be treated with psychotherapy alone.[19]

Despite the rigor of its design, questions have been raised about the adequacy of the implementation of CBT in the TDCRP.[20] Outcomes for CBT varied considerably across the 3 study sites, with CBT performing no better than pill-placebo at the 2 sites with less experienced therapists and as well as ADM at the remaining site, where the cognitive therapists had previous experience with the approach.[21] Subsequent placebo-controlled trials that have implemented CBT more successfully have shown it to be comparable with ADM and each superior to pill-placebo controls. For example, Jarrett and colleagues[22] found CT as efficacious as phenelzine (a monoamine oxidase inhibitor [MAOI]) for the treatment of atypical depression. This group has worked closely with the Beck Institute in Philadelphia to ensure that their cognitive therapists were well trained and had session tapes rated for competence by an off-site consultant expert in the approach. Similarly, MAOIs are the medications of choice for atypical depression and were prescribed at dosage levels that were appropriate.

DeRubeis and colleagues[23] attempted a direct replication of the TDCRP with respect to the comparison between CBT and ADM among more severely depressed patients. Patients who met the TDCRP criterion for moderate to severe depression (scores of 20 or above for 2 consecutive weeks on the Hamilton Depression Rating Scale [HDRS]) were randomly assigned to 16 weeks of either CBT or paroxetine pharmacotherapy or 8 weeks of pill-placebo (a sufficient length of time to establish drug-placebo differences). Paroxetine is generally considered the best of the selective serotonin reuptake inhibitors for dealing with patients with more severe depressions. In addition, patients in the ADM condition who were not fully responsive by the end of 8 weeks of treatment were augmented with either lithium or desipramine through the end of the 16-week trial. This is a more aggressive pharmacotherapy regime than is typically used in short-term treatment trials. The study was conducted at 2 sites, one of which was the original home of CT (University of Pennsylvania), whereas the other had less experienced cognitive therapists (Vanderbilt University). Ratings conducted by experts at the Beck Institute suggested that the less experienced cognitive therapists at Vanderbilt were not performing at the same level of competence as the more experienced cognitive therapists at Penn. Therefore, the Vanderbilt therapists were provided with additional training through the extramural training program at the Beck Institute during the early years of the trail.

CBT and paroxetine pharmacotherapy were superior to pill-placebo across the first 8 weeks of the trial and virtually identical to one another by the end of the full 16-week acute treatment period. There were differences between the sites, with CBT showing a nonsignificant advantage relative to ADM at Penn and ADM performing significantly better than CBT at Vanderbilt. Differences between the sites were more pronounced in the beginning of the trial, with the less experienced cognitive therapists at Vanderbilt catching up with their more experienced colleagues at Penn across time with respect to competence ratings and patient outcomes. There also were indications that patients with comorbid Axis II disorders did better on ADM than they did in CBT, whereas the opposite was true for patients without Axis II disorders.[24] Patients with Axis II disorders constituted a larger portion of the sample at Vanderbilt and differences in patient composition and therapist experience largely explained the differences between the sites. These findings suggest that CBT can be as efficacious as ADM with more severely depressed patients if provided by experienced cognitive therapists who are competent to implement that modality.

Dimidjian and colleagues[25] found a pattern of results in a subsequent placebo-controlled trial that was reminiscent of the one found in the TDCRP, but that might still be consistent with the notion that competence matters with respect to CBT for more severely depressed patients. In that trial, patients with major depression representing a full range of severity were randomly assigned to 16 weeks of CBT, behavioral activation (BA), paroxetine pharmacotherapy (without augmentation), or pill-placebo (8 weeks only). As in the TDCRP, there were no differences between any of the treatment conditions among less severely depressed patients. Among the more severely depressed patients (those with HDRS scores of 20 or greater), ADM and BA were found to be superior to either pill-placebo (at week 8) or CBT (at week 8 and week 16). The advantage of BA compared with CBT was largely a consequence of a subset of patients who showed an extremely poor response to CBT.[26] These patients were severely depressed, functionally impaired, and had problems with their primary support group; most also described themselves as having lifelong depressions. Although Dimidjian and colleagues[25] did not assess the full array of personality disorders (PDs), these patients were similar in many respects to the Axis II patients who did poorly in CBT in the Penn/Vandy trial.[24] There were as many such patients in that earlier study and although they did not do well in CBT, they did not show the extreme nonresponse that they showed in the study by Dimidjian and colleagues. The cognitive therapists started the Dimidjian and colleagues study with about the same level of experience as the less experienced cognitive therapists at the Vanderbilt site in the DeRubeis and colleagues study, but did not have the advantage of the additional training through the Beck Institute during the study proper.

CBT seems to be as efficacious as ADM in the treatment of depression. Two studies found that CBT performed less well than either ADM or an other psychotherapy among more severely depressed patients.[18,25] It is not clear that the cognitive therapists were experienced with the approach in those 2 trials and CBT has performed as well as

ADM in other placebo-controlled trials when therapist experience was not an issue.[22,23] Thus, CBT seems to work as well as ADM for more severely depressed patients, if conducted by well-trained therapists.

It is not clear how much experience and training is necessary to ensure therapist competence but it does seem that much of the variation in the CBT literature is related to the skill with which the modality is implemented. We have emphasized the role played by such variability in determining outcomes in the handful of placebo-controlled trials precisely because they are the most influential studies found in the literature and (one would hope) the most carefully conducted. The bulk of these trials were efficacy studies and it is likely that variability is even greater (and competence less likely to be assured) in the effectiveness literature. Those studies that found the best outcomes for CBT typically selected experienced cognitive therapists (as at the University of Pennsylvania) or provided extended training coordinated with the Beck Institute in Philadelphia (as at the Vanderbilt site in that same study or in the study of atypical depression); studies that depended on more limited training and off-site supervision typically produced less impressive findings relative to alternative interventions (especially medications). These differences were most apparent with severe and complicated patients and it is likely that therapist competence is more an issue with such patients because that is where treatment differences are usually found. How much training and supervision are required and whether it varies as a function of patient difficulty are issues that deserve further exploration.

Cognitive Behavioral Analysis System of Psychotherapy for Chronic Depression

The cognitive behavioral analysis system of psychotherapy (CBASP) was developed specifically for the treatment of chronic depression and combines techniques from cognitive, behavioral, psychodynamic and interpersonal psychotherapies. It shares with CBT its structured approach, the use of homework assignments, and the systematic focus on assessing and changing behaviors or interpretations of a situation. It differs from CBT, however, by its primary focus on interpersonal interaction. Keller and colleagues[27] compared the efficacy of CBASP with that of nefazodone, and with the combination of CBASP and nefazodone, and found that after 12 weeks of acute treatment CBASP and nefazodone resulted in equal response rates (both 48%), whereas combined treatment significantly outperformed both monotreatments (response rate 73%). However, these analyses were based on a modified intention-to-treat in which patients who either did not start treatment or who could not achieve a minimum dose of 300 mg of nefazodone per day by week 3 were dropped from the analyses; it would have been better if the analyses had been conducted on the full intention-to-treat sample.

CBT TO PREVENT RELAPSE AND RECURRENCE

Depression is a chronically recurrent disorder. Although up to two-thirds of all patients respond to acute treatment with ADM (about half of whom fully remit), a sizable number experience a return of symptoms after treatment is over.[28] According to conventions developed in the pharmacotherapy literature, symptom return during the first 6 to 12 months among remitted patients is assumed to represent a return of the treated episode (relapse) and treatment provided during that interval is called continuation treatment. Patients who go more than 12 months without relapse following remission are said to be recovered; symptom return following that interval among recovered patients is said to represent the onset of a wholly new episode (recurrence), and treatment provided after the end of that interval is called maintenance treatment.[29] Although ADM can suppress the expression of symptoms (a purely palliative effect), there is no evidence that it can shorten the duration of the underlying episode or reduce subsequent risk for recurrence,[28] and current medical practice calls for keeping patients with a history of recurrent or chronic depression on medication indefinitely.[19] On the other hand, if CBT has an enduring effect it can be said to be more than purely palliative.[30] Whether it is truly curative depends on how long this enduring effect can be said to last and how and to what extent it prevents subsequent episodes.

Enduring Effects of CBT

There is evidence that CBT has an enduring effect that lasts beyond the end of treatment. Among patients who respond to acute treatment, relapse rates are lower following treatment termination after acute CBT than after acute ADM and also lower for patients treated with combined treatment than for patients treated with ADM alone.[31] This finding suggests that it is not so much the withdrawal of medication that provokes relapse in remitted patients as that previous exposure to CBT prevents it. It remains unclear whether this effect is specific to CBT, because other psychotherapies have rarely been tested against medication withdrawal.

A pair of recent studies found that the magnitude of the enduring effect of CBT was at least as large as keeping patients on continuation ADM.[32,33] In both these studies patients who responded to CBT were essentially withdrawn from that treatment and compared with ADM responders randomized to either ADM continuation or withdrawal onto pill-placebo. CBT responders were significantly less likely to relapse following treatment termination than ADM responders withdrawn from ADM and no more likely to relapse than ADM responders kept on continued medication. Both studies found previous CBT superior to medication withdrawal even after patients were continued on ADM for up to a year after initial response.

Although these results suggest that previous exposure to acute CBT prevents subsequent symptom return, it is possible that these findings may be an artifact of differential mortality. As described by Klein,[34] acute treatment may act as a differential sieve if high-risk patients are more likely to respond to one treatment than another. Although there is no evidence that this was the case in either study, the fact that only about half of the patients initially randomized completed and responded to treatment leaves open the possibility that what seems to be an enduring effect might be nothing more than the differential retention of high-risk patients. Therefore, although the existing evidence is consistent with the notion that CBT has an enduring effect, it is less than wholly conclusive.

Studies that provide CBT following the end of acute treatment are not subject to the possible biasing effects of differential mortality as long as all patients receive the same acute phase treatment. Fava and colleagues[35] found that adding a version of CBT including well-being therapy and lifestyle modification resulted in lower subsequent recurrence rates following medication discontinuation among patients with recurrent depression who were first treated to recovery with ADM, with enduring effects evident up to 6 years later.[36] Similarly, Paykel and colleagues[37] found that adding CBT reduced rates of relapse and subsequent recurrence relative to ADM alone in patients with residual depressive symptoms following initial medication treatment, with enduring effects found up to 3.5 years after the completion of CBT.[38] Bockting and colleagues[39] found that among patients in remission after various types of treatment adding CBT resulted in significantly lower rates of relapse/recurrence than treatment-as-usual (TAU) alone for patients with a history of 5 or more depressive episodes; no such differences were evident for patients with fewer than 5 previous episodes. In a pair of studies, Teasdale and colleagues[40,41] found that adding mindfulness-based CT (MBCT) reduced subsequent rates of relapse/recurrence relative to TAU in a 1-year period for patients with 3 or more previous episodes of depression; no such differences were evident for patients with 2 or fewer previous episodes. MBCT is a group intervention that combines CBT with meditation techniques aimed at teaching patients to relate to depressive thoughts and feelings as mental events, rather than as accurate reflections of reality, to prevent relapse as a result of dysphoric mood. Only Perlis and colleagues[42] failed to find an advantage for adding CBT, but did so in the context of providing ongoing ADM with dose increase for all patients that should have reduced rates of relapse and recurrence regardless of whether CBT was added. These studies suggest that CBT has an enduring effect that is robust to the biasing effects of differential mortality.

CBT as a Continuation and Maintenance Treatment

In addition to the enduring effects of acute CBT treatment, research has focused on the efficacy of keeping patients in CBT after they first respond to that treatment. Jarrett and colleagues[43] focused on whether extending the duration of CBT adds to the efficacy of acute treatment by comparing CBT with and without a continuation phase for CBT responders with a history of recurrent depression. During the ensuing 8 months significantly fewer patients relapsed when CBT was continued than when it was not. Patient characteristics moderated the effects of extending CBT for the full 24-month follow-up period such that patients with an earlier age of depression onset or who showed an unstable pattern of remission were less likely to relapse or recur if provided with continuation/maintenance treatment than if not, whereas extending CBT treatment did not matter for patients with a later age of depression onset or who showed a stable pattern of remission. These findings suggest that extending CBT might be necessary only for patients at higher risk for relapse. Jarrett and colleagues[44] also examined the efficacy of CBT as continuation treatment after acute treatment of patients with atypical depression, but sample sizes were so small that no meaningful conclusions could be drawn.

Klein and colleagues[45] examined the efficacy of CBASP as a maintenance treatment of chronic depression. Treatment responders to 12 weeks of acute and 16 weeks of continuation CBASP treatment in their earlier trial were randomly assigned to CBASP maintenance treatment versus an assessment-only control. Over 52 weeks, CBASP maintenance treatment resulted in lower recurrence rates. Moreover, patients in the CBASP condition experienced a small reduction in depressive symptoms, whereas depressive symptoms increased somewhat for patients in the control condition. This sample consists solely of patients who showed a sustained response to CBASP (all chronically depressed). For this group of patients CBASP maintenance treatment after 28 weeks of acute and continuation phase treatment seems more efficacious than its absence.

Three studies focused on the efficacy of CBT continuation treatment compared with ADM continuation. First, Blackburn and colleagues[46] compared 6 months of continuation treatment with CBT or ADM or their combination for patients who had responded to acute phase treatment in those same modalities. No differences were found across the 6 months of continuation treatment, suggesting a continuation effect of CBT comparable with medication. Across a 2-year follow-up (the last 18 months of which was treatment free) the number of patients who relapsed or recurred was significantly higher following withdrawal from medication alone than for previous CBT with or without medication, suggesting an enduring effect of CBT. However, given that patients were randomized to different treatments during the acute phase, it is possible that acute treatment could have served as a differential sieve that systematically unbalanced the groups of treatment responders and thereby produced a spurious enduring effect that accounted for the results observed. Second, Blackburn and Moore[47] examined the relative efficacy of CBT and ADM maintenance treatments. Patients were randomly assigned to acute ADM followed by maintenance ADM, acute ADM followed by maintenance CBT, and acute CBT followed by maintenance CBT. There were no differences in the reduction of acute phase symptoms and no significant differences between maintenance CBT and maintenance ADM, regardless of whether maintenance CBT followed acute treatment with CBT or with ADM. These results suggest that maintenance CBT can have prophylactic effects similar to maintenance ADM, although it is always treacherous to draw causal inferences from null findings in a small sample, and medication doses were reduced during the maintenance phase. Although maintenance CBT may be as efficacious as maintenance ADM, these studies do little to contribute to our confidence, for the reasons cited.

Kuyken and colleagues[48] compared MBCT plus ADM discontinuation with ADM maintenance treatment in patients with a history of multiple depressive episodes who were fully or partially remitted after initial treatment with ADM. No significant differences in relapse/recurrence rate were found over a 15-month period. Only about three-quarters of the MBCT patients discontinued medications, but that group contained most of the high-risk patients, and comparisons between those in the MBCT group who did discontinue and patients in the ADM maintenance group who were fully compliant also found no differences. Although MBCT might be as efficacious as keeping patients on continuation ADM, methodological problems limit the interpretation of similar findings with regard to CBT.

CBT TO PREVENT RELAPSE IN BIPOLAR DISORDER

Whereas the distinction between relapse and recurrence is relevant to unipolar depression (patients are either in episode and thus at risk for relapse when asymptomatic or not in episode and thus at risk for recurrence), bipolar disorder is thought of as a chronic disorder that never goes away and is marked by periodic symptomatic relapses into mania and depression. Although stabilization on medications is the cornerstone of treatment of bipolar disorder, there has been considerable interest in recent years in using CBT to treat existing symptoms (particularly depression) and to prevent subsequent relapse when euthymic. In addition to such general features as examining the accuracy of dysfunctional beliefs and improving communication and problem-solving skills, CBT also focuses on teaching skills to cope with prodromes (periods when symptoms first emerge but have not yet reached maximum severity) and disruption of routines (especially sleep) that contribute to the onset of an episode in bipolar disorder. These are features that it shares with other promising adjunctive psychosocial interventions like interpersonal social rhythm therapy and family-focused therapy.[49] In a pilot study, Lam and colleagues[50] found that adding CBT reduced the frequency of bipolar episodes across the following year relative to TAU alone in euthymic bipolar I patients who continued to have relapses despite the use of mood stabilizers, but were not currently facing an acute bipolar episode. These investigators subsequently replicated this finding in a larger sample across the course of a 1-year[51] and 2-year follow-up, although the differential relapse prevention effects occurred mainly in the first year after treatment.[52] CBT patients also reported fewer days in episode and better mood ratings, social functioning, and coping with bipolar prodromes. Subsequent studies typically found benefits for CBT compared with TAU in medicated patients, either at the level of a nonsignificant trend[53] or in terms of days free from depression and reductions in medication use.[54]

A recent multicenter trial by Scott and colleagues[55] largely failed to replicate these effects. These investigators studied a more heterogeneous sample, including patients who were currently in episode, and found that the addition of CBT did not result in lower relapse rates or symptom levels for the full sample. Post hoc analyses did suggest an interaction with previous episodes (moderation), such that adding CBT was significantly more effective for patients with fewer than 12 previous episodes, but less efficacious for those with 12 or more previous episodes. This finding led the investigators to conclude that CBT might be helpful for only the minority of bipolar patients with relatively fewer previous episodes, and the investigators of a recent meta-analysis to conclude that CBT was of little use for bipolar patients.[56] However, Lam[57] has criticized this study for including a mixed patient sample; almost one-third of the patients were currently in episode and the focus on acute symptom reduction rather than relapse prevention might have undercut any possible relapse prevention effect. It should be possible to reanalyze the data for only those patients not in episode at the start of the trial to see whether that subsample replicated the effects found in the Lam studies, but that has not yet been done. It also would have been helpful to know whether medication dosing varied between the 2 conditions in the Scott study, because such confounds sometimes obscure the effects of added treatments.[54] More research is needed to determine whether CBT truly has an adjunctive role to play in the treatment or prevention of bipolar disorder and, if so, whether those beneficial effects of CBT (if any) are because of its specific content or because of nonspecific treatment factors like therapist contact and the mobilization of hope and expectation.

PREDICTORS OF CBT EFFICACY

Because different patients respond differently to different treatments, it is important to know who responds best to what with particular reference to CBT. Two types of information are relevant to this question: prognostic information in which you hold treatment constant and allow patient characteristics to vary, and prescriptive information in which you hold patient characteristics constant and allow treatment to vary.[58] Prognostic factors predict outcome to a given treatment (or to treatment in general) and can be used to determine which patients are more likely to respond to CBT relative to other patients. However, although it is useful to know what to expect when starting treatment, prognostic factors are of little use in deciding what treatment to select. On the other hand, prescriptive information (also known as moderators) can detect different patterns of outcomes between different treatments for different types of patients and provide a basis for choosing the best treatment of a given patient.[59]

Demographic Factors

Little research has focused on age, gender, education and other demographic predictors of response to CBT for depression adequately controlling for pretreatment severity.[60] A notable exception is a study by Fournier and colleagues that found that older age and lower intelligence each predicted relatively poor response to CBT and ADM and were therefore purely prognostic factors, whereas being unemployed and having more antecedent life events predicted superior response to CBT relative to ADM and were therefore potentially prescriptive.[58] For whatever reason, married patients seem to do better in CBT than unmarried patients.[61–64] This finding is an example of prognostic information that allows a prediction of likely outcome but does not (on its own) provide a basis for choosing CBT rather than other treatments for such patients. However, Barber and Muenz[65] reanalyzed data from the TDCRP and found that married patients did better in CBT than they did in IPT, whereas unmarried patients showed the opposite pattern. Similarly, Fournier and colleagues[58] found that patients who were married or cohabiting did better in CT than they did in ADM. Both sets of findings are potentially prescriptive and could be used to select CBT rather than either IPT or ADM if replicated. Thus, marital status seems to be prognostic (married patients do better than unmarried patients in CBT) and prescriptive (married patients do better in CBT than they do in at least some other treatments) with respect to CBT efficacy. In addition, more antecedent life events and unemployment are potentially prescriptive factors, associated with better response to CBT relative to ADM.

Illness Characteristics

Chronic depression was found to be prognostic of poor response to either CBT or ADM in one study[58] and brief duration of the current depressive episode, a later age of depression onset, absence of a family history of affective disorder, and a history of more previous episodes of depression predictive of good response to CBT in another.[63] All these indices were purely prognostic and should not be used as a basis for treatment selection. Leykin and colleagues[66] found that the more previous medication exposures that patients had the less well they did in ADM; no such relationship was evident for CBT. Although the investigators did not report tests for treatment differences as a function of number of previous exposures, they did report an effect size favoring CBT rather than ADM for patients with 2 or more previous exposures of sufficient magnitude ($d = 0.46$) to suggest that the difference would have been significant if tested. There is little evidence to support the long-standing belief that patients with melancholic depression would be less responsive to CBT than to ADM.[67] It is also widely assumed that ADM is to be preferred to CBT in the treatment of patients with more severe depressions.[19] In their review, Hamilton and Dobson[60] conclude that depression severity is associated with poor response to CBT (prognostic), but that there is no reason to conclude that alternative treatments such as ADM are any more efficacious than CBT for severely depressed patients (prescriptive). When CBT has failed relative to ADM it has been with patients with more severe depressions,[18,25] but as discussed earlier, questions can be raised about the quality of the CBT in those studies. When CT has been adequately implemented, it seems to be about as efficacious as ADM with such patients.[22,23] In sum, chronicity and severity seem to be prognostic only and melancholia does not seem to be prescriptive, although patients with more previous medication exposures may do better in CBT than on ADM.

Personality Characteristics/Disorders

The presence of a comorbid PD might be relevant from a prognostic and prescriptive perspective. Fournier and colleagues found that depressed patients with Axis II PDs (excluding antisocial, schizotypal, and borderline) were less responsive to CBT than to paroxetine ADM (44% vs 66% response), whereas patients without comorbid Axis II PDs showed the opposite pattern (70% vs 49%).[24] Moreover, only patients with PDs showed a medication discontinuation effect (they were more likely to relapse if withdrawn onto pill-placebo than if continued on active medications); patients without PDs showed no such effect. Patients with PDs who did respond to CT were no more likely to relapse following treatment termination than patients without PDs, suggesting that the patients with PDs who did respond to CT tended to sustain their response. Treatment guidelines published by the American Psychiatric Association suggest that CBT is superior to ADM in the treatment of patients with PDs,[19] but that claim was based on a misreading of findings from the TDCRP that Axis II disorder was predictive of poor response within ADM or IPT but not in CBT. In point of fact, patients with PDs did not do better in CBT than they did in other treatments, but patients without PDs did worse in CBT.[68] Hardy and colleagues[69] similarly found that cluster C PDs predicted differential response within an interpersonal intervention but not within CBT (prognostic). However, the treatment by PD interaction was nonsignificant and the investigators did not conduct the kinds of direct treatment comparisons within patient subgroups required to establish moderation. Barber and Muenz[65] found CBT superior to IPT for patients with avoidant personality traits and IPT superior to CBT for patients with obsessive personality traits. Similarly, McBride and colleagues[70] found that patients with high levels of attachment avoidance (a reluctance to initiate intimate contact and a tendency to withdraw when facing an attachment threat) had better outcomes to CBT than to IPT and Joyce and colleagues[71] found that avoidant and schizoid symptoms predicted poorer response to IPT but not to CBT. Despite the differences in study design and the measures used, these studies approach a conceptual replication of the Barber and Muenz findings with regard to avoidant personality, although Joyce and colleagues did not replicate the finding that IPT might be more efficacious than CBT for patients with obsessive-compulsive traits. In sum, there are consistent indications that presence of PD dimensions may be prescriptive, although the exact nature of that prediction may depend on the specific comparison (CBT may be superior to IPT on some and inferior to ADM on others).

Treatment Preference

Two studies have examined the role of a patient's preference as a moderator of treatment efficacy. Leykin and colleagues[72] found no differences in symptom reduction or likelihood of attrition between patients who received their preferred treatment versus those who did not (CBT vs ADM). On the other hand, Kocsis and colleagues[73] found that patients who preferred either CBT alone or ADM alone had higher rates of remission and fewer depressive symptoms if they received what they preferred than if they received combined treatment. Thus, patient preferences in that study appeared to be driven more by a disaffection for a specific monotherapy than a preference for the other.

Dysfunctional Attitudes

Several studies have reported that high levels of pretreatment dysfunctional attitudes predict poorer response to CBT (prognostic).[62–64,74] Furthermore, Sotsky and colleagues[63] found that patients with lower dysfunctional attitudes did better in CBT (or ADM) than in pill-placebo. Thus, lower levels of dysfunctional attitudes was prescriptive relative to pill-placebo (but not to ADM) in that study. It is unclear whether levels of dysfunctional attitudes are prescriptive relative to other alternative treatments.[60]

MEDIATORS OF CBT EFFICACY

Although CBT has been found to be efficacious in the treatment and prevention of depression, questions remain about precisely how it works (mediation). Such questions are relevant to the identification of the active ingredients in the treatment process and the mechanisms of change within the patient. Cognitive theory posits that negative automatic thoughts and maladaptive information-processing proclivities play a causal role in the cause and maintenance of depression.[7] According to this theory, CBT works by virtue of implementing efforts (process) to correct these errors in thinking (mechanism). To the extent that this is true, efforts to help patients learn how to examine the accuracy of their own beliefs should help ameliorate the level of existing distress and reduce risk for future episodes. Others factors that also are believed to mediate the efficacy of psychotherapy are the quality of the therapeutic relationship and facilitative conditions, such as therapist warmth and empathy. If cognitive theory is correct, then adherence to the specific components of CBT should drive symptom change and subsequent freedom from relapse over and above whatever contribution is made by nonspecific factors common to other therapies.

Treatment Process

Several studies have shown that nonspecific factors are correlated with change across the course of CT.[75–77] Conversely, several studies have found that homework compliance (assessed retrospectively at the end of treatment) was associated with better response to CBT.[61,77,78] However, these studies did not adequately control for reverse causality (that it was symptom change that drove treatment process rather than the other way around); doing so would have required controlling for symptom change up until the point at which homework compliance was measured. Shaw and colleagues[79] found only limited support for the role of therapist competence (it was the ability to structure treatment rather than CBT skills that best predicted outcome), but also did not examine the pattern of temporal relations over time (doing so would have required controlling for previous symptom change at the point at which competence was measured). DeRubeis and Feeley[80,81] revisited these issues in a pair of studies that controlled for symptom change before the assessment of treatment process and then monitored the effects of treatment process on subsequent symptom change. What these investigators found was that after controlling for previous symptom change, the extent to which therapists used concrete symptom-focused CBT methods in an early session predicted subsequent change in depression, whereas nonspecific processes like the helping alliance and facilitative conditions did not. Moreover, ratings of the helping alliance in subsequent sessions were predicted by previous depression change. This finding suggests that concrete symptom-focused techniques may play a causal role in the alleviation of depressive symptoms in CBT, whereas the quality of the therapeutic relationship may be more a consequence than a cause of change. Neither study ruled out possible third variable causality (that some unmeasured patient characteristic facilitated concrete symptom-focused techniques and led to subsequent symptom change with no direct causal link between the two), but they did suggest that specific CBT techniques were predictive of (and possibly causal to) subsequent symptom change in a manner that nonspecific processes were not.

Cognitive Mechanisms

In a similar fashion, early studies assessing whether cognitive change mediated the effects of CBT typically reported that ADM produced as much change in cognition as CBT,[82,83] leading investigators to conclude that cognitive change was more of a nonspecific consequence of change in depression rather than a cause.[83] However, as in the treatment process literature, these early studies did not assess the temporal pattern of change between cognition and subsequent depression and therefore were unable to address the possibility that cognitive change mediated change in depression in one treatment but was a consequence of change in depression in another.[84] DeRubeis and colleagues[85] found that early change in cognition was predictive of subsequent change in depression in CBT but not in ADM despite the fact that both produced comparable change in cognition across the course of treatment, a pattern that is consistent with differential mediation in CBT but not in ADM. Recent studies have extended this line of inquiry by examining the relation between cognitive change and subsequent relapse. Strunk and colleagues[86] found that among treatment responders, patient competence in CBT coping skills and their independent implementation predicted the risk of relapse in the year following treatment termination. Among partially remitted patients, Teasdale and colleagues[87] found that CBT reduced the tendency to use an absolutist, dichotomous thinking style, and that this change (rather than simply becoming more positive) reduced the likelihood of subsequent relapse. Moreover, there is evidence that CBT reduces the extent to which patients think negatively with increased dysphoria (cognitive reactivity)[88] and that this reduction in cognitive reactivity predicts subsequent risk for relapse.[89] Collectively, these studies support the notion of cognitive mediation in CBT by ruling out reverse causality (that cognitive change is caused by change in depression), although as for the process studies they do not rule out third variability causality (that some unmeasured patient factor caused change in cognition and change in depression with no causal link between the two). Thus, some ambiguity still remains as to whether CBT works by virtue of changing cognitions, although the existing evidence is consistent with that notion.

Sudden Gains

Tang and DeRubeis[90] described a pattern of substantial stable decreases in depressive symptoms in CBT with implications for treatment process and the mechanisms of change that they termed sudden gains. Several studies have since replicated the presence of sudden gains during CBT.[91–93] Sudden gains seem to appear in 30% to 50% of patients, accounting for 50% to 60% of the total improvement in these patients. They generally have a magnitude of 10 or more points on the Beck Depression Inventory and appear in the first half of treatment (between sessions 4 and 8). Although the presence of sudden gains during CBT has been consistently associated with better end-of-treatment outcomes, nearly as many patients respond to treatment who show a more gradual course of change.[90–93] Most striking is the finding that sudden gains predict freedom from relapse among treatment responders.[93] Earlier studies had found an inconsistent relation between sudden gains and levels of depression following treatment termination, but had relied on cross-sectional assessments that did not take into account intercurrent relapses that could lead to subsequent treatment.[90,91] Conversely, Vittengl and colleagues[94] found little evidence that sudden gains predicted differential relapse following successful treatment, but used a different definition that allowed modest gains to pass the threshold. Using the original more stringent definition, Tang and colleagues[93] found that sudden gains predicted freedom from subsequent relapse among treatment responders even when controlling for end-of-treatment depression scores, and that that effect disappeared when they applied the less stringent definition used by Vittengl and colleagues. What makes these findings relevant to mediation (and possible process) is that Tang and DeRubeis found more cognitive change in the session preceding the sudden gains than in control sessions from the same patients (with no differences found for other therapeutic factors),[90] and replicated this in a subsequent study.[92] This finding suggests that sudden gains might be triggered by cognitive change, which in turn is likely related to CBT-specific processes on the part of the therapist, as posited by cognitive theory. However, given the correlational nature of this finding, third variable causality cannot be ruled out, and sudden gains also have been found in other types of treatments that are less likely to be mediated by cognitive change.[91,94]

Cognitive Change Versus BA

The studies described here all relied on correlational analyses to identify the causal mechanisms of change in CBT. Jacobson and colleagues[95] used a more experimental approach to dismantle CBT in an effort to identify its active ingredients and came up with a different answer. In that study, the investigators compared the efficacy of 3 different CBT components by comparing (1) BA only, (2) BA plus the activation and modification of dysfunctional thoughts (AT), and (3) BA plus AT plus the identification and modification of core schemes (CT), and found no differences in efficacy between these different components. This finding was surprising because cognitive theory posits that direct efforts to change beliefs are necessary to maximize change in depression and the BA condition did not address those beliefs directly. Moreover, no differences were found on purported mediators hypothesized to be differentially affected by the respective components (pleasant events, automatic thoughts, and attributional style) and early change in cognition was associated with subsequent change in BA (but not in CT) and early change in pleasant events was associated with subsequent change in CT (but not in BA). This study suggests that specific efforts to change beliefs may not be necessary to produce cognitive change, yet at the same time leaving open the possibility that cognitive change (no matter how it is produced) may still play a meditational role in the subsequent reduction of distress. More research is needed in this regard.

SUMMARY

CBT has been found superior to control conditions and as least as efficacious as other psychotherapies and ADM in the acute treatment of depression. When adequately implemented, CBT can be as efficacious as ADM for patients with more severe depressions. CBT may also be of use as an adjunct to medications in the treatment of bipolar disorder, although the evidence there is not so clear or extensive. CBT reduces relapse/recurrence rates, with a magnitude of effect that might be comparable to keeping patients on medications, which is particularly noteworthy in a chronic recurrent disorder. Patients who are married or show low levels of pretreatment dysfunctional attitudes seem to be more likely to respond to CBT than patients who are unmarried or show high levels of dysfunctional attitudes. Unemployment, more antecedent life events and previous ADM exposures, and the absence of Axis II comorbidity are prescriptive factors associated with better response to CBT compared with medications. CBT seems to work through concrete CT-specific strategies and may be mediated by changes in cognition as specified by theory, although it remains unclear whether it is necessary to deal directly with cognition to produce those changes.

REFERENCES

1. Murray CJL, Lopez AD. Global mortality, disability, and the contribution of risk factors: global burden of disease study. Lancet 1997;349(9063):1436–42.
2. Kessler RC, Berglund P, Demler O, et al. The epidemiology of major depressive disorder: results from the national comorbidity survey replication (NCS-R). JAMA 2003;289(23):3095–105.
3. Keller MB. Long-term treatment of recurrent and chronic depression. J Clin Psychiatry 2001;62(Suppl 24):3–5.
4. Rush AJ, Fava M, Wisniewski SR, et al. Sequenced treatment alternatives to relieve depression (STAR*D): rationale and design. Control Clin Trials 2004; 25(1):119–42.
5. DeRubeis RJ, Young PR, Dahlsgaard KK. Affective disorders. In: Bellack AS, Hersen M, editors, Comprehensive clinical psychology, vol. 6. Oxford: Pergamon; 1998. p. 339–66.

6. American Psychiatric Association. Diagnostic and statistical manual of mental disorders, fourth edition, text review. Washington, DC: American Psychiatric Association Press; 2000.

7. Beck AT, Rush AJ, Shaw BF, et al. Cognitive therapy of depression. New York: Guilford Press; 1979.

8. Cuijpers P, van Straten A, Driessen E, et al. Depression and dysthymic disorders. In: Hersen M, Sturmey P, editors. Handbook of evidence-based practice in clinical psychology, vol. II. Adult disorders. Hoboken (NJ): Wiley; in press.

9. Cuijpers P, van Straten A, Warmerdam L. Are individual and group treatments equally effective in the treatment of depression in adults? A meta-analysis. Eur J Psychiatry 2001;22(1):38–51.

10. Gloaguen V, Cottrauxa J, Cucherata M, et al. A meta-analysis of the effects of cognitive therapy in depressed patients. J Affect Disord 1998;49(1):59–72.

11. Wampold BE, Minami T, Baskin TW, et al. A meta-(re)analysis of the effects of cognitive therapy versus 'other therapies' for depression. J Affect Disord 2002; 68(2-3):159–65.

12. Butler AC, Chapman JE, Forman EM, et al. The empirical status of cognitive-behavioral therapy: a review of meta-analyses. Clin Psychol Rev 2006;26(1): 17–31.

13. Rush AJ, Beck AT, Kovacs M, et al. Comparative efficacy of cognitive therapy and pharmacotherapy in the treatment of depressed outpatients. Cognit Ther Res 1977;1(1):17–37.

14. Blackburn IM, Bishop S, Glen AI, et al. The efficacy of cognitive therapy in depression: a treatment trial using cognitive therapy and pharmacotherapy, each alone and in combination. Br J Psychiatry 1981;139(9):181–9.

15. Murphy GE, Simons AD, Wetzel RD, et al. Cognitive therapy and pharmacotherapy. Singly and together in the treatment of depression. Arch Gen Psychiatry 1984;41(1):33–41.

16. Hollon SD, DeRubeis RJ, Evans MD, et al. Cognitive therapy and pharmacotherapy for depression: singly and in combination. Arch Gen Psychiatry 1992; 49(10):774–81.

17. Elkin I, Shea MT, Watkins JT, et al. Treatment of depression collaborative research program: general effectiveness of treatments. Arch Gen Psychiatry 1989;46(11): 971–82.

18. Elkin I, Gibbons RD, Shea MT, et al. Initial severity and differential treatment outcome in the National Institute of Mental Health Treatment of Depression Collaborative Research Program. J Consult Clin Psychol 1995;63(5):841–7.

19. American Psychiatric Association. Practice guideline for the treatment of patients with major depressive disorder [revision]. Am J Psychiatry 2000;157(Suppl 4):1–45.

20. Jacobson NS, Hollon SD. Cognitive behavior therapy vs. pharmacotherapy: now that the jury's returned its verdict, its time to present the rest of the evidence. J Consult Clin Psychol 1996;64(1):74–80.

21. Jacobson NS, Hollon SD. Prospects for future comparisons between drugs and psychotherapy: lessons from the CBT vs. pharmacotherapy exchange. J Consult Clin Psychol 1996;64(1):104–8.

22. Jarrett RB, Schaffer M, McIntire D, et al. Treatment of atypical depression with cognitive therapy or phenelzine: a double-blind, placebo-controlled trial. Arch Gen Psychiatry 1999;56(5):431–7.

23. DeRubeis RJ, Hollon SD, Amsterdam JD, et al. Cognitive therapy vs medications in the treatment of moderate to severe depression. Arch Gen Psychiatry 2005; 62(4):409–16.

24. Fournier JC, DeRubeis RJ, Shelton RC, et al. Antidepressant medications versus cognitive therapy in depressed patients with or without personality disorder. Br J Psychiatry 2008;192(2):124–9.

25. Dimidjian S, Hollon SD, Dobson KS, et al. Randomized trial of behavioral activation, cognitive therapy, and antidepressant medication in the acute treatment of adults with major depression. J Consult Clin Psychol 2006;74(4):658–70.

26. Coffman S, Martell CR, Dimidjian S, et al. Extreme non-response in cognitive therapy: can behavioral activation succeed where cognitive therapy fails? J Consult Clin Psychol 2007;75(4):531–41.

27. Keller MB, McCullough JP, Klein DN, et al. A comparison of nefazodone, the cognitive behavioral-analysis system of psychotherapy, and their combination for the treatment of chronic depression. N Engl J Med 2000;342(20):1462–70.

28. Hollon SD, Thase ME, Markowitz JC. Treatment and prevention of depression. Psychol Sci Publ Interest 2002;3(2):39–77.

29. Frank E, Prien RF, Jarrett RB, et al. Conceptualization and rationale for consensus definitions of terms in major depressive disorder. Remission, recovery, relapse, and recurrence. Arch Gen Psychiatry 1991;48(9):851–5.

30. Hollon SD, Stewart MO, Strunk D. Enduring effects for cognitive behavior therapy in the treatment of depression and anxiety. Annu Rev Psychol 2006;57:285–315.

31. Vittengl JR, Clark LA, Dunn TW, et al. Reducing relapse and recurrence in unipolar depression, a comparative meta-analysis of cognitive-behavioral therapy's effects. J Consult Clin Psychol 2007;75(3):475–88.

32. Hollon SD, DeRubeis RJ, Shelton RC, et al. Prevention of relapse following cognitive therapy vs medications in moderate to severe depression. Arch Gen Psychiatry 2005;62(4):417–22.

33. Dobson KS, Hollon SD, Dimidjian S, et al. Randomized trial of behavioral activation, cognitive therapy, and antidepressant medication in the prevention of relapse and recurrence in major depression. J Consult Clin Psychol 2008;76(3): 468–77.

34. Klein DF. Preventing hung juries about therapy studies. J Consult Clin Psychol 1996;64(1):81–7.

35. Fava GA, Rafanelli C, Grandi S, et al. Prevention of recurrent depression with cognitive behavioral therapy. Arch Gen Psychiatry 1998;55(9):816–20.

36. Fava GA, Ruini C, Rafanelli C, et al. Six-year outcome of cognitive behavior therapy for prevention of recurrent depression. Am J Psychiatry 2004;161(10): 1872–6.

37. Paykel ES, Scott J, Teasdale JD, et al. Prevention of relapse in residual depression by cognitive therapy. A controlled trial. Arch Gen Psychiatry 1999;56(9): 829–35.

38. Paykel ES, Scott J, Cornwall PL, et al. Duration of relapse prevention after cognitive therapy for residual depression: follow-up of controlled trial. Psychol Med 2005;35(1):59–68.

39. Bockting CLH, Schene AH, Spinhoven P, et al. Preventing relapse/recurrence in recurrent depression with cognitive therapy: a randomized controlled trial. J Consult Clin Psychol 2005;73(4):647–57.

40. Teasdale JD, Segal ZV, Williams JMG, et al. Prevention of relapse/recurrence in major depression by mindfulness-based cognitive therapy. J Consult Clin Psychol 2000;68(4):615–23.

41. Ma SH, Teasdale JD. Mindfulness-based cognitive therapy for depression: replication and exploration of differential relapse prevention effects. J Consult Clin Psychol 2004;72(1):31–40.

42. Perlis RH, Nierenberg AA, Alpert JE, et al. Effects of adding cognitive therapy to fluoxetine dose increase on risk of relapse and residual depressive symptoms in continuation treatment of major depressive disorder. J Clin Psychopharmacol 2002;22(5):474–80.
43. Jarrett RB, Kraft D, Doyle J, et al. Preventing recurrent depression using cognitive therapy with and without a continuation phase. A randomized clinical trial. Arch Gen Psychiatry 2001;58(4):381–8.
44. Jarrett RB, Kraft D, Schaffer M, et al. Reducing relapse in depressed outpatients with atypical features: a pilot study. Psychother Psychosom 2000;69(5):232–9.
45. Klein DN, Santiago NJ, Vivian D, et al. Cognitive-behavioral analysis system of psychotherapy as a maintenance treatment for chronic depression. J Consult Clin Psychol 2004;72(4):681–8.
46. Blackburn IM, Eunson KM, Bishop S. A two-year naturalistic follow-up of depressed patients treated with cognitive therapy, pharmacotherapy and a combination of both. J Affect Disord 1986;10(1):67–75.
47. Blackburn IM, Moore RG. Controlled acute and follow-up trial of cognitive therapy and pharmacotherapy in outpatients with recurrent depression. Br J Psychiatry 1997;171(10):328–34.
48. Kuyken W, Byford S, Taylor RS, et al. Mindfulness-based cognitive therapy to prevent relapse in recurrent depression. J Consult Clin Psychol 2008;76(6):966–78.
49. Miklowitz DJ, Otto MW, Frank E, et al. Psychosocial treatments for bipolar disorder: a 1-year randomized trial from the Systematic Treatment Enhancement Program. Arch Gen Psychiatry 2007;64(4):419–27.
50. Lam DH, Bright J, Jones S, et al. Cognitive therapy for bipolar illness – a pilot study of relapse prevention. Cognit Ther Res 2000;24(5):503–20.
51. Lam DH, Watkins ER, Hayward P, et al. A randomized controlled study of cognitive therapy for relapse prevention for bipolar affective disorder. Arch Gen Psychiatry 2003;60(2):145–52.
52. Lam DH, Hayward P, Watkins ER, et al. Relapse prevention in patients with bipolar disorder: cognitive therapy outcome after 2 years. Am J Psychiatry 2005;162(2):324–9.
53. Ball JR, Mitchell PB, Corry JC, et al. A randomized controlled trial of cognitive therapy for bipolar disorder: focus on long-term change. J Clin Psychiatry 2006;67(2):277–86.
54. Zaretzky A, Lancee W, Miller C, et al. Is cognitive-behavioural therapy more effective than psychoeducation in bipolar disorder? Can J Psychiatry 2008;53(7):441–8.
55. Scott J, Paykel E, Morriss R, et al. Cognitive-behavioral therapy for severe and recurrent bipolar disorders. Randomised controlled trial. Br J Psychiatry 2006;188(5):313–20.
56. Lynch D, Laws KR, McKenna PJ. Cognitive behavioural therapy for major psychiatric disorder: does it really work? A meta-analytic review of well-controlled trials. Psychol Med 2010;40(1):9–24.
57. Lam D. What can we conclude from studies on psychotherapy in bipolar disorder? Invited commentary on: cognitive-behavioral therapy for severe and recurrent bipolar disorders. Br J Psychiatry 2006;188(4):321–2.
58. Fournier JC, DeRubeis RJ, Shelton RC, et al. Prediction of response to medication and cognitive therapy in the treatment of moderate to severe depression. J Consult Clin Psychol 2009;77(4):775–87.
59. Kraemer HC, Wilson T, Fairburn CG, et al. Mediators and moderators of treatment effects in randomized clinical trials. Arch Gen Psychiatry 2002;59(10):877–83.

60. Hamilton KE, Dobson KS. Cognitive therapy of depression: pretreatment patient predictors of outcome. Clin Psychol Rev 2002;22(6):875–93.
61. Burns DD, Spangler DL. Does psychotherapy homework lead to improvements in depression in cognitive-behavioral therapy or does improvement lead to increased homework compliance? J Consult Clin Psychol 2000;68(1):46–56.
62. Jarrett RB, Eaves GG, Granneman BD, et al. Clinical, cognitive, and demographic predictors of response to cognitive therapy for depression: a preliminary report. Psychiatry Res 1991;37(3):245–60.
63. Sotksy SM, Glass DR, Shea MT, et al. Patient predictors of response to psychotherapy and pharmacotherapy: findings in the NIMH Treatment of Depression Collaborative Research Program. Am J Psychiatry 1991;148(8):997–1008.
64. Thase ME, Simons A, McGeary J, et al. Severity of depression and response to cognitive behavior therapy. Am J Psychiatry 1991;148(6):784–9.
65. Barber JP, Muenz LR. The role of avoidance and obsessiveness in matching patients to cognitive and interpersonal psychotherapy: empirical findings from the treatment for depression collaborative research program. J Consult Clin Psychol 1996;64(5):951–8.
66. Leykin Y, Amsterdam JD, DeRubeis RJ, et al. Progressive resistance to a selective serotonin reuptake inhibitor but not to cognitive therapy in the treatment of major depression. J Consult Clin Psychol 2007;75(2):267–76.
67. Hollon SD, Jarrett RB, Nierenberg AA, et al. Psychotherapy and medication in the treatment of adult and geriatric depression: which monotherapy or combined treatment? J Clin Psychiatry 2005;66(4):455–68.
68. Shea MT, Pilkonis PA, Beckham E, et al. Personality disorders and treatment outcome in the NIMH Treatment of Depression Collaborative Research Program. Am J Psychiatry 1990;147(6):711–8.
69. Hardy GE, Barkham M, Shapiro DA, et al. Impact of cluster C personality disorders on outcome of contrasting brief psychotherapies for depression. J Consult Clin Psychol 1995;63(6):997–1004.
70. McBride C, Atkinson L, Quilty LC, et al. Attachment moderator of treatment outcome in major depression: a randomized control trial of interpersonal psychotherapy versus cognitive behavior therapy. J Consult Clin Psychol 2006;74(6):1041–54.
71. Joyce PR, McKenzie JM, Carter JD, et al. Temperament, character and personality disorders as predictors of response to interpersonal psychotherapy and cognitive-behavioral therapy for depression. Br J Psychiatry 2007;190(6):503–8.
72. Leykin Y, DeRubeis RJ, Gallop R, et al. The relation of patients' treatment preference to outcome in a randomized clinical trial. Behav Ther 2007;38(3):209–17.
73. Kocsis JH, Leon AC, Markowitz JC, et al. Patient preference as a moderator of outcome for chronic forms of major depressive disorder treated with nefazodone, cognitive behavioral analysis system of psychotherapy, or the combination. J Clin Psychiatry 2009;70(3):354–61.
74. Keller KE. Dysfunctional attitudes and the cognitive therapy for depression. Cognit Ther Res 1983;7(5):437–44.
75. Castonguay LG, Goldfried MG, Wiser S, et al. Predicting the effect of cognitive therapy for depression: a study of unique and common factors. J Consult Clin Psychol 1996;64(3):497–504.
76. Krupnick JL, Sotsky SM, Simmens S, et al. The role of the therapeutic alliance in psychotherapy and pharmacotherapy outcome: findings in the National Institute of Mental Health Treatment of Depression Collaborative Research Program. J Consult Clin Psychol 1996;64(3):532–9.

77. Burns DD, Nolen-Hoeksema D. Therapeutic empathy and recovery from depression in cognitive-behavioral therapy: a structural equation model. J Consult Clin Psychol 1992;60(3):441–9.
78. Burns DD, Nolen-Hoeksema D. Coping styles, homework compliance, and the effectiveness of cognitive-behavioral therapy. J Consult Clin Psychol 1991; 59(2):305–11.
79. Shaw BF, Elkin I, Yamaguchi J, et al. Therapist competence ratings in relation to clinical outcome in cognitive therapy for depression. J Consult Clin Psychol 1999; 67(6):837–46.
80. DeRubeis RJ, Feeley M. Determinants of change in cognitive therapy for depression. Cognit Ther Res 1990;14(5):469–82.
81. Feeley M, DeRubeis RJ, Gelfand LA. The temporal relation of adherence and alliance to symptom change in cognitive therapy for depression. J Consult Clin Psychol 1999;67(4):578–82.
82. Imber SD, Pilkonis PA, Sotsky SM, et al. Mode-specific effects among three treatments for depression. J Consult Clin Psychol 1990;58(3):352–9.
83. Simons AD, Garfield SL, Murphy GE. The process of change in cognitive therapy and pharmacotherapy for depression. Arch Gen Psychiatry 1984;41(1):45–51.
84. Hollon SD, DeRubeis RJ, Evans MD. Causal mediation of change in treatment for depression: discriminating between nonspecificity and noncausality. Psychol Bull 1987;102(1):139–49.
85. DeRubeis RJ, Evans MD, Hollon SD, et al. How does cognitive therapy work? Cognitive change and symptom change in cognitive therapy and pharmacotherapy for depression. J Consult Clin Psychol 1990;58(6):862–9.
86. Strunk DR, DeRubeis RJ, Chiu AW, et al. Patients' competence in and performance of cognitive therapy skills: relation to the reduction of relapse risk following treatment for depression. J Consult Clin Psychol 2007;75(4):523–30.
87. Teasdale JD, Scott J, Moore RG, et al. How does cognitive therapy prevent relapse in residual depression? Evidence from a controlled trial. J Consult Clin Psychol 2001;69(3):347–57.
88. Beevers CG, Miller IW. Unlinking negative cognition and symptoms of depression: evidence of a specific treatment effect for cognitive therapy. J Consult Clin Psychol 2005;73(1):68–77.
89. Segal ZV, Kennedy S, Gemar M, et al. Cognitive reactivity to sad mood provocation and the prediction of depressive relapse. Arch Gen Psychiatry 2006;63(7): 749–55.
90. Tang TZ, DeRubeis RJ. Sudden gains and critical sessions in cognitive-behavioral therapy for depression. J Consult Clin Psychol 1999;67(6):894–904.
91. Hardy GE, Cahill J, Stiles WB, et al. Sudden gains in cognitive therapy for depression: a replication and extension. J Consult Clin Psychol 2005;73(1):59–67.
92. Tang TZ, DeRubeis RJ, Beberman R, et al. Cognitive changes, critical sessions, and sudden gains in cognitive-behavioral therapy for depression. J Consult Clin Psychol 2005;73(1):168–72.
93. Tang TZ, DeRubeis RJ, Hollon SD, et al. Sudden gains in cognitive therapy of depression and depression relapse/recurrence. J Consult Clin Psychol 2007; 75(3):404–8.
94. Vittengl JR, Clark LA, Jarrett RB. Validity of sudden gains in acute phase treatment of depression. J Consult Clin Psychol 2005;73(1):173–82.
95. Jacobson NS, Dobson KS, Truax PA, et al. A component analysis of cognitive-behavioral treatment for depression. J Consult Clin Psychol 1996;64(2): 295–304.

Efficacy of Cognitive Behavioral Therapy for Anxiety Disorders: A Review of Meta-Analytic Findings

Bunmi O. Olatunji, PhD[a],*, Josh M. Cisler, MA[b],
Brett J. Deacon, PhD[c]

KEYWORDS

- Anxiety disorders • Cognitive behavioral therapy
- Exposure • Meta-analysis

Anxiety disorders are characterized by excessive fear and subsequent avoidance, typically in response to a specified object or situation and in the absence of true danger. Anxiety disorders have the highest overall prevalence rate among psychiatric disorders, with 12-month and lifetime rates of 18.1% and 28.8%, respectively.[1,2] Untreated anxiety also represents a significant economic burden, and associated functional impairments have a substantial negative impact on quality of life.[3,4] Descriptive and experimental research have been instrumental in delineating the structure of anxiety and the core psychosocial and biological mechanisms that contribute to the development and maintenance of these disorders.[5] For example, information-processing studies have shown automatic attentional biases toward threat-relevant stimuli across the anxiety disorders.[6] Conditioning research has also shown that elevated sensitivity to danger and safety cues is characteristic of many anxiety disorders, with resulting avoidance behaviors negatively reinforcing the persistence of the

The authors have nothing to disclose.
[a] Department of Psychology, Vanderbilt University, 301 Wilson Hall, 111 21st Avenue South, Nashville, TN 37203, USA
[b] Department of Psychiatry and Behavioral Sciences, National Crime Victims Research and Treatment Center, Medical University of South Carolina, PO Box 250852, 65 Cannon Street, Charleston, SC 29425, USA
[c] Department of Psychology, University of Wyoming, Dept 3415, 1000 East University Avenue, Laramie, WY 82071, USA
* Corresponding author.
E-mail address: olubunmi.o.olatunji@vanderbilt.edu

Psychiatr Clin N Am 33 (2010) 557–577
doi:10.1016/j.psc.2010.04.002
0193-953X/10/$ – see front matter ©2010 Published by Elsevier Inc.

anxiety.[7] This combined body of research serves as the foundation for the development of empirically supported treatments for anxiety disorder symptoms.

Cognitive and behavioral interventions are the most widely studied psychological interventions for addressing the information processing biases and avoidance behaviors that are characteristic of the anxiety disorders.[8] Cognitive behavioral therapy (CBT) is a collaborative, structured, skill-building, time-limited, and goal-oriented intervention designed to target core components of a given disorder.[9] Numerous randomized controlled trials have shown that CBT is effective in reducing symptoms of psychopathology, and stronger effects are often reported for the treatment of anxiety disorders relative to other conditions.[10] Meta-analysis is the primary means through which researchers have synthesized the results from multiple treatment trials examining the efficacy of CBT. Although the use of meta-analytic data is not without limitations, this approach has proven useful in characterizing the general effectiveness of CBT in the treatment of anxiety.

Numerous meta-analyses on the effectiveness of various treatments for the anxiety disorders have been conducted, suggesting the need for succinct qualitative analysis of this large quantitative literature. In a previous review, Deacon and Abramowitz[11] examined the results of 10 years of meta-analyses on psychotherapies for the anxiety disorders with the primary goal of delineating the relative effectiveness of cognitive versus behavioral treatments (**Table 1**). These authors concluded that the relative efficacy of cognitive versus behavioral treatment for some anxiety disorders remains an open question. Addressing this question through meta-analysis is admittedly complicated by the observation that behavioral and cognitive treatments emphasize similar techniques (exposure vs behavioral experiments), with the only difference being the proposed mechanism for the observed benefits (eg, extinction in the case of exposure vs belief change). Another complication is that the therapeutic procedure (eg, exposure vs cognitive restructuring) should not be confused with the mediating mechanism of change (eg, fear extinction vs expectancy and appraisal modification). For example, one qualitative review suggests that minimal evidence exists that cognitive treatments enhance the efficacy of behavioral approaches for anxiety disorders.[12] However, even if this is true, changes in cognitive processes may still be the mechanism through which behavioral treatments work.[13] Accordingly, it is important to consider which therapeutic procedure leads to better outcomes, and the mechanisms through which the treatment actually works.

One popular view is that combined CBT approaches for some anxiety disorders are more effective than either cognitive or behavior therapy alone, and many clinicians likely use a combination of cognitive and behavioral therapeutic methods in the real world. Although the relative efficacy of cognitive versus behavioral treatments for anxiety disorders must be further addressed in future research, the incremental efficacy of their combination (CBT) over other bona fide treatments remains unclear and continues to be heavily debated.[14] Given these observations, this article synthesizes the results of meta-analytic studies published since the Deacon and Abramowitz[11] review examining the efficacy of CBT for various anxiety disorders. The article highlights the efficacy of CBT relative to other treatment approaches when data are available and concludes with a discussion of current and future directions in the enhancement and dissemination of CBT for the anxiety disorders.

PANIC DISORDER

CBT for panic disorder typically involves education about the nature and physiology of the panic response, cognitive therapy techniques designed to modify catastrophic misinterpretations of panic symptoms and their consequences, and graduated exposure to panic-related body sensations (ie, interoceptive exposure) and avoided situations. Some CBT approaches[15] also include arousal-reduction techniques, such as diaphragmatic breathing or progressive muscle relaxation.

Several published meta-analyses have examined the relative efficacy of CBT for treating panic disorder. Siev and Chambless[16] contrasted the effects of CBT and relaxation training for patients with panic disorder without severe agoraphobia. Studies of CBT for panic disorder with severe agoraphobia were excluded, because treatment for these patients typically emphasizes in vivo exposure and differs from the standard application of CBT for less-agoraphobic patients. Five studies were located that directly compared the efficacy of CBT to relaxation training. None of the CBT interventions in these studies included a relaxation component. Taken together, results of these studies showed the superiority of CBT on a range of outcomes. The percentage of patients who no longer experienced panic attacks after treatment was significantly higher with CBT (77%) than with relaxation training (53%). Similar between-group differences in rates of clinically significant change (72% vs 50%) were observed. Drop-out rates (12% and 14% for CBT and relaxation treatments, respectively) were comparable between the treatments.

Notably, compared with patients undergoing relaxation training, those receiving CBT were less afraid of anxiety ($g = 0.64$) and endorsed significantly fewer catastrophic cognitions at posttreatment ($g = 0.48$). These findings indicate that CBT is superior to relaxation training in modifying catastrophic misinterpretations of anxiety and panic symptoms, a key cognitive process in cognitive behavioral models of panic disorder.[17] In contrast, CBT and relaxation training did not differ with respect to improvement in secondary measures such as general anxiety and depressive symptoms. Unfortunately, follow-up data on the maintenance of gains in these two treatments were not available. Overall, these findings highlight CBT as an efficacious treatment for panic disorder and suggest that relaxation training is less effective. Given that none of the CBT approaches analyzed by Siev and Chambless[16] incorporated a relaxation component, and component control dismantling studies also suggest the lack of additive value of relaxation training to standard CBT,[18] it seems that neither relaxation training nor breathing retraining produce incremental benefits beyond those achieved with traditional CBT techniques in panic disorder.

Mitte[19] conducted a comprehensive meta-analysis of CBT for panic disorder. Compared with no-treatment and placebo psychotherapy control groups, CBT was associated with significantly greater improvement on measures of anxiety, depression, and quality of life. Both CBT and behavior therapy without an explicit cognitive component were effective in reducing anxiety; however, CBT was superior to behavior therapy in reducing depressive symptoms and improving quality of life. Compared with behavior therapy, CBT was also associated with somewhat lower rates of attrition (12.7% vs 18.3%). Therapist-administered CBT was more effective than CBT administered in a self-help format. The investigator concluded that the combined CBT approach is the preferential psychological treatment for panic disorder.

SPECIFIC PHOBIA

CBTs for specific phobia[20] generally focus on exposure to the phobia-relevant stimuli. Exposure may be conducted either in vivo (ie, direct confrontation to actual phobic stimuli/situations) or imaginal (ie, imagery-based representations). Recent technologic advances have also allowed for the use of virtual reality exposures to phobic stimuli that may be otherwise difficult to create in the standard treatment setting (eg, flight

Table 1
Summary of review of meta-analyses on psychotherapies for anxiety disorders[11]

Anxiety Disorder	Meta-Analyses	Psychological Treatment Findings	Pharmacologic Findings
Panic disorder			
	Clum et al, 1993[88]	• ES ranking: psychological coping = exposure > flooding = combination treatments • However, NSD between in vivo exposure, flooding, or psychological coping	Antidepressants most effective
	van Balkom et al, 1997[89]	• In vivo exposure effective reducing panic/agoraphobia • Greater effects on avoidance in agoraphobia than on panic attacks	
	Bakker et al, 1998[90]	In vivo exposure ≈ psychological panic management with exposure	
	Gould et al, 1995[91]	• C-B treatments had largest ES • C-B had less drop-outs (vs pharmacologic or combination pharmapsychological) • Within C-B those combining cognitive restructuring with interoceptive exposure had strongest ES • C-B suggested to have best long term outcomes	NSD between antidepressants and benzodiazepines
	Oei et al, 1999[92]	C-B therapy is effective for panic with agoraphobia	
	Westen and Morrison, 2001[93]	Improvements were significant and maintained for cognitive behavioral treatments	
	Cox et al, 1992[94]	Exposure was significantly effective for phobia variables, further exposure had strong effect sizes consistently	Imipramine = ineffective for most variables; Alprazolam = improvements for panic and anxiety variables

Social phobia		
	Feske and Chambless, 1995[95]	Exposure = C-B interventions in potency
	Taylor, 1996[96]	• C-B therapies are effective • Effectiveness is improved by adding cognitive restructuring • Pre- to posttreatment: all psychological treatments were superior to placebo and follow-ups were maintained across treatments
	Gould et al, 1997[97]	Exposure alone and cognitive restructuring were more effective than restructuring alone
	Fedoroff and Taylor, 2001[98]	• Cognitive therapy alone or combined with exposure were both effective but NSD from each other • Exposure alone was no more effective than wait list Deacon and Abramowitz[11] suggest this is caused by reliance on confidence intervals
Posttraumatic stress disorder		
	van Etten and Taylor, 1998[99]	C-B treatments are effective for symptom reduction
	Sherman, 1998[100]	Psychological treatments have moderate effects on symptoms compared with wait list, supportive counseling, and dynamic therapy
Generalized anxiety disorder		
	Gould et al, 1997[101]	• ES rank: combined > anxiety management > relaxation > cognitive therapy > behavior therapy > relaxation with biofeedback • Only significant ES comparison was combined treatment > relaxation with biofeedback
	Westen and Morrison, 2001[93]	• C-B treatments were effective for GAD • Because of small number of studies, individual treatments not compared
	Borkovec and Whisman, 1996[102]	• All psychological treatments superior to wait-list • ES rank: behavioral > cognitive therapy • Highest ES incorporated combination of behavioral and cognitive

(continued on next page)

Table 1
(continued)

Anxiety Disorder Meta-Analyses	Psychological Treatment Findings	Pharmacologic Findings
Obsessive–compulsive disorder		
van Balkom et al, 1994[103]	• No direct comparisons between treatments were conducted • However, ES for behavioral > cognitive therapy • Combination treatments were better than serotonergic antidepressants alone	All serotonergic antidepressants and combination with serotonergic antidepressant were more effective than placebo
Abramowitz, 1997[104]	• Exposure more effective than cognitive approaches • Particularly ERP	Clomipramine = most effective serotonergic medications in reducing symptoms
Abramowitz et al, 2002[105]	• ERP and cognitive therapies better than no treatment control • ES rank: ERP ≈ cognitive therapies	

Abbreviations: C-B, cognitive behavioral; ERP, exposure response prevention; ES, effect size; NSD, no significant difference; ≈, equal.

phobia[21]). In addition to exposure-based protocols, some treatments also incorporate cognitive restructuring to address beliefs and expectancies that may contribute to the phobic anxiety.

Only one meta-analysis of specific phobia treatment outcome exists, synthesizing findings from 33 outcome studies.[22] Treatments were classified as either exposure-based (ie, included at least some procedure that involved confronting the feared stimuli), non–exposure-based (ie, treatments theorized to be active, but not involving exposure, such as relaxation and cognitive restructuring), placebo treatments (ie, procedures in which patients were given a credible rationale but not provided an intervention known to remediate specific phobia, such as education), or wait-list controls. The effect sizes for posttreatment comparisons against wait-list-control groups were 1.05, 0.98, and 0.57 for exposure-based, non–exposure-based, and placebo treatments, respectively. The effect size for comparisons between exposure-based treatments and placebo treatments was 0.48 at posttreatment and 0.8 at follow-up. The effect size for comparisons between exposure-based protocols and non–exposure based protocols was 0.44 at posttreatment, and 0.35 at follow-up. In vivo exposure protocols also outperformed non–in vivo based protocols at posttreatment (Cohen's $d = 0.38$) but not at follow-up. No significant differences were seen between exposure-based protocols that last 1 session versus 5. However, length of treatment was found to moderate the effect sizes of exposure-based interventions versus wait-list controls, with longer treatments tending to produce larger effect sizes. No significant differences were seen between exposure-only approaches and those that also included cognitive therapy elements. Differences in the type of phobia also did not moderate treatment outcome.

This meta-analysis concludes that in vivo exposure is the preferred treatment for specific phobia. Although non–exposure-based approaches provide large effect sizes, the effect sizes for exposure-based interventions were significantly larger when directly compared. In vivo exposure produced larger effect sizes than non–in vivo exposure at posttreatment, but not at follow-up. Some evidence showed that longer-lasting treatments tended to produce larger effects, although single-session exposure treatments also produced comparably large effect sizes to five-session exposure treatments. Finally, exposure-based protocols outperformed placebo treatments, showing that exposure principles add incremental efficacy above those achieved through nonspecific treatment factors.

SOCIAL PHOBIA

CBT for social phobia typically emphasizes cognitive restructuring and in vivo exposure to feared social situations. Patients are instructed in identifying and challenging their beliefs about their social competence and the probability of experiencing negative social evaluation and consequences. In vivo exposures provide opportunities to confront feared and avoided social encounters and to practice social skills. CBT for social phobia is often delivered and studied in group format.[23] Compared with individual therapy, group CBT conveniently allows in vivo exposures to be conducted in the therapy setting using group members as confederates or audience members, and provides opportunities for patients to receive immediate support, feedback, and reinforcement from other group members.

A recent meta-analysis examined the effectiveness of psychotherapy for social phobia and social anxiety under various conditions.[24] Twenty-nine studies were located that involved comparisons between a bona fide psychotherapy and a wait-list or psychological placebo control group. Most studies used CBT techniques such as exposure, cognitive restructuring, social skills training, relaxation, or a combination of these elements. Overall, CBT interventions produced controlled effect sizes in the 0.70 to 0.80 range on measures of social anxiety, general anxiety, and depression. Effect sizes were higher in studies that were compared with wait-list control groups and when analog socially anxious participants were treated. Specific therapy techniques, such as exposure and cognitive restructuring, were not associated with higher effect sizes. However, given the substantial heterogeneity in the samples and treatment approaches used in the studies, it is difficult to make firm conclusions about the relative efficacy of different CBT techniques. Furthermore, studies comparing the effects of different CBT approaches with more clinically representative populations seem warranted.[25]

Segool and Carlson[26] conducted a meta-analysis of CBT studies in socially phobic children and adolescents. The authors identified seven group studies of CBT, defined as exposure plus cognitive restructuring, in youths aged 5 to 18 years (mean age, 10.5), with the average number of therapy sessions equaling 11.9. Within-group effect size estimates were calculated to quantify the degree of improvement from pretreatment to posttreatment. CBT produced large and statistically significant improvement in social anxiety symptoms ($d = 0.86$), general anxiety symptoms ($d = 0.75$), and impairment ($d = 1.56$). Seven studies of selective serotonin reuptake inhibitor (SSRI) medications were also located, with SSRIs producing significantly greater improvement than CBT on each outcome variable. Unfortunately, the authors did not examine the possible influence of publication bias on the apparent efficacy of SSRI medications. The authors concluded that both CBT and SSRI medications are effective in the treatment of children with social phobia.

OBSESSIVE–COMPULSIVE DISORDER

The development of exposure and response prevention (ERP)[27] challenged previously held notions that obsessive–compulsive disorder (OCD) is unresponsive to psychotherapy. It is now widely accepted that ERP is an efficacious treatment of OCD,[28] and regarded as a first-line treatment for this condition.[29] Cognitive interventions that derive from Beck's[30] cognitive model of depression have also been applied to the treatment of OCD. The addition of cognitive elements to the treatment of OCD has raised important questions regarding the incremental efficacy of cognitive and ERP approaches.[11] The effect sizes for ERP, CBT, and CT interventions for OCD were similar across these modalities, although slightly stronger for ERP and CBT conditions.[31] Across all treatments, approximately two thirds of the patients who completed treatment improved (range, 33%–78%), whereas only one third met recovery criteria (range, 27%–47%). Among the intent-to-treat sample (including patients who chose not to complete), about one half of patients improved (range, 25%–74%), compared with only one fourth who recovered (range, 22%–33%). Findings were again stronger for ERP relative to the other conditions. ERP posttreatment OCD symptom levels were also generally lower than the poststreatment outcomes for CBT and CT.

The efficacy of CBT in pediatric OCD samples has also been investigated.[32,33] A recent meta-analysis included only investigations using randomized, controlled methodology for OCD participants aged 19 years and younger.[34] A comprehensive literature review yielded 13 randomized controlled trials containing 10 pharmacotherapy to control comparisons and 5 CBT to control comparisons. A statistically significant pooled effect size that was robust against publication bias was found for only pharmacotherapy and CBT, with CBT yielding a stronger effect size (1.45) over pharmacotherapy (0.48).

However, the durability of the effects of CBT for pediatric OCD remains largely unknown. In a recent review of the long-term outcome of OCD among youth in general,

Stewart and colleagues[35] found 22 studies with follow-up periods ranging between 1 and 15.6 years. At follow-up, rates of persistent full OCD (range, 13%–87%; pooled mean, 41%) and subclinical OCD (range, 17%–46%; pooled mean, 19%) were reported to be lower than expected.

Cost-effectiveness considerations have motivated the application of CBT interventions for OCD in a group format. In a meta-analysis of 13 trials examining the efficacy of group CBT for OCD, Jonsson and Hougaard[36] reported overall a pre- to posteffect size of 1.18 and between-group effect size of 1.12 when compared with wait-list control conditions.[36] Furthermore, group CBT achieved better results than pharmacological treatment in two studies included in the meta-analysis. Although one study in this meta-analysis found no significant differences between individual and group CBT, Eddy and colleagues[31] found that pre- versus posttreatment effect sizes were slightly higher for individual therapy (1.48) than for group therapy (1.17). Furthermore, patients who completed individual therapy had a greater percentage of those meeting recovery criteria (mean, 44%) relative to those participating in the group format (mean, 28%). Among the intent-to-treat sample, 37% of patients in individual therapy recovered, compared with only 22% of those in group-based approaches.

Contemporary meta-analyses continue to support the efficacy of interventions for OCD that are based on empirically supported behavioral and cognitive principles. Specifically, these findings clearly indicate that ERP, CBT, and cognitive therapy have strong effects in the treatment of OCD. In fact, a recent meta-analysis suggests that the strongest effect sizes for CBT across the anxiety disorders are generally observed for OCD.[37] Furthermore, ERP seems to be more efficacious than cognitive approaches. Although cost-effectiveness concerns may warrant the implementation of group CBT approaches, empirical findings support the superiority of individual over group interventions for OCD.

An important issue that must be further addressed in these randomized controlled trials is that of sustained efficacy.[31] Although some evidence shows that the long-term persistence of OCD after treatment may be lower than previously thought,[35] additional research is needed to adequately determine the extent to which CBT produces lasting symptom changes for patients with OCD. This assessment will require future studies to include substantially longer follow-up intervals (ie, ≥1 year posttreatment) so more definite inferences can be made regarding the durability of CBT for OCD.

POSTTRAUMATIC STRESS DISORDER

CBTs for posttraumatic stress disorder (PTSD) typically include three components: (1) psychoeducation about the nature of fear, anxiety, and PTSD; (2) controlled, prolonged exposure to stimuli related to the traumatic event; and, (3) cognitive restructuring, processing, or challenging of maladaptive beliefs/appraisals. Relaxation training or breathing retraining components are periodically included in some treatment packages. The most-studied CBT approaches are prolonged exposure[38] and cognitive processing therapy.[39]

A meta-analysis of PTSD is particularly notable because it coded for many relevant variables pertaining to clinical utility and external validity beyond just reporting treatment outcome effect sizes.[40] The authors noted, however, that approximately 40% of studies failed to report inclusion/exclusion rates. Most studies excluded participants because of psychosis (85%), organic disorders (77%), suicide risk (46%), alcohol or drug abuse or dependence (62%), and unspecified concerns of serious comorbidity (62%). Comorbidity data were also sparsely reported for both axis I (42%) and II (12%) disorders. Nonetheless, these data allow for some important inferences regarding to whom the treatment outcome effect size results can be generalized.

Bradley and colleagues[40] report treatment outcome effect size estimates for exposure therapy, eye movement desensitization and reprocessing (EMDR) therapy, exposure therapy plus cognitive restructuring, and CBT. In this meta-analysis, CBT referred to all forms of CBT that did not include exposure or EMDR (eg, cognitive restructuring–only was considered CBT); 79% of participants who entered a treatment study completed it. The pre- versus posttreatment effect sizes were as follows: exposure (1.57); CBT (1.65); exposure plus cognitive restructuring (1.66); EMDR (1.43); wait-list control (0.35); and, supportive control (0.59). The effect sizes for the active treatments compared with wait-list controls were 1.26, 1.26, 1.53, and 1.25 for exposure, CBT, exposure plus cognitive restructuring, and EMDR, respectively. The effect sizes for the active treatments compared with supportive control conditions were 0.84, 1.01, 0.99, and 0.75 for exposure, CBT, exposure plus cognitive restructuring, and EMDR, respectively. The rates of change in diagnostic status (ie, no longer meeting criteria for PTSD) across the treatment conditions among the intent-to-treat samples were best for EMDR (60%), followed by exposure plus cognitive restructuring (54%), exposure (53%), CBT (46%), supportive control (36%), and wait-list control (14%). The rates of change in diagnostic status across the treatment conditions among the treatment-completer samples were most favorable for exposure plus cognitive restructuring (70%), followed by exposure (68%), EMDR (65%), CBT (56%), supportive control (39%), and wait-list control (16%). Because few studies reported follow-up data of at least 6 months, the authors were only able to provide effect sizes confidence intervals (CIs) for pretreatment versus follow-up comparisons for exposure (95% CI = 0.92–2.57), CBT (95% CI = –0.11–3.01), and exposure plus cognitive restructuring (95% CI = 1.58–2.55).

Finally, Bradley and colleagues[40] also reported on variables that moderate treatment outcome. Year of publication was positively associated with pre- versus posttreatment effect sizes and treatment versus wait-list control effect sizes. Number of exclusion criteria was positively associated with pre- versus posttreatment effect sizes, such that studies with more exclusion criteria tended to have greater effect sizes. Completion rate was negatively associated with pre- versus posttreatment effect sizes, such that greater dropout rate was associated with greater effect sizes. Type of trauma also moderated treatment outcome, with combat-related trauma groups yielding smaller effect sizes than those for mixed trauma or sexual assault.

Other meta-analyses of PTSD treatment outcome have similarly found evidence for the efficacy of CBT. Bisson and colleagues[41,42] compared CBT treatments (which they called *trauma-focused treatments*, indicating any treatment that focused directly on trauma-related memories, such as exposure or cognitive restructuring), EMDR, and non–trauma focused treatments (eg, stress management). The authors found that the treatment versus wait-list effect sizes were 1.4, 1.5, and 1.1 for CBT, EMDR, and stress management, respectively. The relative risk for retaining the diagnosis of PTSD in the treatment conditions relative to the control groups was lowest (ie, implying that participants no longer met PTSD diagnostic criteria) in CBT (0.44), followed by EMDR (0.49), and stress management (0.64). This meta-analysis also examined the effects of treatment on general anxiety and depression. For depression, effect sizes for the treatment versus control group were 1.26, 1.48, and 0.73 for CBT, EMDR, and stress management, respectively. For anxiety, effect sizes for the treatment versus control group were 0.99, 1.20, and 0.73 for CBT, EMDR, and stress management, respectively.

In another meta-analysis, Seidler and Wagner[43] compared the efficacies of CBT (which they referred to as *trauma-focused CBT*) and EMDR. Seven studies that directly compared CBT with EMDR were included. The effect size for the CBT versus EMDR post-treatment comparison was 0.28, favoring CBT, although the CI overlapped with zero and thus was not considered to be significant. The effect size for the CBT versus EMDR follow-up comparison was 0.13, again favoring CBT, but the CI again overlapped with zero and was considered nonsignificant. True comparisons between the efficacies of CBT (and its components) and EMDR have not been without controversy. Several authors[44,45] and dismantling studies[46] suggest that the active element of EMDR is imaginal exposure, a known active factor in exposure-based treatments, and eye movements are an additive, yet nonactive component in therapy. Based on these findings, caution is warranted in comparing CBT and EMDR in PTSD treatment outcome studies.

Meta-analyses have also been conducted on randomized controlled trials of treatments aimed at preventing the onset of PTSD after initial traumatic event exposure.[47,48] Roberts and colleagues[48] conducted a meta-analysis of 25 studies investigating the prevention of PTSD for individuals exposed to a traumatic event within the past 3 months. Effect sizes suggested that posttreatment symptoms of PTSD were not lower for psychoeducation or structured writing treatments relative to control groups. By contrast, trauma-focused CBT (ie, interventions that focused on the traumatic memories, including exposure and cognitive therapy elements) resulted in lower risk for PTSD diagnoses compared with wait-list control at 3 months follow-up (relative risk, 0.64), and lower risk for PTSD diagnoses compared with supportive counseling at 3 to 6 months (relative risk, 0.37) and 3 to 4 years (relative risk, 0.28) posttreatment. Trauma-focused CBT also resulted in fewer PTSD symptoms relative to supportive counseling at posttreatment ($d = 0.95$), 3 to 6 months follow-up, ($d = 0.62$), and 2 to 4 years follow-up ($d = 0.85$).

The meta-analysis conducted by Kornor and colleagues[47] included studies of individuals with acute stress disorder or initial symptoms of PTSD. The seven comparative studies included supportive counseling for trauma-focused CBT, defined as an intervention that consisted of any of the following components: exposure, stress inoculation, cognitive processing, assertiveness, biofeedback, or relaxation training. The relative risks for being diagnosed with PTSD at 3 to 6 months, 9 months, and 36 to 48 months posttreatment were 0.49, 1.09, and 0.73, respectively, with all effect sizes favoring trauma-focused CBT. The only statistically significant effect was at 3 to 6 months posttreatment.

These meta-analyses show that CBT procedures are efficacious in the treatment and prevention of PTSD. The qualitative review of these studies highlights the significant heterogeneity with the combination of treatment elements that fall under the umbrella term *CBT*. Furthermore, CBT outperforms both wait-list controls and supportive counseling controls, showin that CBT procedures provide incremental efficacy above and beyond the efficacy provided by nonspecific factors. The effect sizes for primarily exposure-based protocols were not substantially different from those of primarily cognitively based protocols or the combination of exposure and cognitive therapy. Accordingly, clinicians can confidently use any of one these CBT procedures.

GENERALIZED ANXIETY DISORDER

Generalized anxiety disorder (GAD) is marked by excessive and uncontrollable worry. However, the unspecified nature of worry cues and the often diverse and fluctuating nature of the worry content complicates the application of specific treatments. GAD has been well documented as one of the most difficult anxiety disorders to treat,[49] yielding lower treatment response relative to other anxiety disorders. However, the combination of various CBT-based approaches for treating GAD has produced promising results. These CBT interventions vary considerably in the relative combination of specific techniques used, such as self-monitoring, relaxation training, cognitive therapy, worry exposure, and the rehearsal of new learned relaxation and cognitive coping responses.

In a meta-analysis examining a total of 65 CBT and pharmacological studies for GAD, Mittes[50] found a significant medium-to-large effect size for CBT compared with wait-list and psychological/pill placebo. Significant symptom improvement as a function of CBT compared with wait-list was observed for anxiety and depression (effect sizes, 0.82 and 0.76, respectively) and psychological/pill placebo (effect sizes, 0.57 and 0.52, respectively). Direct comparison of CBT and pharmacotherapy showed a significantly greater effect for CBT among studies that examined the efficacy of both treatment approaches. Although the incremental efficacy of CBT compared with pharmacotherapy was no longer observed after controlling for study-specific parameters, attrition rates were lower for CBT. These finding are similar to those of Haby and colleagues,[51] who report an effect size of 0.64 for the efficacy of CBT relative to controls. However, an important conclusion from this study is that these effect size estimates seem to be contingent on the type of control group used and the baseline severity of patients included in the randomized controlled trials.

A comprehensive examination of the GAD treatment outcome literature by Hunot and colleagues[52] found that 46% of patients assigned to CBT showed clinical response at posttreatment, in contrast with 14% in wait-list/treatment-as-usual groups. Furthermore, those undergoing CBT were more likely to show reduction in anxiety and depression symptoms than those undergoing analytic therapy at posttreatment and at 6-month follow-up. CBT treatment completers also showed a greater reduction in depression symptoms at posttreatment relative to patients who completed supportive therapy. Although evidence for the incremental efficacy of some treatments for GAD versus others is limited to a small number of studies, the general consensus of the available literature is that a cognitive behavioral approach seems to be more effective than non-CBT modalities in maximizing treatment gains. However, the question remains as to which CBT interventions are most effective for treating GAD.

Siev and Chambless[16] recently examined the question of the specificity of treatment effects of cognitive therapy and relaxation training for GAD. The findings showed that the weighted average percentage of patients meeting criteria for clinically significant change at posttreatment was 44% for cognitive therapy and 45% for relaxation training, suggesting that the treatment groups did not differ in the relative odds of achieving clinically significant change at posttreatment. Furthermore, no difference was seen between the treatment groups in anxiety, anxiety-related cognitions, and depression.

Meta-analytic investigations have also examined the efficacy of CBT for chronic worry among patients with GAD. For example, Covin and colleagues[53] found a large effect size when comparing CBT with a control group (–1.15). Subsequent analysis showed that the average weighted effect size was larger (–1.69) for young adults than for older adults (–0.82), suggesting that CBT for GAD may not be as effective in older adults. However, treatment gains made by patients of all ages after CBT were largely maintained for up to 1-year follow-up. This finding suggests that CBT may yield longer-term benefits toward preventing symptom relapse in GAD. Meta-analytic findings also suggest superiority of individual CBT (effect size, –1.72) over group CBT (effect size, –0.91) in reducing chronic and uncontrollable worry symptoms in GAD.

Although more recent meta-analyses continue to support the efficacy of CBT for GAD, effect sizes for GAD are lower than those observed in other anxiety disorders.[54] This observation has reinforced the need for additional techniques that can be incorporated into standard CBT for GAD to maximize efficacy. Emotion regulation models of GAD posit that cognitive avoidance strategies in GAD, such as worry, are largely used to avoid the experience of negative emotions. Accordingly, effective treatment of GAD should provide patients with the tools to (1) identify, differentiate, and describe emotions, even in their most intense form; (2) increase acceptance of affective experience and ability to adaptively manage emotions when necessary; (3) decrease use of worry and other emotional avoidance strategies; and, (4) increase ability to use emotional information in identifying needs, making decisions, guiding thinking, motivating behavior, and managing interpersonal relationships and other contextual demands.[55] Researchers have begun to consider incorporating specific techniques in the management of GAD and worry, such as learning to identify emotions and their possible evolutionary functions, creating an emotion hierarchy to systematically address different emotions, using imaginal exposure to increase tolerance to different emotions, and eliminating behavioral avoidance of emotional experiences.[56]

FUTURE DIRECTIONS IN COGNITIVE BEHAVIORAL THERAPY FOR ANXIETY DISORDERS
Enhancing Efficacy

Contemporary meta-analytic findings support the efficacy of CBT for treating anxiety disorders, with CBT being more efficacious than other bona fide treatments for specific anxiety disorders. Although these data are consistent with the view held by many that CBT is the gold standard psychosocial treatment for anxiety, CBT interventions are by no means 100% effective. For example, one study found that 27% of patients that were panic-free after a trial of CBT underwent additional panic treatment over a 2-year follow-up period.[57] The questionable durability of CBT for treating anxiety disorders has encouraged researchers to examine augmenting approaches, such as pharmacotherapy, to enhance its effectiveness. Unfortunately, clinical trials have generally failed to show a consistent benefit of augmenting CBT with either anti-anxiety or antidepressant medications.[29,58,59]

Other lines of research have focused on supplementing exposure-based interventions with biological agents that enhance learning and facilitate fear extinction. D-cycloserine (DCS), a drug approved by the U.S. Food and Drug Association for treating tuberculosis, has been shown in animal studies to enhance the consolidation of learning processes that underlie fear extinction.[60] The use of DCS to augment exposure therapy is fundamentally different from combination treatment with traditional pharmacological agents because the sole purpose of DCS is to enhance the effects of exposure, rather than produce a general state of sedation or correct a presumed biological dysfunction.

In the first anxiety study of DCS, Ressler and colleagues[61] randomly assigned 27 adults with acrophobia to undergo two sessions of virtual reality exposure combined with either pill placebo, 50 mg of DCS, or 500 mg of DCS. The DCS or placebo was ingested 2 to 4 hours before each exposure session. Patients in each group had equivalent levels of fear during the first exposure session. However, during the second exposure session, 1 week later, and at 3-month follow-up, patients who had received either dose of DCS were less afraid during the exposures than patients who received placebo. The beneficial effects of DCS extended beyond the virtual world, with patients receiving DCS reporting fewer real-world acrophobic symptoms than those receiving placebo at each assessment.

Clinical trials have examined the effects of combining DCS with exposure in the treatment of social phobia, panic disorder, OCD, and specific phobias.[62] In nearly all studies, augmenting exposure therapy with DCS produced substantial benefits at both posttreatment and follow-up compared with placebo augmentation. In addition to DCS, other potential cognitive-enhancer agents also seem to facilitate fear extinction in exposure therapy. Augmenting exposure for claustrophobia with yohimbine, a selective competitive α_2-adrenergic receptor antagonist, has been shown to substantially improve outcomes in comparison with placebo augmentation.[63] Similarly, administration of the glucocorticoid cortisone before exposure tasks produced significantly improved outcomes for patients with social phobia and spider phobia.[64] Future cutting-edge research on combining exposure therapy with these nontraditional pharmacological agents holds significant promise for improving the efficacy of CBT and may help reduce the total number of sessions to achieve desirable treatment outcomes.

Enhancing Dissemination

Despite the efficacy of CBT, considerable evidence shows that most individuals with anxiety disorders do not receive this empirically supported intervention. In 1996, psychodynamic therapy was the most common psychosocial treatment for patients with GAD, panic disorder, and social phobia.[65] More recent work has shown that half or more of doctoral-level licensed therapists who treat OCD do not use ERP, the empirically supported preferred treatment.[66] Furthermore, only half of the licensed psychotherapists who treat patients with PTSD use imaginal exposure.[67] Evidence also shows that when CBT approaches are used to treat anxiety disorders, they are often being delivered suboptimally. For example, 60% of a small sample of patients with OCD who reported undergoing CBT did not meet defined minimal criteria for adequacy.[68] The limited availability and poor delivery of CBT for anxiety are strong indicators of inadequate dissemination.

Fortunately, the dissemination (targeted distribution of information on evidence-based health interventions) and implementation (adaptation and application of these interventions over time) of CBT interventions for anxiety have become a focus of recent research.

Population-based dissemination efforts, such as computerized CBT delivery for primary care patients with anxiety disorders, have yielded promising findings.[69] For example, Craske and colleagues[70] examined the acceptance and effectiveness of a computer-assisted CBT program designed to support the delivery of CBT for panic disorder, PTSD, GAD, and social anxiety disorder in primary care. The program was rated as very helpful by clinicians. Results indicate that the patients fully participated (ie, attendance and homework compliance), understood the program material, and acquired CBT skills. Furthermore, patients with anxiety disorder reported significant improvements in self-rated anxiety and depression. The effectiveness of this computerized approach highlights a potential role of Web-based technologies in increasing the efficiency of CBT dissemination for anxiety disorders. Internet delivery of CBT components for anxiety disorders has increased rapidly over recent years, and treatment outcome research examining the efficacy of this approach has found large effect sizes for some anxiety disorders.[71]

ATTENTION RETRAINING TREATMENT FOR ANXIETY DISORDERS

A large body of research suggests that attention is biased toward threat-relevant stimuli in anxiety.[72] More recently, research has shown that this bias may actually causally influence anxiety vulnerability. Macleod and colleagues[73] found that nonanxious individuals who were trained to attend toward threatening stimuli in a computerized attentional bias task showed greater emotional reactivity during a subsequent frustrating anagram task compared with individuals in a control condition. Subsequent studies then examined whether training attention away from threat would lead to decreases in symptoms of anxiety disorders.

Attention retraining treatment procedures are computerized tasks that typically modify the "dot probe" attentional bias task.[74] Participants see two stimuli displayed above and below a fixation cross on a computer screen. One stimulus is threatening, the other stimulus is neutral. The stimuli disappear after 500 ms and a probe appears in either the top or bottom of the screen. The participants' task is to determine the location (top or bottom) of the probe stimulus as quickly as possible. In the attention retraining protocol, the probe always occurs in the location previously occupied by the neutral stimulus. Thus, over time, the participant learns to attend to the neutral stimulus, as the neutral stimulus signals the impending location of the probe. This training counters the anxious individual's tendency to attend to the threatening stimulus; therefore, the attention retraining protocols are theorized to correct attentional biases toward threat. In control procedures, the location of the probe is randomized and occurs equally in locations previously occupied by the threat and neutral stimuli. Randomized controlled trials have found that the attention retraining protocols reduce symptoms of social phobia[75–77] and GAD[78,79] compared with the control conditions. These data show that attention retraining procedures may be effective stand-alone treatments for anxiety disorders. Furthermore, attention retraining procedures seem to be well-suited for Internet delivery, which could help disseminate effective treatments to many individuals experiencing anxiety.

Although preliminary data examining the efficacy of attention retraining as an intervention component for anxiety disorders are promising, research along these lines have not been entirely consistent. For example, one study found that attention retraining only led to reductions in symptoms on one of three measures of social phobia.[80] Additionally, Klumpp and Amir[81] found that two groups of socially anxious individuals who underwent either one session of attention training toward threat or attention training away from threat both displayed reduced anxiety during a subsequent social stressor relative to a control group. Although the authors argued that these data are consistent with the notion that attention training improves attentional control, which subsequently reduces social anxiety, the fact that training attention toward threat reduces symptoms of anxiety disorders calls into question the notion that attentional biases causally increase or maintain anxiety,[73] which was the foundation for this line of research. The mechanisms producing attentional biases are only beginning to be elucidated,[82–84] and the mechanisms through which reduction of these biases leads to improvements in anxiety are even less clear. However, future research delineating the mechanisms of action of attention retraining and their incremental efficacy to existing CBT treatments may offer more definitive data regarding this computerized treatment approach.

SUMMARY

This article summarizes recent meta-analytic findings supporting the efficacy of CBT for anxiety disorders. However, the exact mechanisms of change in these treatments remain unclear. Prior work suggests that behavioral interventions in the form of exposure during CBT may constitute the dominant, active ingredient in the treatment of some anxiety disorders, particularly OCD and social phobia.[11] Although some form of exposure may be necessary and sufficient for the treatment of OCD and social phobia, the extent to which this is true for other anxiety disorders remains unclear. More randomized controlled trials using dismantling designs (ie, studies that take apart the multiple components of a given treatment) will be necessary to better determine the specific active features of CBT. Constructing the appropriate combination of components relative to nonspecific control conditions will facilitate multiple component comparisons. These comparisons allow for strong experimental tests of the effects of alternative treatment components, key components, and the combined treatment components of CBT.[85]

Dismantling randomized controlled trials of CBT will also help identify the necessary (and perhaps sufficient) components of CBT that should be the focus of further enhancement and dissemination. A general consensus exists that exposure is a central feature of CBT for all anxiety disorders,[86] and the form of exposure varies depending on the core feature of the anxiety disorder. Exposure therapy may consist of systematic and repeated approach to feared external (agoraphobic situations) and internal (bodily sensations) stimuli. Imaginal exposure is also an empirically supported treatment of trauma memories in PTSD. Virtual reality exposure is also being increasingly used to treat phobias, social anxiety disorder, and PTSD. Augmenting exposure delivery with cognitive enhancer agents also holds promise in improving the efficiency of treatment delivery. Advancing the efficacy and dissemination of CBT for anxiety disorders will continue to require systematic investigation with basic research models in fear learning and extinction.[87]

ACKNOWLEDGMENTS

The authors thank Bethany G. Ciesielski for her administrative assistance with this paper and the special issue.

REFERENCES

1. Kessler RC, Berglund P, Demler O, et al. Lifetime prevalence and age-of-onset distributions of DSM-IV disorders in the National Comorbidity Survey Replication. Arch Gen Psychiatry 2005;62:593–602.
2. Kessler RC, Chiu WT, Demler O, et al. Prevalence, severity, and comorbidity of 12-month DSM-IV disorders in the National Comorbidity Survey Replication. Arch Gen Psychiatry 2005;62:617–27.
3. DuPont RL, Rice DP, Miller LS, et al. Economic costs of anxiety disorders. Anxiety 1996;2:167–72.
4. Olatunji BO, Cisler JM, Tolin DF. Quality of life in the anxiety disorders: a meta-analytic review. Clin Psychol Rev 2007;27:572–81.
5. Craske MG, Rauch SL, Ursano R, et al. What is an anxiety disorder? Depress Anxiety 2009;26:1066–85.
6. Mathews A, MacLeod C. Cognitive vulnerability to emotional disorders. Annu Rev Clin Psychol 2005;1:167–95.
7. Lovibond PF, Mitchell CJ, Minard E, et al. Safety behaviours preserve threat beliefs: protection from extinction of human fear conditioning by an avoidance response. Behav Res Ther 2009;47:716–20.
8. Barlow DH. Anxiety and its disorders: the nature and treatment of anxiety and panic. 2nd edition. New York: Guilford Press; 2002.
9. Hollon SD, Beck AT. Cognitive and cognitive behavioral therapies. In: Lambert MJ, editor. Bergin and Garfield's handbook of psychotherapy and behavior change. 5th edition. Hoboken (NJ): Wiley; 2004. p. 447–92.

10. Butler AC, Chapman JE, Forman EM, et al. The empirical status of cognitive-behavioral therapy: a review of meta-analyses. Clin Psychol Rev 2006;26: 17–31.
11. Deacon BJ, Abramowitz JS. Cognitive and behavioral treatments for anxiety disorders: a review of meta-analytic findings. J Clin Psychol 2004;60:429–41.
12. Longmore RJ, Worrell M. Do we need to challenge thoughts in cognitive behavior therapy? Clin Psychol Rev 2007;27:173–87.
13. Hofmann SG. Common misconceptions about cognitive mediation of treatment change: a commentary to Longmore and Worrell (2007). Clin Psychol Rev 2008; 28:67–70 [discussion: 71–4].
14. Benish SG, Imel ZE, Wampold BE. The relative efficacy of bona fide psychotherapies for treating post-traumatic stress disorder: a meta-analysis of direct comparisons. Clin Psychol Rev 2008;28:746–58.
15. Barlow DH, Craske MG. Mastery of your anxiety and panic: therapist guide. 4th edition. New York: Oxford University Press; 2007.
16. Siev J, Chambless DL. Specificity of treatment effects: cognitive therapy and relaxation for generalized anxiety and panic disorders. J Consult Clin Psychol 2007;75:513–22.
17. Clark DM. A cognitive approach to panic. Behav Res Ther 1986;24:461–70.
18. Schmidt NB, Woolaway-Bickel K, Trakowski J, et al. Dismantling cognitive-behavioral treatment for panic disorder: questioning the utility of breathing retraining. J Consult Clin Psychol 2000;68:417–24.
19. Mltte K. A meta-analysis of the efficacy of psycho- and pharmacotherapy in panic disorder with and without agoraphobia. J Affect Disord 2005;88:27–45.
20. Antony MM, Swinson RP. Phobic disorders and panic in adults: a guide to assessment and treatment. Washington, DC: American Psychological Association; 2000.
21. Rothbaum BO, Hodges L, Smith S, et al. A controlled study of virtual reality exposure therapy for the fear of flying. J Consult Clin Psychol 2000;68:1020–6.
22. Wolitzky-Taylor KB, Horowitz JD, Powers MB, et al. Psychological approaches in the treatment of specific phobias: a meta-analysis. Clin Psychol Rev 2008;28: 1021–37.
23. Heimberg RG, Liebowitz MR, Hope DA, et al. Cognitive behavioral group therapy vs phenelzine therapy for social phobia: 12-week outcome. Arch Gen Psychiatry 1998;55:1133–41.
24. Acarturk C, Cuijpers P, van Straten A, et al. Psychological treatment of social anxiety disorder: a meta-analysis. Psychol Med 2009;39:241–54.
25. Hofmann SG. Cognitive mediation of treatment change in social phobia. J Consult Clin Psychol 2004;72:393–9.
26. Segool NK, Carlson JS. Efficacy of cognitive-behavioral and pharmacological treatments for children with social anxiety. Depress Anxiety 2008;25:620–31.
27. Meyer V. Modification of expectations in cases with obsessional rituals. Behav Res Ther 1966;4:273–80.
28. Franklin ME, Abramowitz JS, Kozak MJ, et al. Effectiveness of exposure and ritual prevention for obsessive-compulsive disorder: randomized compared with nonrandomized samples. J Consult Clin Psychol 2000;68:594–602.
29. Foa EB, Franklin ME, Moser J. Context in the clinic: how well do cognitive-behavioral therapies and medications work in combination? Biol Psychiatry 2002;52:987–97.
30. Beck AT. Cognitive therapy and the emotional disorders. New York: International Universities Press; 1976.

31. Eddy KT, Dutra L, Bradley R, et al. A multidimensional meta-analysis of psychotherapy and pharmacotherapy for obsessive-compulsive disorder. Clin Psychol Rev 2004;24:1011–30.

32. Abramowitz JS, Whiteside SP, Deacon BJ. The effectiveness of treatment for pediatric obsessive-compulsive disorder: a meta-analysis. Behav Ther 2005;36: 55–63.

33. Freeman JB, Choate-Summers ML, Moore PS, et al. Cognitive behavioral treatment for young children with obsessive-compulsive disorder. Biol Psychiatry 2007;61:337–43.

34. Watson HJ, Rees CS. Meta-analysis of randomized, controlled treatment trials for pediatric obsessive-compulsive disorder. J Child Psychol Psychiatry 2008; 49:489–98.

35. Stewart SE, Geller DA, Jenike M, et al. Long-term outcome of pediatric obsessive-compulsive disorder: a meta-analysis and qualitative review of the literature. Acta Psychiatr Scand 2004;110:4–13.

36. Jonsson H, Hougaard E. Group cognitive behavioural therapy for obsessive-compulsive disorder: a systematic review and meta-analysis. Acta Psychiatr Scand 2009;119:98–106.

37. Hofmann SG, Smits JA. Cognitive-behavioral therapy for adult anxiety disorders: a meta-analysis of randomized placebo-controlled trials. J Clin Psychiatry 2008; 69:621–32.

38. Foa EB, Rothbaum BO, Riggs DS, et al. Treatment of posttraumatic stress disorder in rape victims: a comparison between cognitive-behavioral procedures and counseling. J Consult Clin Psychol 1991;59:715–23.

39. Resick PA, Schnicke MK. Cognitive processing therapy for sexual assault victims. J Consult Clin Psychol 1992;60:748–56.

40. Bradley R, Greene J, Russ E, et al. A multidimensional meta-analysis of psychotherapy for PTSD. Am J Psychiatry 2005;162:214–27.

41. Bisson JI, Ehlers A, Matthews R, et al. Psychological treatments for chronic posttraumatic stress disorder. Systematic review and meta-analysis. Br J Psychiatry 2007;190:97–104.

42. Bisson J, Andrew M. Psychological treatment of post-traumatic stress disorder (PTSD). Cochrane Database Syst Rev 2007;3:CD003388.

43. Seidler GH, Wagner FE. Comparing the efficacy of EMDR and trauma-focused cognitive-behavioral therapy in the treatment of PTSD: a meta-analytic study. Psychol Med 2006;36:1515–22.

44. Herbert JD, Lilienfeld SO, Lohr JM, et al. Science and pseudoscience in the development of eye movement desensitization and reprocessing: implications for clinical psychology. Clin Psychol Rev 2000;20:945–71.

45. McNally RJ. EMDR and Mesmerism: a comparative historical analysis. J Anxiety Disord 1999;13:225–36.

46. Pitman RK, Orr SP, Altman B, et al. Emotional processing during eye movement desensitization and reprocessing therapy of Vietnam veterans with chronic post-traumatic stress disorder. Compr Psychiatry 1996;37:419–29.

47. Kornor H, Winje D, Ekeberg O, et al. Early trauma-focused cognitive-behavioural therapy to prevent chronic post-traumatic stress disorder and related symptoms: a systematic review and meta-analysis. BMC Psychiatry 2008;8:81.

48. Roberts NP, Kitchiner NJ, Kenardy J, et al. Systematic review and meta-analysis of multiple-session early interventions following traumatic events. Am J Psychiatry 2009;166:293–301.

49. Gould RA, Safren SA, O'Neill Washington D, et al. Cognitive-behavioral treatments: a meta analytic review. In: Heimberg RG, Turk CL, Mennin DS, editors. Generalized anxiety disorder: advances in research and practice. New York: Guilford Press; 2004. p. 248–64.
50. Mitte K. Meta-analysis of cognitive-behavioral treatments for generalized anxiety disorder: a comparison with pharmacotherapy. Psychol Bull 2005;131:785–95.
51. Haby MM, Donnelly M, Corry J, et al. Cognitive behavioural therapy for depression, panic disorder and generalized anxiety disorder: a meta-regression of factors that may predict outcome. Aust N Z J Psychiatry 2006;40:9–19.
52. Hunot V, Churchill R, Silva de Lima M, et al. Psychological therapies for generalised anxiety disorder. Cochrane Database Syst Rev 2007;1:CD001848.
53. Covin R, Ouimet AJ, Seeds PM, et al. A meta-analysis of CBT for pathological worry among clients with GAD. J Anxiety Disord 2008;22:108–16.
54. Newman MG, Castonguay LG, Borkovec TD, et al. An open trial of integrative therapy for generalized anxiety disorder. Psychotherapy 2008;45:135–47.
55. Mennin DS. Emotion regulation therapy: an integrative approach to treatment resistant anxiety disorders. J Contemp Psychother 2006;36:95–105.
56. Huppert JD, Alley AC. The clinical application of emotion research in generalized anxiety disorder: some proposed procedures. Cogn Behav Pract 2001; 11:387–92.
57. Brown TA, Barlow DH. Long-term outcome in cognitive-behavioral treatment of panic disorder: clinical predictors and alternative strategies for assessment. J Consult Clin Psychol 1995;63:754–65.
58. Deacon BJ. The effect of pharmacotherapy on the effectiveness of exposure therapy. In: Richard DCS, Lauterbach D, editors. Comprehensive handbook of the exposure therapies. New York: Academic Press; 2007. p. 311–33.
59. Otto MW, Smits JA, Reese HE. Combined psychotherapy and pharmacotherapy for mood and anxiety disorders in adults: review and analysis. Clin Psychol Sci Pract 2005;27:572–81.
60. Ledgerwood L, Richardson R, Cranney J. Effects of D-cycloserine on extinction of conditioned freezing. Behav Neurosci 2003;117:341–9.
61. Ressler KJ, Rothbaum BO, Tannenbaum L, et al. Cognitive enhancers as adjuncts to psychotherapy: use of D-cycloserine in phobic individuals to facilitate extinction of fear. Arch Gen Psychiatry 2004;61:1136–44.
62. Norberg MM, Krystal JH, Tolin DF. A meta-analysis of D-cycloserine and the facilitation of fear extinction and exposure therapy. Biol Psychiatry 2008;63: 1118–26.
63. Powers MB, Smits JA, Otto MW, et al. Facilitation of fear extinction in phobic participants with a novel cognitive enhancer: a randomized placebo controlled trial of yohimbine augmentation. J Anxiety Disord 2009;23:350–6.
64. Soravia LM, Heinrichs M, Aerni A, et al. Glucocorticoids reduce phobic fear in humans. Proc Natl Acad Sci U S A 2006;103:5585–90.
65. Goisman RM, Warshaw MG, Keller MB. Psychosocial treatment prescriptions for generalized anxiety disorder, panic disorder, and social phobia, 1991–1996. Am J Psychiatry 1999;156:1819–21.
66. Freiheit S, Vye C, Swan R, et al. Cognitive-behavioral therapy for anxiety: is dissemination working? The Behavior Therapist 2004;27:25–32.
67. Becker CB, Zayfert C, Anderson E. A survey of psychologists' attitudes towards and utilization of exposure therapy for PTSD. Behav Res Ther 2004;42:277–92.
68. Stobie B, Taylor T, Quigley A, et al. 'Contents may vary': a pilot study of treatment histories of OCD patients. Behav Cogn Psychother 2007;35:273–82.

69. Craske MG, Roy-Byrne PP, Stein MB, et al. Treatment for anxiety disorders: efficacy to effectiveness to implementation. Behav Res Ther 2009;47:931–7.

70. Craske MG, Rose RD, Lang A, et al. Computer-assisted delivery of cognitive behavioral therapy for anxiety disorders in primary-care settings. Depress Anxiety 2009;26:235–42.

71. Andersson G. Using the Internet to provide cognitive behaviour therapy. Behav Res Ther 2009;47:175–80.

72. Bar-Haim Y, Lamy D, Pergamin L, et al. Threat-related attentional bias in anxious and nonanxious individuals: a meta-analytic study. Psychol Bull 2007;133:1–24.

73. MacLeod C, Rutherford E, Campbell L, et al. Selective attention and emotional vulnerability: assessing the causal basis of their association through the experimental manipulation of attentional bias. J Abnorm Psychol 2002;111:107–23.

74. MacLeod C, Mathews A, Tata P. Attentional bias in emotional disorders. J Abnorm Psychol 1986;95:15–20.

75. Amir N, Beard C, Taylor CT, et al. Attention training in individuals with generalized social phobia: a randomized controlled trial. J Consult Clin Psychol 2009; 77:961–73.

76. Amir N, Weber G, Beard C, et al. The effect of a single-session attention modification program on response to a public-speaking challenge in socially anxious individuals. J Abnorm Psychol 2008;117:860–8.

77. Schmidt NB, Richey JA, Buckner JD, et al. Attention training for generalized social anxiety disorder. J Abnorm Psychol 2009;118:5–14.

78. Amir N, Beard C, Burns M, et al. Attention modification program in individuals with generalized anxiety disorder. J Abnorm Psychol 2009;118:28–33.

79. Hazen RA, Vasey MW, Schmidt NB. Attentional retraining: a randomized clinical trial for pathological worry. J Psychiatr Res 2009;43:627–33.

80. Li S, Tan J, Qian M, et al. Continual training of attentional bias in social anxiety. Behav Res Ther 2008;46:905–12.

81. Klumpp H, Amir N. Preliminary study of attention training to threat and neutral faces on anxious reactivity to a social stressor in social anxiety. Cognit Ther Res, in press.

82. Bishop SJ. Neurocognitive mechanisms of anxiety: an integrative account. Trends Cogn Sci 2007;11:307–16.

83. Bishop SJ. Neural mechanisms underlying selective attention to threat. Ann N Y Acad Sci 2008;1129:141–52.

84. Cisler JM, Koster EHW. Mechanisms of attentional bias towards threat in anxiety disorders: an integrative review. Clin Psychol Rev 2010;26:203–16.

85. Lohr JM, DeMaio C, McGlynn FD. Specific and nonspecific treatment factors in the experimental analysis of behavioral treatment efficacy. Behav Modif. 2003; 27:322–68.

86. Arch JJ, Craske MG. First-line treatment: a critical appraisal of cognitive behavioral therapy developments and alternatives. Psychiatr Clin North Am 2009;32: 525–47.

87. Schiller D, Monfils MH, Raio CM, et al. Preventing the return of fear in humans using reconsolidation update mechanisms. Nature. 2010;463:49–53.

88. Clum GA, Clum GA, Surls R. A meta-analysis of treatments for panic disorder. J Consult Clin Psych 1993;61:317–26.

89. van Balkom AJLM, Bakker A, Spinhoven P, et al. A meta-analysis of the treatment of panic disorder with or without agoraphobia: a comparison of psychopharmacological, cognitive-behavioral, and combination treatments. J Nerv Ment Dis 1997;185:510–6.

90. Bakker A, van Balkom AJ, Spinhoven P, et al. Follow-up on the treatment of panic disorder with or without agoraphobia: a quantitative review. J Nerv Ment Dis 1998;186:414–9.

91. Gould RA, Otto MW, Pollack MH. A meta-analysis of treatment outcome for panic disorder. Clin Psychol Rev 1995;8:819–44.

92. Oei TPS, Llamas M, Devilly GJ. The efficacy and cognitive processes of cognitive Behav Ther in the treatment of panic disorder with agoraphobia. Behav Cogn Psychoth 1999;27:63–88.

93. Westen D, Morrison K. A multidimensional meta-analysis of treatments for depression, panic, and generalized anxiety disorder: an empirical examination of the status of empirically supported therapies. J Consult Clin Psych 2001;69: 875–99.

94. Cox BJ, Endler NS, Lee PS, et al. A meta-analysis of treatments for panic disorder with agoraphobia: imipramine, alprazolam, and in vivo exposure. J Behav Ther Exp Psy 1992;23:175–82.

95. Feske U, Chambless DL. Cognitive behavioral versus exposure only treatment for social phobia: a meta-analysis. Behav Ther 1995;26:695–720.

96. Taylor S. Meta-analysis of cognitive-behavioral treatments for social phobia. J Behav Ther Exp Psy 1996;27:1–9.

97. Gould RA, Buckminster S, Pollack MH, et al. Cognitive-behavioral and pharmacological treatment for social phobia: a meta-analysis. Clin Psychol: Sci and Pract 1997;4:291–306.

98. Fedoroff IC, Taylor S. Psychological and pharmacological treatments of social phobia: a meta-analysis. J Clin Psychopharm 2001;21:311–24.

99. van Etten M, Taylor S. Comparative efficacy of treatments for posttraumatic stress disorder: a meta-analysis. Clin Psychol Psychot 1998;5:126–45.

100. Sherman JJ. Effects of psychotherapeutic treatments for PTSD: a meta-analysis of controlled clinical trials. J Trauma Stress 1998;11:413–35.

101. Gould RA, Otto MW, Pollack MH, et al. Cognitive behavioral and pharmacological treatment of generalized anxiety disorder: a preliminary meta-analysis. Behav Ther 1997;28:285–305.

102. Borkovec TD, Whisman MA. Psychosocial treatment for generalized anxiety disorder. In: Mavissakalian M, Prien R, editors. Long-term treatment of anxiety disorders. Washington, DC: American Psychiatric Association; 1996.

103. van Balkom AJLM, van Oppen P, Vermeulen AWA, et al. A meta-analysis on the treatment of obsessive compulsive disorder: a comparison of antidepressants, behavior, and cognitive therapy. Clin Psychol Rev 1994;14:359–81.

104. Abramowitz JS. Effectiveness of psychological and pharmacological treatments for obsessive-compulsive disorder: a quantitative review. J Consult Clin Psych 1997;65:44–52.

105. Abramowitz JS, Franklin ME, Zoellner LA, et al. Treatment compliance and outcome in obsessive-compulsive disorder. Behav Modif 2002;26:447–63.

Cognitive Behavioral Therapy for Somatoform Disorders

Lesley A. Allen, PhD[a],*, Robert L. Woolfolk, PhD[b,c]

KEYWORDS

- Somatoform disorders • Somatization
- Conversion disorder • Hypochondriasis
- Body dysmorphic disorder • Cognitive behavioral therapy

OVERVIEW

Somatoform disorders are characterized by physical symptoms that suggest a medical condition but are not fully explained by a medical condition.[1] Physical symptoms with uncertain etiologies are some of the most common presentations in primary care. As many as 25% of visits to primary care physicians are prompted by physical symptoms that lack any clear organic pathology.[2] Patients presenting with medically unexplained physical (somatoform) symptoms provide significant challenges to health care providers. These patients tend to overuse health care services, derive little benefit from treatment, and experience protracted impairment, often lasting many years.[3] Often, patients with somatoform symptoms are dissatisfied with the medical services they receive and repeatedly change physicians.[4] Likewise, physicians of these treatment-resistant patients often feel frustrated by patients' frequent complaints and dissatisfaction with treatment.[4,5] Because standard medical care has been unsuccessful in treating somatoform disorders, alternative treatments have been developed. Cognitive behavioral therapy (CBT) has been the most widely studied alternative treatment for these disorders. This article summarizes the research on the efficacy of CBT for somatoform disorders.

Funded, in part, by NIH grant P20 MH074634.

[a] Department of Psychiatry, Robert Wood Johnson Medical School, University of Medicine and Dentistry of New Jersey, 671 Hoes Lane, Piscataway, NJ 08854, USA
[b] Department of Psychology, Rutgers University, NJ, USA
[c] Department of Psychology, Princeton University, 18 Turner Court, Princeton, NJ 08540, USA
* Corresponding author.
E-mail address: allenla@umdnj.edu

Psychiatr Clin N Am 33 (2010) 579–593
doi:10.1016/j.psc.2010.04.014
0193-953X/10/$ – see front matter © 2010 Elsevier Inc. All rights reserved.

psych.theclinics.com

SOMATIZATION DISORDER AND SUBTHRESHOLD SOMATIZATION
Overview of Disorder

Diagnostic criteria and prevalence

According to the current *Diagnostic and Statistical Manual of Mental Disorders* (Fourth Edition) *(DSM-IV)*[1] somatization disorder is characterized by a lifetime history of at least 4 unexplained pain complaints (eg, in the back, chest, joints), 2 unexplained nonpain gastrointestinal complaints (eg, nausea, bloating), 1 unexplained sexual symptom (eg, sexual dysfunction, irregular menstruation), and 1 pseudoneurological symptom (eg, seizures, paralysis, numbness). For a symptom to be counted toward the diagnosis of somatization disorder, its presence must be medically unexplained or its degree of severity be substantially in excess of the associated medical pathology. Also, symptoms counted toward the diagnosis must either prompt the seeking of medical care or interfere with patients' functioning. In addition, at least some of the somatization symptoms must have occurred before the patients' thirtieth birthday.[1] The course of somatization disorder tends to be characterized by symptoms that wax and wane, remitting only to return later or be replaced by new unexplained physical symptoms. Thus, somatization disorder is a chronic, polysymptomatic disorder whose requisite symptoms need not be manifested concurrently.

Epidemiological research suggests that somatization disorder is rare. The prevalence of somatization disorder in the general population has been estimated to be 0.1% to 0.7%.[6–8] When patients in primary care, specialty medical, and psychiatric settings are assessed, the rate of somatization is higher than in the general population, with estimates ranging from 1.0% to 5.0%.[9–13]

Although somatization disorder is classified as a distinct disorder in *DSM-IV*, it has been argued that somatization disorder represents the extreme end of a somatization continuum.[14,15] The number of unexplained physical symptoms reported correlates positively with the patients' degree of emotional distress and functional impairment.[16] A broadening of the somatization construct has been advocated by those wishing to underscore the many patients encumbered by unexplained symptoms that are not numerous or diverse enough to meet criteria for full somatization disorder.[14–16]

DSM-IV includes a residual diagnostic category for subthreshold somatization cases. *Undifferentiated somatoform disorder* is a diagnosis characterized by 1 or more medically unexplained physical symptoms lasting for at least 6 months.[1] Long considered a category that is too broad because it includes patients with only 1 unexplained symptom *and* those with many unexplained symptoms, undifferentiated somatoform disorder never has been well validated or widely applied.[17]

As an alternative to the wide-ranging category of undifferentiated somatoform disorder, 2 groups of researchers have suggested alternative categories for subthreshold somatization using criteria less restrictive and requiring less extensive symptomatology than the *DSM-IV* standards for full somatization disorder. Escobar and colleagues[14] proposed the label, *abridged somatization*, to be applied to men experiencing 4 or more unexplained physical symptoms or to women experiencing 6 or more unexplained physical symptoms. Kroenke and colleagues[15] suggested the category of *multisomatoform disorder* to describe men or women currently experiencing at least 3 unexplained physical symptoms and reporting a 2-year history of somatization.

Both of these subthreshold somatization categories appear to be significantly more prevalent than is *somatization disorder* as defined by *DSM-IV*. Abridged somatization has been observed in 4% of community samples[14] and 16% to 22% of primary care samples.[2,9,18] The occurrence of multisomatoform disorder has been estimated at 8% of primary care patients.[15,19]

Demographic and clinical characteristics
Gender, ethnicity, race, and education have been associated with somatization disorder and subthreshold somatization. Epidemiological research has shown that patients with somatization are more likely to be women, nonwhite, and less educated than nonsomatizers.[2,7] In the Epidemiological Catchment Area (ECA) study, the ratio of women to men who met criteria for somatization disorder was 10:1.[20] Higher rates of occurrence in women, though not as extreme, also have been found in some studies employing subthreshold somatization categories, such as Escobar's abridged somatization or Kroenke's multisomatoform disorder.[15,20] Findings on ethnicity have been less consistent across studies. In the ECA study, Hispanics in the community were no more likely to meet criteria for somatization disorder than were non-Hispanics in the community.[21] The World Health Organization's Cross National study, which was conducted in primary care offices across 14 different countries, revealed a higher incidence of somatization, as defined by either the *International Classification of Diseases, Tenth Revision (ICD-10)* or Escobar's abridged criteria, in primary care practices in Latin American countries than in the United States.[2] Perhaps, Hispanic somatizers are more likely to seek treatment than are non-Hispanic somatizers.

Much attention has focused on the illness behavior of patients with somatization and the resulting impact of that behavior on the health care system. These patients disproportionately use and misuse health care services. When standard diagnostic evaluations fail to uncover organic pathology, patients with somatization tend to seek additional medical procedures, often from several different physicians. Patients may even subject themselves to unnecessary hospitalizations and surgeries, which introduce the risk for iatrogenic illness.[22] One study found that patients with somatization disorder, on average, incurred 9 times the per capita health care cost of the United States.[3] Abridged somatization and multisomatoform disorder also have been associated with significant health care use.[15,23,24]

The abnormal illness behavior of patients with somatization extends beyond medical offices and hospitals to patients' workplaces and households. Somatizers withdraw from productive and pleasurable activities because of discomfort, fatigue, or fears of exacerbating their symptoms. Estimates of unemployment among patients with somatization disorder range from 36% to 83%.[3,25,26] Whether working outside their homes or not, these patients report substantial functional impairment. Some investigators have found that patients with somatization disorder report being bedridden for 2 to 7 days per month.[3,16] Likewise, high levels of functional impairment have been associated with subthreshold somatization.[2,15,19,24,27]

In addition to their physical complaints, many patients with somatization complain of psychiatric distress. As many as 80% of patients meeting criteria for somatization disorder or subthreshold somatization meet *DSM* criteria for another lifetime Axis I disorder, usually an anxiety or mood disorder.[3,7] When investigators consider only current psychiatric diagnoses, rates of psychiatric comorbidity associated with somatization are closer to 50%.[27,28] Also, overall severity of psychological distress, defined as the number of psychological symptoms reported, correlates positively with the number of functional somatic symptoms reported.[16,28]

Empirical studies on cognitive behavioral therapy for somatization
Three studies have compared the efficacy of individually administered CBT with standard medical care for patients manifesting a diverse set of unexplained physical symptoms. Only 1 study has been published treating patients meeting *DSM-IV* criteria for full somatization disorder.[25] Two studies were conducted in primary care settings

with patients who were diagnosed with subthreshold somatization, defined as abridged somatization in 1 study[29] and defined as 5 or more unexplained physical symptoms in the other.[30]

All 3 studies showed that individual CBT coincided with greater reductions in somatic complaints than did standard medical care.[25,29,30] Allen and colleagues[25] found that 40% of their subjects treated with CBT, versus 7% of the control group, were judged to have achieved clinically significant improvement defined as being very much improved or much improved on a clinician-rated scale of somatization severity. Also, CBT was associated with enhanced physical functioning in 1 study[25] and with reduced health care use in 2 studies.[25,30] Long-term maintenance of symptom relief was demonstrated in 2 studies; 1 showed significant differences in somatization symptomatology 6 months after treatment completion[29] and the other showed that symptom improvement lasted for 12 months after the treatment phase of the study.[25]

Two groups of investigators have conducted controlled treatment trials assessing the efficacy of CBT with a less severely disturbed group of subjects, those complaining of at least 1 psychosomatic symptom. In 1 study, subjects treated with individual CBT showed greater improvement in their psychosomatic complaints than did subjects treated with standard medical care.[31] The other study found group CBT, led by a trained physician, superior to a waiting-list control condition in reducing physical symptoms and hypochondriacal beliefs.[32] In both studies improvements were observed after treatment and 6 months later.[31,32] Lidbeck's CBT participants seemed to maintain reductions in somatization and hypochondriacal beliefs 18 months after treatment.[33]

CONVERSION DISORDER
Overview of Disorder

Diagnostic criteria and prevalence
Conversion symptoms, also described as pseudoneurological symptoms, are abnormalities or deficits in voluntary motor or sensory function that are medically unexplained. Some of the most common pseudoneurological symptoms are pseudoseizures, pseudoparalysis and psychogenic movement disorders. According to DSM-IV, conversion disorder is characterized by the presence of 1 or more pseudoneurological symptoms that are associated with psychological stressors or conflicts.[1] The diagnosis of conversion disorder requires a thorough psychiatric evaluation and a physical examination to rule out organic neurological illness. Patients presenting with conversion symptoms typically have normal reflexes and normal muscle tone.

The course of conversion disorder appears to be different from that of somatization disorder, which tends to be chronic.[34] The onset and course of conversion disorder often take the form of an acute episode. Symptoms may remit within a few weeks of an initial episode and they may recur in the future. Some research indicates that a brief duration of symptoms before treatment is associated with a better prognosis.[35–37]

Estimates of the prevalence of conversion disorder have varied widely, ranging from 0.01% to 0.3% in the community.[6,38] As is the case with the other somatoform disorders, conversion disorder is much more common in medical and psychiatric practices than in community samples. As many as 25% of patients at neurology clinics may present for treatment of a medically unexplained neurological symptom.[39,40]

Demographic and clinical characteristics
The demographic characteristics of conversion disorder have not been investigated extensively. Nevertheless, there is some evidence that conversion disorder is more

common among women,[6,41] nonwhites,[38] and individuals from lower socioeconomic classes.[38,42] Comorbid psychiatric distress in patients with pseudoneurological symptoms is high; it has been estimated that 30% to 90% of patients seeking treatment for pseudoneurological symptoms also meet criteria for at least 1 other psychiatric disorder, typically somatoform disorders, affective disorders, anxiety disorders, or personality disorders.[35,43–45] A comorbid personality disorder diagnosis has been found to indicate poor prognosis of conversion disorder.[46]

Like somatization disorder, conversion disorder is costly to the health care system, especially when symptoms are chronic.[46] Patients with long-standing conversion symptoms are likely to submit themselves to unnecessary diagnostic and medical procedures. Martin and colleagues[47] reported an average of $100,000 being spent per year per patient with conversion disorder.

Empirical studies on cognitive behavioral therapy for conversion disorder
To date there have been no controlled trials examining the efficacy of CBT for conversion disorder.

PAIN DISORDER
Diagnostic Criteria and Prevalence

According to *DSM-IV*, pain disorder is characterized by clinically significant pain in 1 or more anatomical sites. Also, psychological factors must be deemed important in the onset, severity, exacerbation, or maintenance of that pain.[1] Little research has been conducted that addresses pain disorder as defined by *DSM-IV* (or its *DSM-III-R* [Third Edition Revised] counterpart, somatoform pain disorder) as a discrete diagnostic category. Instead, researchers have tended to formulate research based on the anatomical site and the chronicity of the pain. Thus, there is voluminous literature on distinct pain conditions, (eg, back pain, chest pain, pelvic pain, headaches) in which investigators make no attempt to distinguish between pain that was apparently affected by psychological factors and pain that was apparently not. The existing literatures on *DSM-III-R* somatoform pain disorder and *DSM-IV* pain disorder, in which psychological factors have been considered to be influential, are reviewed here.

Estimates of the prevalence of somatoform pain disorder have ranged from 0.6% to 5.4% in the community.[6,48] The discrepancy between these 2 figures is likely to be attributable in part to differences between the 2 studies' raters (ie, physicians vs trained nonmedical interviewers). The study employing physician interviewers, who were presumably better able to rule out organic causes of pain, resulted in a much lower prevalence rate.[6] Prevalence rates of pain disorder appear to be higher in medical practices than in the community.[49]

Demographic and Clinical Characteristics

There is little research on the demographic or clinical characteristics of individuals meeting criteria for somatoform pain disorder. Two studies have found pain disorder to be more prevalent among women than men.[6,48] A third study found no difference in prevalence rates between men and women.[49]

Empirical Studies on Cognitive Behavioral Therapy for Pain Disorder

To date there have been no controlled trials examining the efficacy of CBT for pain disorder.

HYPOCHONDRIASIS
Overview of Disorder

Diagnostic criteria and prevalence

According to DSM-IV, hypochondriasis is defined as a "preoccupation with fears of having, or the idea that one has, a serious disease based on the person's misinterpretation of bodily symptoms".[1(p462)] This preoccupation must persist despite medical evaluation and physician reassurance and cause significant distress or impairment in one's functioning.[1] Thus, unlike in somatization where the distress and dysfunction experienced is due to the physical symptoms themselves, in hypochondriasis the distress and dysfunction is due to the patient's interpretation of the meaning of his or her symptoms. The course of hypochondriasis is often chronic: As many as 50% of patients meeting DSM criteria for hypochondriasis have excessive health concerns for many years.[50,51]

There are only a few epidemiological studies that have examined the prevalence of hypochondriasis. Studies that have used a clinical interview to assess prevalence have suggested that hypochondriasis occurs rarely in the general population. Such estimates range from 0.02–4.5%.[6,52,53] In primary care, estimates range from 0.8%–6.3%.[49,50,54,55]

Demographic and clinical characteristics

Unlike somatization disorder, hypochondriasis does not appear to be related to gender.[51,52,54] Men are as likely to meet DSM criteria for hypochondriasis as are women. Findings have been inconsistent on whether hypochondriasis is related to education, socio-economic status, and ethnicity.[51,54]

Like patients with somatization disorder and sub-threshold somatization, those with hypochondriasis exhibit abnormal illness behavior. They over-use health care, subjecting themselves to multiple physician visits and multiple diagnostic procedures.[52,54] They report great dissatisfaction with their medical care.[56,57] In addition, patients diagnosed with hypochondriasis report substantial physical impairment and functional limitations related to employment.[52,54,55,57] Also, hypochondriasis frequently co-occurs with other Axis I disorders, such as mood, anxiety, or other somatoform disorders.[54,58]

Empirical studies on CBT for hypochondriasis

Cognitive behavioral types of treatment for hypochondriasis have been examined in six randomized controlled trials.[59–64] The interventions in all six studies were theoretically grounded in social learning theory and were administered on an individual basis. The labels applied to these treatments, the specific techniques employed, and their durations have varied sufficiently to warrant a more comprehensive description of each.

The first intervention to be examined in a controlled trial, labeled by Warwick, Clark and colleagues as CBT, focused on identifying and challenging patients' misinterpretations of physical symptoms and constructing more realistic interpretations of them. Also included in Warwick's and colleagues[59] original CBT were graded exposure to avoided illness-related situations and response prevention of bodily checking and reassurance seeking. Two years later, Clark and colleagues[60] examined the efficacy of a treatment condition that "was essentially the same as in Warwick and colleagues (1996)," but called it cognitive therapy (CT). It included cognitive techniques as well as exposure and response prevention.[60] The only apparent difference between Warwick and colleagues[59] and Clark and colleagues[60] treatments was that the former was administered in 16 1-hour sessions, whereas Clark and colleagues allowed for

3 additional booster sessions over the 3-month interval following the initial 16 sessions. A third study investigated the efficacy of a similar treatment condition comprising cognitive procedures as well as exposure and response prevention.[61] Greeven and colleagues[61] labeled this treatment CBT and administered it in 6–16 sessions.

Visser and Bouman dismantled the multifaceted cognitive behavioral treatment described above into two separate treatments: (1) cognitive therapy (CT) involving rational disputation of thoughts and (2) exposure and response prevention (ERP).[62] Visser and Bouman's CT and ERP each consisted of 12 weekly sessions, each presumably lasting 1 hr, though session duration was not indicated.[62]

Barsky and Ahern also identify their intervention as CBT.[63] In it Barksy and Ahern emphasize restructuring dysfunctional illness cognitions, reducing patients' tendency to amplify physical symptoms, and altering patients' illness behaviors.[63] Exposure and response prevention were not included in Barsky's treatment. Barsky and Ahern's treatment entailed six 90-min sessions.[63]

Each of the above-mentioned CT and CBT interventions for hypochondriasis was associated with significantly greater reductions in hypochondriacal symptoms than was the comparable waiting list control condition.[59–63] Barsky and Ahern's study was the only one that examined long-term differences between the waiting list group and the treated group: Ten months after treatment completion patients enrolled in CBT reported a greater decline in hypochondriacal cognitions than did controls.[63] Also, Barsky and Ahren's CBT-treated patients reported a significantly greater increase in daily activities than did controls, even 10 months after treatment.[63]

The one study comparing CBT, that is a combination of cognitive restructuring and exposure plus response prevention, with a pharmacological intervention for hypochondriasis demonstrated that CBT was more effective than a placebo pill, but no more effective than paroxetine, in reducing hypochondriacal beliefs.[61] Despite the statistical significance of these findings, the clinical significance of changes observed in this study suggests that patients experienced only modest improvement. Instead of using Jacobson's recommendation of a change of 1.96 standard deviations from the pretreatment mean as an index of clinically significant change,[65] the investigators judged as clinically significant a change of 1.0 standard deviation. Using this more lenient criterion, only 45% of CBT recipients and 30% of paroxetine recipients versus 14% of waiting list controls responded to treatment at clinically significant levels.[61]

As an alternative to and comparison treatment for CT or CBT, Clark and colleagues[60] developed a psychosocial intervention that did not directly address hypochondriacal concerns and labeled it behavioral stress management (BSM). BSM was intended to address anxiety related to hypochondriasis by training patients in relaxation, problem-solving, assertiveness training, and time management. BSM entailed 16 individual sessions plus as many as three booster sessions. Clark and colleagues[60] found BSM significantly more effective in alleviating hypochondriacal concerns than was a waiting list. Clark and colleagues[60] also compared this treatment to their CT described earlier. At post-treatment CT-treated participants experienced greater reductions in their hypochondrical cognitions than did BSM-treated participants. Nevertheless, 12 months after the post-treatment assessment, these differences were not observed.

Finally, Fava and colleagues[64] examined the efficacy of explanatory therapy for hypochondriasis, in hopes of identifying a beneficial treatment that is less complex and easier to administer than CBT. Explanatory therapy is a physician-administered individual therapy consisting of eight 30-minute sessions of patient education, reassurance, and training in selective attention (ie, reducing somatic attention). Like the cognitive and behavioral treatments described above, explanatory therapy appeared to result in greater reductions in worry about illness than did the waiting list.[64] Although explanatory therapy was also associated with greater reductions in physician visits than was the control group, the mean reduction in visits was minimal (3 visits) considering the treatment group received 8 additional visits as part of their explanatory therapy.[64] Methodological problems with this study hinder the interpretation of its results.

A recent meta-analysis of the psychosocial intervention literature on hypochondriasis is consistent with our assessment of the research.[66] In their meta-analysis assessing the efficacy of all forms of psychotherapy studied in randomized controlled trials (ie, combining the results of the studies described above except Barsky and Ahern's which did not include a post-treatment assessment point), Thomson and Page found the psychotherapy conditions to outperform the waiting list conditions (SMD (random) [95% CI] = −0.86 [−1.25 to −0.46]).[66] An internal analysis of the data from this meta-analysis revealed that the total amount of time with a therapist was highly correlated with the effect size as measured by standardized mean difference ($r^2 = 0.93$, $r = 0.090$ (95% CI 0.056–0.124) $P = .002$).[66] The authors suggested that despite the methodological problems with some of the literature (eg, some investigators failed to use adequate sample sizes, intention-to-treat statistical analyses, and validated hypochondriasis scales), "psychotherapy using cognitive therapy, exposure plus response prevention, cognitive behavioral therapy or behavioral stress management approaches are effective in reducing symptoms of hypochondriasis".(p12)

BODY DYSMORPHIC DISORDER
Overview of Disorder

Diagnostic criteria and prevalence
Body dysmorphic disorder (BDD) is characterized by a preoccupation with an imagined defect in appearance. If a slight physical irregularity is present, the person's concern must be excessive to meet criteria for BDD. Also required for a diagnosis of BDD is significant distress or impairment caused by this preoccupation.[1] Typically, patients are concerned about their skin or complexion, the size of their nose or head, or the attractiveness of their hair; however, the preoccupation may concern any body part. BDD tends to be chronic; in one study Phillips at al. found only a .09 probability of full remission and .21 probably of partial remission over the course of a year.[67]

The prevalence of BDD is uncertain. Research conducted in community settings has produced varying estimates: a prevalence of 0.7% in a community setting in Italy,[6] 1.7% in a national survey of German adolescents and adults,[68] and 2.4% in a telephone survey of U.S. adults.[69] The prevalence of BDD in medical practices has been found to be substantially higher than that found in the general population: 4% of general medicine patients,[70] 3%–16% of cosmetic surgery patients,[71] and 8%–15% of dermatology patients.[71]

Demographic and clinical characteristics
Very little research has been conducted on sex and cultural differences in BDD. Phillips and Diaz found that women and men were equally likely to meet criteria for BDD.[72] We are aware of no systematic investigation of race and culture in BDD, though the condition has been described in various cultures around the world.[70]

Patients meeting criteria for BDD have been shown to have substantial functional impairment.[73] Negative thoughts about one's appearance interfere with concentration at work and the social lives of patients. In addition, individuals with BDD are so afraid of exposing their flaw to others that they go to great lengths to hide it. They may spend substantial amounts of time camouflaging their perceived defect or avoiding activities in which they will be conspicuous.[74] Avoidance of social activities and work is common.[74]

Health care use associated with BDD tends to be directed toward seeking various appearance enhancing medical treatments, especially cosmetic surgery and dermatological procedures. For patients with BDD these treatments typically fail to alleviate distress.[75,76] Investigators have found that 48% to 76% of patients with BDD sought cosmetic surgery, dermatological treatment, or dental procedures[75–77] and 26% received multiple procedures.[77]

Patients meeting criteria for BDD experience an enormous amount of emotional distress and psychiatric co-morbidity.[77,78] Depression and suicidal thoughts are frequent.[79,80] Also common is alcohol abuse and dependence, social phobia and obsessive compulsive disorder.[79,81] Often, compulsions are related to the perceived physical defect, such as checking mirrors or brushing one's hair.

Many patients preoccupied with an imagined defect in their physical appearance have such inaccurate perceptions of their appearance that they meet DSM-IV criteria for delusional disorder, somatic type. About 50% of clinical samples meeting criteria for BDD also meet criteria for delusional disorder, somatic type[82]; however, instead of considering this somatic type of delusional disorder a co-morbid condition with BDD, a growing body of research suggests psychotic variants of BDD are simply a more severe form of non-psychotic BDD and are, therefore, best conceived as on the same continuum. It seems that non-psychotic and psychotic BDD share the same demographic characteristics, clinical characteristics, and response to treatment.[83] Further evidence suggests that the cognitions of BDD patients involving such matters as the degree of conviction with which these patients hold their beliefs are more indicative of a dimensional rather than a categorical structure.[83] Thus, the research data suggest a dimensional model of BDD with varying levels of insight indicating severity of the condition.

EMPIRICAL STUDIES ON CBT FOR BDD

Only two randomized controlled trials have been published on the efficacy of psychosocial treatment for BDD.[84,85] Both assessed the efficacy of CBT involving the restructuring dysfunctional beliefs about one's body and exposure to avoided situations plus response prevention, for example, preventing checking behavior and reassurance seeking. Rosen and colleagues'[84] treatment was administered in 8 2-hour group sessions, whereas Veale and colleagues[85] administered treatment in 12 weekly individual sessions. Both groups of investigators compared the effects of CBT with those of a waiting list control condition.

Both studies provided strong evidence for the short-term efficacy of CBT for BDD. Rosen and colleagues[84] found that 81.5% of treated participants but only 7.4% of control participants experienced clinically significant improvement, in that their scores on the Body Dysmorphic Disorder Examination (BDDE) dropped more than two standard deviations and they no longer met criteria for BDD. The effect size on the BDDE was substantial ($d = 2.81$). Follow-up assessment, occurring 4.5 months after post-treatment, was conducted with only CBT participants, 74% of whom continued to have achieved clinically meaningful gains.[84] Veale and colleagues[85] reported that at post-treatment 77.8% of the treatment group either had absent or sub-clinical BDD symptomatology whereas all waiting list participants still met criteria for BDD. Furthermore, Veale's effect size on the BDDE and on a BDD-modified Yale Brown Obsessive

Compulsive Scale were also noteworthy ($d = 2.65$ and 1.81, respectively). Follow-up was not investigated in this study.

In all, CBT appears to be an empirically supported treatment for BDD. Although the potency of the treatments described in these two well-designed controlled trials is noteworthy, a number of questions remain about the efficacy of CBT for BDD. No additional RTCs have been published. CBT has not been compared with alternative treatments nor with an attention control. It is unclear whether treatment gains reported above could be attributable to nonspecific aspects of therapy. Also, long-term follow-up has not been adequately studied. Other important outcomes, such as physical and social functioning and health care use, have not been assessed. Finally, the generalizability of these findings is unclear. Between the two studies only 36 patients have been treated. Rosen and colleagues[84] sample consisted of women, 83% of whom had body weight and shape concerns. Veale and colleagues[85] sample specifically excluded potential participants with body weight and shape concerns.

SUMMARY

An evaluation of the empirical research on CBT for somatoform disorders suggests effect sizes are respectable, relative to other medical or quasi-medical interventions. Although the literature on the specific somatoform disorders is relatively small, a few global conclusions can be posited. CBT for somatization, hypochondriasis, and BDD has been empirically supported, probably with some lasting effects; however, there is little data on the impact of treatment on health care use, especially when the cost of a psychosocial intervention such as those described above is factored in to the equation. There is inadequate data on the treatment of conversion disorder or of pain disorder to make any conclusion. The data on CBT's efficacy on BDD is the most powerful. Effect sizes are large and the vast majority of patients appear to have made clinically meaningful gains from treatment; however, the two groups of investigators who have systematically studied CBT's efficacy in BDD acknowledge residual symptoms persist and argue for a longer, more intensive treatment before these patients are likely to resolve their difficulties. Longer term treatments for other somatoform disorders have been recommended by others as well.[86]

We have very little data on the mechanisms by which CBT may have its impact upon somatoform disorders. There are many reasons for this. First, the mediators and moderators style of research has not been extensively applied to research on these disorders. Second, the treatments studied have not been disassembled into discrete components and those constituents systematically assessed. Evidence that might shed some light on this issue, that pertaining to differential efficacy of treatment, is also scant.

Somatoform researchers as a whole recommend treatment for these conditions be administered in primary care settings. It has been estimated that 50%–80% of patients with somatoform disorders, who are referred for mental health services, fail to seek mental health treatment.[18] Barriers to following through with psychiatric referrals occur at both the systemic level (eg, lack of collaboration between and proximity of primary care physicians and mental health practitioners, lack of mental health training for primary care physicians, inadequate mental health insurance) and individual level (eg, concerns about the stigma of having a psychiatric disorder, resistance to psychiatric diagnosis, health beliefs that lead to somatic presentations, pessimism, and fatigue).[87] The efficacy of CBT conducted in primary care has not been studied adequately for hypochondriasis or BDD.

The treatment of somatoform disorders via psychosocial methods is very much in its infancy. The methodological quality of the early research has been uneven. Nevertheless, there is sufficient evidence to believe that cognitive behavioral interventions have therapeutic value for a number of the disorders. For somatization, hypochondriasis, and BDD, CBT is likely the treatment of choice by default in that no other intervention has demonstrated efficacy.

REFERENCES

1. American Psychiatric Association. Diagnostic and statistical manual of mental disorders. 4th edition. Washington, DC: American Psychiatric Association; 1994.
2. Gureje O, Simon GE, Ustun T, et al. Somatization in cross-cultural perspective: a World Health Organization study in primary care. Am J Psychiatry 1997;154: 989–95.
3. Smith GR, Monson RA, Ray DC. Patients with multiple unexplained symptoms: their characteristics, functional health, and health care utilization. Arch Intern Med 1986;146:69–72.
4. Lin EH, Katon W, VonKorff M, et al. Frustrating patients: physician and patient perspectives among distressed high users of medical services. J Gen Intern Med 1991;6:241–6.
5. Hahn SR. Physical symptoms and physician-experienced difficulty in the physician-patient relationship. Ann Intern Med 2001;134:897–904.
6. Faravelli C, Salvatori S, Galassi F, et al. Epidemiology of somatoform disorders: a community survey in Florence. Soc Psychiatry Psychiatr Epidemiol 1997;32:24–9.
7. Robins LN, Reiger D. Psychiatric disorders in America: the epidemiological catchment area study. New York: Free Press; 1991.
8. Weissman MM, Myers JK, Harding PS. Psychiatric disorders in a U.S. urban community: 1975–1976. Am J Psychiatry 1978;135:459–62.
9. Kirmayer LJ, Robbins JM. Three forms of somatization in primary care: prevalence, co-occurrence, and sociodemographic characteristics. J Nerv Ment Dis 1991;179:647–55.
10. Peveler R, Kilkenny L, Kinmonth AL. Medically unexplained physical symptoms in primary care: a comparison of self-report screening questionnaires and clinical opinion. J Psychosom Res 1997;42:245–52.
11. Fink P, Steen Hansen M, Sondergaard L. Somatoform disorders among first-time referrals to a neurology service. Psychosomatics 2005;46:540–8.
12. Fabrega H, Mezzich J, Jacob R, et al. Somatoform disorder in a psychiatric setting: systematic comparisons with depression and anxiety disorders. J Nerv Ment Dis 1988;176:431–9.
13. Altamura AC, Carta MG, Tacchini G, et al. Prevalence of somatoform disorders in a psychiatric population. An Italian nationwide survey. Eur Arch Psychiatry Clin Neurosci 1998;248:267–71.
14. Escobar JI, Burnam MA, Karno M, et al. Somatization in the community. Arch Gen Psychiatry 1987;44:713–8.
15. Kroenke K, Spitzer RL, de Gruy FV, et al. Multisomatoform disorder: an alternative to undifferentiated somatoform disorder for the somatizing patient in primary care. Arch Gen Psychiatry 1997;54:352–8.
16. Katon W, Lin E, VonKorff M, et al. Somatization: a spectrum of severity. Am J Psychiatry 1991;148:34–40.
17. Kroenke K, Sharpe M, Sykes R. Revising the classification of somatoform disorders: key questions and preliminary recommendations. Psychosomatics 2007; 48:277–85.

18. Escobar JI, Waitzkin H, Silver RC, et al. Abridged somatization: a study in primary care. Psychosom Med 1998;60:466–72.
19. Jackson JL, Kroenke K. Prevalence, impact, and prognosis of multisomatoform disorder in primary care: a 5-year follow-up study. Psychosom Med 2008;70:430–4.
20. Swartz M, Landermann R, George L, et al. Somatization. In: Robins LN, Reiger D, editors. Psychiatric disorders in America. New York: Free Press; 1991. p. 220–57.
21. Escobar JI, Rubio-Stipec M, Canino G, et al. Somatic Symptom Index (SSI): a new and abridged somatization construct. J Nerv Ment Dis 1989;177:140–6.
22. Fink P. Surgery and medical treatment in persistent somatizing patients. J Psychosom Res 1992;36:439–47.
23. Barsky AJ, Orav EJ, Bates DW. Somatization increases medical utilization and costs independent of psychiatric and medical comorbidity. Arch Gen Psychiatry 2005;62:903–10.
24. Escobar JI, Golding JM, Hough RL, et al. Somatization in the community: relationship to disability and use of services. Am J Public Health 1987;77(7):837–40.
25. Allen LA, Woolfolk RL, Escobar JI, et al. Cognitive-behavioral therapy for somatization disorder: a randomized controlled trial. Arch Intern Med 2006;166:1512–8.
26. Yutzy SH, Cloninger R, Guze SB, et al. DSM-IV field trial: testing a new proposal for somatization disorder. Am J Psychiatry 1995;152:97–101.
27. Allen LA, Gara MA, Escobar JI, et al. Somatization: a debilitating syndrome in primary care. Psychosomatics 2001;42:63–7.
28. Simon GE, VonKorff M. Somatization and psychiatric disorder in the NIMH Epidemiologic catchment area study. Am J Psychiatry 1991;148:1494–500.
29. Escobar JI, Gara MA, Diaz-Martinez AM, et al. Effectiveness of a time-limited cognitive behavior therapy type intervention among primary care patients with medically unexplained symptoms. Ann Fam Med 2007;5:328–35.
30. Sumathipala A, Hewege S, Hanwella R, et al. Randomized controlled trial of cognitive behaviour therapy for repeated consultations for medically unexplained complaints: a feasibility study in Sri Lanka. Psychol Med 2000;30:747–57.
31. Speckens AEM, van Hemert AM, Spinhoven P, et al. Cognitive behavioural therapy for medically unexplained physical symptoms: a randomised controlled trial. BMJ 1995;311:1328–32.
32. Lidbeck J. Group therapy for somatization disorders in general practice: effectiveness of a short cognitive-behavioural treatment model. Acta Psychiatr Scand 1997;96:14–24.
33. Lidbeck J. Group therapy for somatization disorders in primary care: maintenance of treatment goals of short cognitive-behavioural treatment one-and-a-half-year follow-up. Acta Psychiatr Scand 2003;107:449–56.
34. Kent DA, Tomasson K, Coryell W. Course and outcome of conversion and somatization disorder. A four-year follow-up. Psychosomatics 1995;36:138–44.
35. Crimlisk HL, Bhatia K, Cope H, et al. Slater revisited: 6-year follow-up study of patients with medically unexplained motor symptoms. BMJ 1998;316:582–6.
36. Hafeiz HB. Hysterical conversion: a prognostic study. Br J Psychiatry 1980;136:548–51.
37. Ron M. The prognosis of hysteria/somatization disorder. Contemporary approaches to the study of hysteria. Oxford (UK): Oxford University Press; 2001.
38. Stefansson JG, Messina JA, Meyerowitz S. Hysterical neurosis, conversion type: clinical and epidemiological considerations. Acta Psychiatr Scand 1979;53:119–38.
39. Creed F, Firth D, Timol M, et al. Somatization and illness behaviour in a neurology ward. J Psychosom Res 1990;34:427–37.

40. Perkin GD. An analysis of 7,836 successive new outpatient referrals. J Neurol Neurosurg Psychiatr 1989;52:447–8.
41. Deveci A, Taskin O, Dinc G, et al. Prevalence of pseudoneurological conversion disorder in an urban community in Manisa, Turkey. Soc Psychiatry Psychiatr Epidemiol 2007;42:857–64.
42. Folks DG, Ford CV, Regan WM. Conversion symptoms in a general hospital. Psychosomatics 1984;25:285–95.
43. Binzer M, Andersen PM, Kullgren G. Clinical characteristics of patients with motor disability due to conversion disorder: a prospective control group study. J Neurol Neurosurg Psychiatr 1997;63:83–8.
44. Sar V, Akyuz G, Kundakci T, et al. Childhood trauma, dissociation, and psychiatric co-morbidity in patients with conversion disorder. Am J Psychiatry 2004;161:2271–6.
45. Mokleby K, Blomhoff S, Malt UF, et al. Psychiatric comorbidity and hostility in patients with psychogenic nonepileptic seizures compared with somatoform disorders and healthy controls. Epilepsia 2002;43:193–8.
46. Mace CJ, Trimble MR. Ten-year prognosis of conversion disorder. Br J Psychiatry 1996;169:282–8.
47. Martin R, Bell B, Hermann B, et al. Non epileptic seizures and their costs: the role of neuropsychology. In: Pritigano GP, Pliskin NH, editors. Clinical neuropsychology and cost outcome research: a beginning. New York: Psychology Press; 2003. p. 235–58.
48. Grabe HJ, Meyer C, Hapke U, et al. Somatoform pain disorder in the general population. Psychother Psychosom 2003;72:88–94.
49. Toft T, Fink P, Oernboel E, et al. Mental disorders in primary care: prevalence and co-morbidity. results from the functional illness in primary care (FIP) study. Psychol Med 2005;35:1175–84.
50. Barsky AJ, Fama JM, Bailey ED, et al. A prospective 4- to 5-year study of DSM-III-R hypochondriasis. Arch Gen Psychiatry 1998;55:737–44.
51. Barsky AJ, Wyshak G, Klerman GL, et al. The prevalence of hypochondriasis in medical outpatients. Soc Psychiatry Psychiatr Epidemiol 1990;25:89–94.
52. Looper KJ, Kirmayer LJ. Hypochondriacal concerns in a community population. Psychol Med 2001;31:577–84.
53. Martin A, Jacobi F. Features of hypochondriasis and illness worry in the general population in Germany. Psychosom Med 2006;68:770–7.
54. Gureje O, Ustun TG, Simon GE. The syndrome of hypochondriasis: a cross-national study in primary care. Psychol Med 1997;27:1001–10.
55. Escobar JI, Gara M, Waitzkin H, et al. DSM-IV hypochondriasis in primary care. Gen Hosp Psychiatry 1998;20:155–9.
56. Barsky AJ. Hypochondriasis: medical management and psychiatric treatment. Psychosomatics 1996;37:48–56.
57. Noyes R, Kathol RG, Fisher MM, et al. The validity of DSM-III-R hypochondriasis. Arch Gen Psychiatry 1993;50:961–70.
58. Noyes R, Kathol RG, Fisher MM, et al. Psychiatric comorbidity among patients with hypochondriasis. Gen Hosp Psychiatry 1994;16:78–87.
59. Warwick HM, Clark DM, Cobb AM, et al. A controlled trial of cognitive-behavioural treatment of hypochondriasis. Br J Psychiatry 1996;169:189–95.
60. Clark DM, Salkovskis PM, Hackmann A, et al. Two psychological treatments for hypochondriasis: a randomized controlled trial. Br J Psychiatry 1998;173:218–25.
61. Greeven A, van Balkom AJ, Visser S, et al. Cognitive behavior therapy and paroxetine in the treatment of hypochondriasis: a randomized controlled trial. Am J Psychiatry 2007;164:91–9.

62. Visser S, Bouman TK. The treatment of hypochondriasis: exposure plus response prevention vs. cognitive therapy. Behav Res Ther 2001;39:423–42.

63. Barsky AJ, Ahern DK. Cognitive behavior therapy for hypochondriasis: a randomized controlled trial. JAMA 2004;291:1464–70.

64. Fava GA, Grandi S, Rafanelli C, et al. Explanatory therapy in hypochondriasis. J Clin Psychiatry 2000;61:317–22.

65. Jacobson NS, Truax P. Clinical significance: a statistical approach to defining meaningful change in psychotherapy research. J Consult Clin Psychol 1991;59: 12–9.

66. Thomson AB, Page LA. Psychotherapies for hypochondriasis. Cochrane Database Syst Rev 2007;4:CD006520.

67. Phillips KA, Pagano ME, Menard W, et al. A 12-month follow-up study of the course of body dysmorphic disorder. Am J Psychiatry 2006;163:907–12.

68. Rief W, Buhlmann U, Wilhelm S, et al. The prevalence of body dysmorphic disorder: a population-based survey. Psychol Med 2006;36:877–85.

69. Koran LM, Abujaoude E, Large MD, et al. The prevalence of body dysmorphic disorder in the United States adult population. CNS Spectrums 2008;13: 316–22.

70. Phillips KA. The broken mirror: understanding and treating body dysmorphic disorder. New York: Oxford University Press; 1996.

71. Sarwer DB, Crerand CE. Body dysmorphic disorder and appearance enhancing medical treatments. Body Image 2008;5:50–8.

72. Phillips KA, Diaz S. Gender differences in body dysmorphic disorder. J Nerv Ment Dis 1997;185:570–7.

73. Phillips KA. Quality of life for patients with body dysmorphic disorder. J Nerv Ment Dis 2000;188:170–5.

74. Phillips KA, McElroy SL, Keck PE Jr, et al. Body dysmorphic disorder: 30 cases of imagined ugliness. Am J Psychiatry 1993;150:302–8.

75. Crerand CE, Phillips KA, Menard W, et al. Nonpsychiatric medical treatment of body dysmorphic disorder. Psychosomatics 2005;46:549–55.

76. Phillips KA, Grant J, Siniscalchi J, et al. Surgical and nonpsychiatric medical treatment of patients with body dysmorphic disorder. Psychosomatics 2001;42: 504–10.

77. Veale D, Boocock A, Goumay E, et al. Body dysmorphic disorder. A survey of fifty cases. Br J Psychiatry 1996;169:196–201.

78. Phillips KA, Menard W, Fay C, et al. Demographic characteristics, phenomenology, comorbidity, and family history in 200 individuals with body dysmorphic disorder. Psychosomatics 2005;46:317–25.

79. Gunstad J, Phillips KA. Axis I comorbidity in body dysmorphic disorder. Compr Psychiatry 2003;44:270–6.

80. Phillips KA, Menard W. Suicidality in body dysmorphic disorder: a prospective study. Am J Psychiatry 2006;163:1280–2.

81. Grant JE, Menard W, Pagano ME, et al. Substance use disorders in individuals with body dysmorphic disorder. J Clin Psychiatry 2005;66:309–16.

82. Phillips KA, McElroy SL, Keck PE Jr. A comparison of delusional and nondelusional body dysmorphic disorder in 100 cases. Psychopharmacol Bull 1994;30: 179–86.

83. Phillips KA. Psychosis in body dysmorphic disorder. J Psychiatr Res 2004;38: 63–72.

84. Rosen JC, Reiter J, Orosan P. Cognitive-behavioral body image therapy for body dysmorphic disorder. J Consult Clin Psychol 1995;63:263–9.

85. Veale D, Gournay K, Dryden W, et al. Body dysmorphic disorder: a cognitive be-havioural model and pilot randomised controlled trial. Behav Res Ther 1996;34: 717–29.
86. Woolfolk RL, Allen LA. Treating somatization: a cognitive-behavioral approach. New York: Guilford Press; 2007.
87. Pincus HA. The future of behavioral health and primary care: drowning in the mainstream or left on the bank? Psychosomatics 2003;44:1–11.

Cognitive Behavioral Therapy for Sexual Dysfunctions in Women

Moniek M. ter Kuile, PhD[a],*, Stephanie Both, PhD[a],
Jacques J.D.M. van Lankveld, PhD[b]

KEYWORDS

- Sexual dysfunctions • Women • CBT treatment

The *Diagnostic and Statistical Manual of Mental Disorders,* fourth edition (DSM-IV-TR)[1] classifies female sexual dysfunctions into disorders of desire, arousal, orgasm, and pain (including genital pain and vaginismus). As the cognitive behavioral treatment procedures differ among most these sexual disorders we review the treatments for each disorder separately. For each sexual disorder, diagnostic issues are discussed before treatment issues are presented. There is a growing consensus about female sexual (dys)functioning and about shortcomings in the traditional nosology of women's sexual disorders. An international consensus conference concluded that the DSM-IV-TR definitions of female sexual dysfunction are unsatisfactory and developed a revised classification system[2] that is discussed in this article for each disorder separately. In light of the upcoming publication of the DSM-5, it is likely that the current diagnostic criteria for these disorders will change.[3] In the context of the current issue of the *Psychiatric Clinics of North America,* we focus on cognitive behavioral therapy (CBT) for sexual dysfunctions only. When discussing the degree of evidence of a treatment, we follow the criteria of Chambless and Hollon.[4]

HYPOACTIVE SEXUAL DESIRE DISORDER AND FEMALE SEXUAL AROUSAL DISORDER
Definitions and Epidemiology

In DSM-IV-TR, the condition of low or reduced sexual desire is referred to as hypoactive sexual desire disorder (HSDD) and is described as "Persistent or recurrent deficiency (or absence) of sexual fantasies and desire for sexual activity. This disturbance causes marked distress or interpersonal difficulty".[1(p541)] Sexual desire

---

[a] Outpatient Clinic for Psychosomatic Gynecology and Sexology (VRSP), Leiden University Medical Center, Poortgebouw-Zuid, P.O. Box 9600, 2300 RC Leiden, The Netherlands
[b] Faculty of Psychology & Neuroscience, Department of Clinical Psychological Science, Maastricht University, P.O. Box 616, 6200 MD, Maastricht, The Netherlands
* Corresponding author.
E-mail address: m.m.ter_kuile@lumc.nl

Psychiatr Clin N Am 33 (2010) 595–610
doi:10.1016/j.psc.2010.04.010
0193-953X/10/$ – see front matter © 2010 Elsevier Inc. All rights reserved.

and interest deal with the individual experience of wanting to become or to continue being sexual. Sexual desire may include erotic fantasies and thoughts and may be expressed as the initiative to engage in self- or other-directed sexual behavior. Absent or low sexual interest is not intrinsically pathological, but may become problematic in the context of interpartner sexual desire discrepancy.[5]

Female sexual arousal disorder (FSAD) is defined in the DSM-IV-TR as "a persistent or recurrent inability to attain or to maintain until completion of sexual activity an adequate genital lubrication-swelling response of sexual excitement that causes marked distress or interpersonal difficulty".[1(p502)] The DSM-IV-TR definition of FSAD has been criticized as it focuses exclusively on the genital response, whereas the absence of or markedly diminished feelings of subjective sexual arousal, sexual excitement, and sexual pleasure are not mentioned.[2] In the few studies that measured genital responding under laboratory conditions, it is found that medically healthy women diagnosed with FSAD responded with an increase of vaginal vasocongestion comparable with the response of women without sexual problems[2]; however, women with FSAD reported less positive affect and often more negative affect in response to these sexual stimuli than women without sexual problems.[6] These studies indicate that medically healthy women with FSAD are equally capable of genital responding as women without sexual problems to explicit erotic stimuli suggesting that these sexual arousal problems may be related to inadequate erotic stimulation in daily life or negative evaluation of the sexual situation.[7] Thus, it is highly problematic that the current definition of FSAD neglects the most important aspect of subjective sexual arousal.[8]

Overall, the prevalence of desire complaints varies from 10% to 40% and for arousal difficulties from 10% to 30%. When the assessment of distress is included, the prevalence of these complaints drops approximately by half.[8] There is high comorbidity of desire complaints and arousal difficulties. In a study including women (n = 588) with HSDD as the primary diagnosis, in 41% of these women at least one other diagnosis of FSAD or orgasmic disorder was appropriate. In 18% of the women all 3 disorders could be diagnosed.[9]

Mood and anxiety disorders have been associated with sexual desire and arousal difficulties. Some theorists suggest that the high comorbidity of sexual problems such as HSDD and FSAD at the one hand and anxiety and depression at the other might suggest that sexual dysfunctions may conceptually belong to a broad latent internalizing dimension.[10] There are indications that CBT that focuses on disorders such as depression and anxiety also decreases symptom severity of the comorbid sexual problem.[11] Furthermore, childhood sexual abuse disrupts adult sexual functioning[12] but the effects of sexual traumatization on sexual desire are not consistent.[13] Higher levels of marital distress are found in women with HSDD and FSAD. Meston and Bradford[14] stated that although factors within the individual woman may contribute to sexual desire and arousal difficulties, it is valuable to conceptualize these problems in the context of the relationship with the sexual partner.

Circular Sexual Response Model

Sexual desire and arousal are governed by both biological and psychological factors. Here we address psychological factors. The term "hypoactive sexual desire" appears to imply that sexual desire possesses an intrinsically activating or motivating quality, independent of other aspects of sexual functioning. This notion can also be found in linear models of the sexual response in which desire is considered as a phase in the sexual response cycle, independent of, and preceding sexual arousal and orgasm.[15,16] However, recently it has been stated that to understand women's sexual desire, one should move from a focus on spontaneous desire to a response cycle model in which the seeking of, or receptivity to, sexual stimuli leads to feelings of arousal and desire.[17,18] Basson and colleagues[3,17] presented a circular sexual response model in which the need for intimacy in a relationship is an important motive to be receptive to sexual stimuli. Women may decide to engage in sexual behavior as a result of a large array of sexual and nonsexual motives including the wish to experience physical pleasure, to show affection, to please or pacify a partner, to feel strong or desirable, to dispel boredom, to distract from negative preoccupations, to continue a longstanding habit, or to meet a felt obligation.[19] When engaging in sexual behavior, processing of sexual stimuli may result in responsive sexual arousal and desire. The rewarding quality of the sexual experience will facilitate future receptivity. Consequently, cognitive processes that interfere with obtaining reward from sexual activity will also impair sexual desire, including ruminative, worrisome ideation,[20,21] low outcome expectancy,[22] displaced focus of attention,[23] general insufficient attentional capacity,[24,25] and level of propensity to sexual excitation versus sexual inhibition.[26]

In recognition of the empirical research suggesting a lack of differentiation between sexual desire and arousal in women and the high degree of comorbidity between FSAD and HSDD, the proposal for the DSM-5 is to merge these two diagnostic categories and the suggested name for the disorder is sexual interest/arousal disorder.[27,28]

Treatment

The treatment literature focuses primarily on HSDD, with little apparent work directed specifically at FSAD. However, the treatment ingredients for HSDD, as discussed here, may be as effective for FSAD as they are for HSDD.

The circular model of sexual desire implies that low sexual desire is a consequence of problematic functioning in other domains of sexuality, the partner relationship, or the physical and psychological condition of the female client or her partner. It also implies that treatment should focus on helping the client to increase the rewards necessary to experience stronger motivation to engage in sexual activity, including other aspects of the woman's sexual functioning, such as her sexual arousal response and lubrication during sexual stimulation, ability to experience orgasm, or reduction of pain during sex. Treatment might also help to improve her partner's or her own skills of erotic stimulation and relieve her partner's sexual dysfunction. Treatment might also aim to increase the rewards and reducing punishment that the woman experiences within nonsexual domains of her relationship. In a CBT treatment of HSDD, interventions based on the sensate focus approach are often combined with other CBT interventions.

Sensate focus therapy or sex therapy was first described by Masters and Johnson.[29] When starting treatment, the rationale of treatment is explained, sexual education is given, and a temporary ban on intercourse is suggested. The partners then follow a program of homework exercises, including mutual nongenital and genital pleasuring, communication exercises, and exercises aimed at reducing performance demand and the resulting anxiety. For example, Trudel and colleagues[30] developed a cognitive behavioral group program for HSDD. Treatment was administered in 2-hour, weekly group sessions of couple sex therapy over 12 weeks. Group interventions included sex education; couple sexual intimacy–enhancing exercises; sensate focus; communication skills training; emotional communication skills training; sexual fantasy training; cognitive restructuring; and various homework assignments, including reading a manual. In some formats, orgasm consistency training has been added to the treatment.[31,32] Orgasm consistency training includes (1) an introduction to directed masturbation; (2) instructing the couple to allow the woman to reach orgasm during sexual interaction before the male partner climaxes and before intercourse is initiated (the "ladies come first" rule); and (3) the coital alignment technique to ensure direct clitoral stimulation by the penis during intercourse. Until now there are only 4 controlled studies published that investigated the effect of CBT in women with HSDD.[30–33] Based on the results of these 4 studies we can conclude that CBT in group format,[30–32] including orgasm consistency training[31,32] is a promising approach,[4] with large effect sizes.[34] CBT in a bibliotherapy format for women with HSDD seems not effective in the long run.[33]

FEMALE ORGASMIC DISORDER
Definition and Epidemiology

In the DSM-IV-TR female orgasmic disorder (FOD) is described as a persistent or recurrent delay in, or absence of, orgasm following a normal sexual excitement phase, that causes marked distress or interpersonal difficulty.[1] The DSM-IV-TR describes subtypes of FOD as (1) lifelong (primary) versus acquired (secondary), and (2) generalized (never experiencing orgasm) versus situational (reaching orgasm only with specific stimulation). The DSM acknowledges that women exhibit wide variability in the type and intensity of stimulation that triggers orgasm.[1] The diagnosis of the disorder is based on the clinician's judgment that the women's capacity to orgasm is less than would be reasonable for her age, sexual experience, and adequacy of sexual stimulation. However, a definition of orgasm or indications of what is a reasonable capacity are not provided. Recently, an international expert committee stated that a woman who can obtain orgasm through intercourse with manual stimulation but not through intercourse alone would not meet the criteria for clinical diagnosis.[35]

Following the definition of DSM-IV-TR, FOD is diagnosed only when there is a normal sexual excitement phase that is not followed by orgasm; however, many women with lifelong, generalized anorgasmia experience little sexual excitement or report problems maintaining sexual excitement. Thus, the diagnosis orgasmic disorder may be made when, according to DSM-IV-TR criteria, FSAD would be more accurate. Some women with HSDD have a history of sexual excitement problems and anorgasmia, resulting in a lack of sexually rewarding experiences. Thus, orgasmic problems often involve sexual arousal problems, and desire problems can be caused by arousal and orgasmic problems. Unsurprisingly, there is often comorbidity of anorgasmia, FSAD, and HSDD.[9] Some theorists have suggested that most female sexual difficulties reflect disruptions in sexual arousal.[7,36]

Simons and Carey[37] reported a pooled current and 1-year prevalence estimate of 7% to 10% for FOD. A precise estimate of the prevalence of orgasmic disorder in women is, however, difficult to determine because few well-designed studies have been conducted and definitions of orgasmic disorder differ between studies.[35]

Education level seems to be related to FOD, with women who have graduated from college being half as likely to experience problems achieving orgasm as women who have not graduated from high school.[38] Perhaps more educated women have more liberal views on sexuality and are more inclined to seek pleasure as a goal of sexual activity.[14] Medical conditions including damage to the central nervous system, the spinal cord, or the peripheral nerves caused by trauma or multiple sclerosis can result in orgasmic difficulties.[39] Drugs that increase serotonergic activity (eg, antidepressants; paroxitine, fluoxetine, sertraline) or decrease dopaminergic activity (eg, antipsychotics) are reported to delay or inhibit orgasm in women.[14]

Treatment

Cognitive behavioral approaches for FOD focus on promoting changes in attitudes and thoughts, decreasing anxiety, and increasing orgasmic ability and sexual satisfaction. The approaches generally include behavioral exercises like systemic desensitization, sensate focus, and directed masturbation (DM). DM has been developed by LoPicolo and Lobitz[40] specifically for orgasmic disorder in women and is based on the sex therapy format introduced by Masters and Johnson.[29] They designed a 9-step DM program for anorgasmic women that consisted of education, self-exploration and body awareness, masturbation exercises, and sensate focus exercises.[40] Initially the program involved both partners but later, Barbach[41] transformed the masturbation program to a group treatment format for women without their partners, the so called "preorgasmic" women's groups. The use of the word *preorgasmic* stressed the view that anorgasmia was thought to be mainly the result of an inadequate learning process. In this view, women who never experienced orgasm missed a history of discovery of their own sexuality, which was supposed to be repaired through learning of adequate masturbation skills that resulted in sexual arousal and orgasm. DM is characterized by the prescription of homework exercises that focus initially on body awareness and body acceptance, and on visual and tactile exploration of the body. Women are then instructed in masturbation techniques, to use fantasy and imagery to increase sexual excitement, and to use topical lubricants and vibrators; erotic literature or film is often recommended. Frequently Kegel[42] exercises, involving contraction and relaxation of the pelvic floor muscles, are prescribed because they may increase the woman's awareness of genital sensations and sexual arousal. For women who are inhibited in achieving orgasm because of fear of losing control, role play of orgasmic experience is recommended.[43]

Based on the results of 13 randomized controlled trials (RCTs) for FOD it was concluded that DM is a successful treatment for women with primary orgasmic disorder.[44,45] High success rates are reported, with 60% to 90% of women being able to experience orgasm by masturbation, and a lower percentage (33%–85%) being able to experience orgasm with coitus. Generally, treatment effects are maintained or even improved at follow-up. The treatment is successful in different settings like group, individual, and couple therapy and the treatment duration varied between 10 and 20 sessions.[44,45] One study reported success of written or videotaped masturbation assignments with minimal therapist contact, indicating that self-directed masturbation training may be a valuable and cost-effective treatment format.[46]

Learning how to become orgasmic during masturbation does not necessarily generalize to being orgasmic during sexual activity with a partner. In cases of situational anorgasmia, when a woman is able to attain orgasm through masturbation but not with her partner, couple treatment with a focus on communication, adequate clitoral stimulation, and engaging in intercourse using positions that maximize clitoral stimulation, seem to be more effective than DM. Hurlbert and Apt[47] compared the effectiveness of DM with coital alignment technique in women with secondary orgasmic disorder. Coital alignment is a technique in which the woman assumes the female supine posture, and the man positions himself up forward on the women, higher than in the conventional missionary position. Hurlbert and Apt[47] found that coital alignment resulted in a 56% increase in frequency of coital orgasm, compared with 27% with DM.

Most outcome studies applied a combination of education, systematic desensitization, sensate focus, communication training, and DM. There are very few studies that investigated the independent contribution of different treatment components. Comparison of DM alone with systemic desensitization alone shows equal success rates for DM and systemic desensitization in women with primary orgasmic disorder.[48] Comparison of sensate focus with or without DM in a couple format showed better results for the combination treatment.[49] Thus, for the treatment of primary orgasmic disorder, sensate focus alone seems less appropriate; masturbation exercises are an important component. Regarding the frequently prescribed Kegel exercises, Roughan and Kunst[50] found no difference in orgasmic ability between women who received treatment including Kegel exercises and women who received relaxation therapy or no treatment, which suggests that Kegel exercises alone are not sufficient to treat anorgasmia.

It can be concluded that DM is an empirically validated and efficacious treatment for women with primary orgasmic disorder.[44,45] For women with secondary orgasmic disorder DM may be helpful; however, for women who can reach orgasm alone through masturbation but not with coitus, a couples approach, including communication training and adequate clitoral stimulation techniques like coital alignment technique, may be more beneficial.

SEXUAL PAIN DISORDER: DYSPAREUNIA
Definition and Epidemiology

Dyspareunia is defined in DSM-IV-TR as recurrent genital pain associated with sexual intercourse that causes distress and interpersonal problems. Dyspareunia should not be diagnosed if it is caused exclusively by vaginismus, lack of lubrication, or a medical condition.[1] In practice, the latter criteria may be limiting and difficult to establish, as sexual pain is frequently associated with lack of sexual arousal/lubrication and the persistent difficulty to allow vaginal entry of a penis. It is difficult to judge the causes of the different complaints. Accordingly, an international consensus committee recommended the following more inclusive revision of the definition of dyspareunia: "Persistent or recurrent pain with attempted or completed vaginal entry and/or penile vaginal intercourse".[2(p226)] Although not a formal aspect of the definition, dyspareunia is typically described as either superficial (eg, associated with the vulva and/of vaginal entrance) or deep (perceived as located in the abdominal or internal organs, often associated with penile thrusting).[14] As the etiology of deep dyspareunia is nearly always somatic (eg, endometriosis) and because most of the cases involve superficial dyspareunia, we focus on the last category. Provoked vestibulodynia disorder (PVD), formerly referred to as vulvar vestibulitis syndrome, is thought to be the most frequent type of superficial dyspareunia in premenopausal women. PVD is defined as burning or pain that is localized strictly to the vestibule of the vulva and is provoked by pressure or friction in the vestibule.[51] Its etiology is unknown and the presence or absence of inflammation in the vestibular tissue is debated. Generalized vulvodynia is diagnosed when pain is located on the whole vulva, not only on the vestibulum. It can be triggered by physical contact (provoked) or the discomfort occurs spontaneously, without a specific physical trigger.[52] Generalized vulvodynia is rare, compared with provoked vestibulodynia, and is diagnosed as a chronic pain problem rather than a sexual problem.[53] Women who have provoked vestibulodynia are mostly premenopausal and generalized vulvodynia is more commonly observed in older women.[53]

Prevalence estimates for dyspareunia range from 6.5% to 45.0% in older women and from 14% to 34% in younger women, depending on geographic location and setting.[54]

Women with dyspareunia report higher levels of anxiety and depression, although the data are inconsistent. Sexual traumatization appears not to play a significant role. Women with dyspareunia experience more difficulties with sexual arousal and lubrication during partnered sexual activities as compared with masturbation. They are more erotophobic, reflecting negative and conservative attitudes toward sex. Women with PVD are found to have more catastrophic thoughts about intercourse pain, to be more sensitive to thermal and tactile stimulation, reflected in lowered thresholds for sensitivity and the experience of pain on stimulation.[54]

Circular Cognitive Behavioral Model

Already more than 30 years ago, Spano and Lamont[55] introduced the first circular CB-model of dyspareunia. This model was the starting point for the development of the current CB model for PVD (**Fig. 1**).[56] It is assumed that pain during penetration, or catastrophic memories of that pain, lead to fear of pain and hypervigilance in new intercourse situations. The fear of penetration and hypervigilance result in decreased sexual arousal during sexual activity and thus in vaginal dryness and/or increased pelvic floor muscle tone (as a protective reaction to anticipated or actual pain). The combination of vaginal dryness and increased pelvic floor muscle tone, causing friction between the penis and vulvar skin, may result in pain and even tissue damage. This damage may in itself result in pain or may further increase already existing pain. According to this model, diminished sexual response and/or increased pelvic floor muscle tone can be a cause, as well as a consequence of the genital pain complaint.[56] Elements of this CBT model have received some empirical support.[57–70] However, more research is necessary in understanding the mechanism by which these factors relate in maintaining the pain problem.

Treatment

In attempts to relieve pain, a variety of medical and nonmedical interventions have been used. Medical interventions include local temporary use of inert or

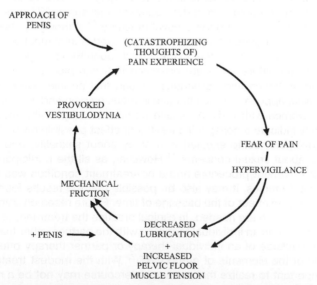

Fig. 1. Circular cognitive behavioral model of provoked vestibulodynia (PVD).

corticosteroid ointments, surgical excision of the painful vestibular tissue (vestibulectomy), and behavioral interventions focusing on the pelvic muscle-tension (ie, biofeedback training), and CBT focusing on pain and sexuality. For an extensive review of controlled and uncontrolled outcome studies we refer to Landry and colleagues.[71]

Until now there have been 9 RCTs evaluating the effect of medical and nonmedical interventions for women with dyspareunia. Most of these studies (n = 7) included only women with PVD.[72–78] Two studies have been conducted in a combined sample of women with provoked and nonprovoked vestibulodynia.[79,80] Five studies examined the effect of CBT.[72,75,76,79,80]

The purpose of CBT is to achieve pain control by the woman themselves. It focuses on reducing catastrophic fear of pain and reestablishing satisfying sexual functioning (eg, nonpenetrative sex), with an aim of reducing muscle contraction in the pelvic floor and promoting lubrication during sexual activity. The ultimate goal is pain reduction in the sexual situation. CBT is often delivered in a group format, with 8 to 10 sessions over a 10- to 12-week period. The treatment package includes (1) education and information about vestibulodynia and how dyspareunia affects desire and arousal, (2) education concerning a multifactorial view of pain, (3) education about sexual anatomy, (4) progressive muscle relaxation, (5) abdominal breathing, (6) Kegel exercises, (7) vaginal dilatation, (8) distraction techniques focusing on sexual imagery, (9) rehearsal of coping self-statements, (10) communication skills training, and (11) cognitive restructuring.

A behavioral intervention that focuses on pelvic muscle tension, using biofeedback electromyography (EMG) with visual feedback, was introduced by Glazer and colleagues.[81] Women are trained to use a vaginal EMG sensor and a biofeedback device in the clinic and are then asked to complete a standard pelvic floor training program at home twice a day consisting of pelvic floor contraction exercises of various durations, separated by prescribed rest periods. Participants receive 8, 45-minute sessions over 12 weeks.

Both the behavioral intervention (EMG, biofeedback training) and CBT (mostly in a group format) have effects comparable to surgery[72,82] and to pharmacological treatments,[75,76] and on some secondary outcome measures CBT was found superior to medication[76,80] or supportive psychotherapy.[79] Although patients reported significantly less pain during intercourse and improved sexual functioning, the effect sizes were modest. It is notable that in the 2 medication RCTs, large placebo effects were found and no differences were observed between placebo and active treatment.[73,74] Also, Petersen and colleagues[78] found that an injection of either Botox or placebo (saline) appeared to be effective in reducing pain and in improving sexual functioning in women with PVD. As active treatment and placebo results are very similar, this may indicate a nonspecific treatment effect possible owing to expectancies for improvement, being enrolled in a study about sexuality, and/or talking to a professional about sexual concerns.[14] However, as all the participants improved irrespective of treatment procedure and a no-treatment condition was not included in one of the RCT studies, it may also be possible that the results found in these 9 studies are merely an effect of the passage of time. Future research using RCTs with a wait-list control group are needed. In clinical practice the treatment of dyspareunia is often implemented in an individual format or with the partner rather than in a group. The treatment package of an individual therapy or partner therapy often resembles a combination of the elements of group CBT.[72] With the modest treatment effects found, it is important to realize that painless intercourse may not be a realistic therapeutic goal for many women.

SEXUAL PAIN DISORDER: VAGINISMUS
Definition and Epidemiology

Vaginismus is defined in DSM IV-TR as an involuntary contraction of the musculature of the outer third of the vagina interfering with intercourse, causing distress and interpersonal difficulty.[1] This definition has received considerable criticism. For example, the only unique diagnostic criterion for vaginismus is "vaginal spasm" that interferes with intercourse but that has never been validated.[59] An international consensus committee has suggested revised criteria, recommending that vaginismus be defined as "persistent difficulties to allow vaginal entry of a penis, a finger, and/or any object, despite the woman's expressed wish to do so. There is variable involuntary pelvic muscle contraction, (phobic) avoidance and anticipation/fear/experience of pain. Structural or other physical abnormalities must be ruled out/addressed".[2(p226)] Vaginismus can be classified as either lifelong (primary) or acquired (secondary). Lifelong vaginismus occurs when the woman has never been able to have intercourse. In acquired vaginismus, a woman loses the ability to have intercourse after a nonsymptomatic period of time. Acquired vaginismus can develop as a sequel to dyspareunia.

The DSM-IV-TR prohibits coexisting diagnoses of vaginismus and dyspareunia.[1] In practice however, it is often problematic for clinicians to differentiate these two disorders because patients often present with features of both. In fact, there are a number of studies that have attempted and failed to differentiate vaginismus from dyspareunia. Overall, there is no current empirical evidence that dyspareunia can be reliably differentiated from vaginismus.[83,84] For the DSM-5, it is proposed that the diagnoses of vaginismus and dyspareunia be collapsed into a single diagnostic entity called genito-pelvic pain/penetration disorder. This diagnostic category is defined according to different dimensions, ie, percentage success of vaginal penetration; pain with vaginal penetration; fear of vaginal penetration.[83,84]

Because many epidemiological studies excluded questions about vaginismus, the prevalence of vaginismus is not well established, although it is estimated to vary between 1% and 6%.[85]

Women with vaginismus were found to have increased comorbid anxiety disorders, while depression rates were not found to be increased. A history of sexual trauma has been linked with vaginismus, although the data are inconsistent. Vaginismus is unrelated to marital distress.[54]

Circular Cognitive Behavioral Model

Based on the fear-avoidance model of Vlaeyen and Linton,[86] a circular fear-avoidance model is proposed for vaginismus (**Fig. 2**). This model provides an explanation of why

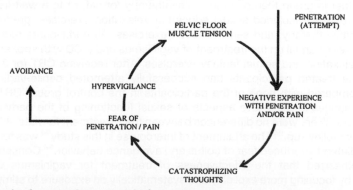

Fig. 2. Circular fear-avoidance model of vaginismus.

vaginistic problems develop in a minority of the women who experience discomfort or pain during vaginal penetration. The basic tenet of the model is that the catastrophic interpretation of vaginal penetration may lead to a vicious circle.[87] These dysfunctional interpretations give rise to vaginal penetration–related fear. To cope with the fear, a woman may avoid all activities related to vaginal penetration or she may be hypervigilant for pain-related stimuli. The latter can result in exaggerated attention to physical sensations and psychological arousal facilitating sensations of pain. Attempts at vaginal penetration are met with a defensive pelvic floor muscle contraction. Increased muscle tonus results in painful or impossible attempts. Not being able to "achieve" penetration in turn contributes to negative experiences and confirms negative expectations. By reducing avoidance behavior and increasing successful penetration behavior, erroneous cognitions can be disconfirmed.[87–89] Some of the elements of the cycle have received empirical support.[57–60,69,88,90]

Treatment

The use of gradual exposure and applied relaxation (systematic desensitization) has a relatively long history in the treatment of vaginismus, but has surprisingly little empirical support.[14,91] Gradual exposure exercises are assigned for homework, with gradual habituation to vaginal touch and penetration, usually beginning with the woman's fingers or artificial devices specifically designed for this purpose. These core elements are often part of a broader approach involving cognitive restructuring, education, and sex therapy.[92]

There are only 4 RCTs investigating the effect of behavior therapy and CBT in the treatment of vaginismus.[90,93–95] Schnyder and colleagues[93] investigated the effect of 2 types of systematic dezensitization in 44 women with vaginismus, 19 with lifelong vaginismus. Both groups received information and relaxation exercises. In the first group, the physician introduced the dilator. In the second group, the physician provided verbal instruction for introducing the dilator. Four sizes of vaginal dilators made of silicon were used with a lubricant. Therapy sessions were conducted every 2 weeks to support progress made in home-based treatment, to reduce resistance, and to use larger dilators. There were no differences between the groups at the end of the treatment period: 43 of 44 participants reported successful penetrative sexual intercourse suggesting that common elements of the therapies used were successful. At follow-up, 18 (50%) of 36 participants reported that the vaginismus had altogether disappeared, whereas 17 (48%) reported that they were improved. The mean number of treatment sessions was 6.

In the second study, 117 women with lifelong vaginismus were randomly assigned to CBT, either in group therapy or in a bibliotherapy format, or to a wait-list control group.[94] Treatment included sexual education, relaxation exercises, gradual exposure, cognitive therapy, and sensate focus exercises. All participants received the same self-help manual on the treatment of vaginismus and a CD with spoken instructions for relaxation and sexual fantasy exercises. After receiving CBT for 3 months, 18% of the treated participants had successfully attempted penile-vaginal intercourse, compared with none of the participants in the control group. CBT did not produce changes in subjective aspects of sexual functioning of the participants or their partners. There were no differences between the 2 treatment formats at 3 months and at 1 year follow-up.[94] The attainment of intercourse in this study[94] was found to be partly mediated by reduced fear of coitus and avoidance behavior.[88] Consequently, it was hypothesized that the effectiveness of treatment for vaginismus could be enhanced by focusing more explicitly and systematically on exposure to stimuli feared during penetration.

To test this hypothesis, a prolonged and therapist-aided exposure therapy was developed that took place both in a hospital setting and at home[90] Exposure at the hospital was self-controlled, ie, the participant performed the vaginal penetration-exercises by herself, while a female therapist gave her directions how to do the exercises and motivated her to expose herself to the anxiety-provoking penetration stimuli. Exposure at the hospital constituted of a maximum of 3, 2-hour sessions during 1 week. After each session, the participant and her partner were given a number of specific exposure homework assignments in which penetration exercises with the partner were also involved. To investigate the effectiveness of therapist-aided exposure for lifelong vaginismus, a replicated randomized single-subject experimental AB-phase design was used. Ten women with lifelong vaginismus participated. Nine of the 10 participants reported having had intercourse after treatment and in 5 of these 9, intercourse was possible within the first week of treatment. The results were maintained at 1-year follow-up. Furthermore, exposure was found to be successful in decreasing fear and negative penetration beliefs at posttreatment and 1-year follow-up. Although 90% of them reported intercourse, for more than half of the participants the questionnaire scores for vaginismus were still not within the normal range of sexually functional women, indicating that these participants still reported some discomfort during intercourse.[90] Recently, these results were replicated in a multicenter, waiting-list controlled trial including 70 women with lifelong vaginismus.[95]

The success rates (90%) found in the controlled studies of Schnyder and colleagues[93] and Ter Kuile and colleagues[90,95] are comparable with effects sizes reported in earlier, uncontrolled outcome studies[14,91,92] and much larger than the success rates found in an RCT of self-controlled, home-based exposure therapy, where only 18% of the women were able to have intercourse after 3 months of CBT treatment.[94] We conclude that focusing explicitly and systematically on exposure to stimuli feared during penetration, while reducing avoidant behavior by intensive therapist guidance appears to be an effective treatment for lifelong vaginismus.

SUMMARY

Twenty-six studies investigated the effect of CBT treatment for women with sexual dysfunction, 16 of which were conducted between mid-1980 and 1995. In 1997, Heiman and Meston's review[44] concluded that only DM for primary anorgasmia fulfilled the criteria of well-established treatments, and that DM for secondary anorgasmia fell within the category of probably efficacious treatments. This conclusion is still valid today. Orgasm consistency training, and coital alignment,[31,32] including sensate focus exercises, are promising approaches in the treatment of HSDD. There are no evidence-based CBT treatments for FSAD, but directed masturbation or comparable approaches may be as effective for FSAD as they are for FOD or HSDD, although we await the empirical evidence on this possibility. There are no well-established CBT treatments for dyspareunia and vaginismus; however, CBT in a group format and individual EMG biofeedback are promising treatment procedures for dyspareunia. Focusing explicitly and systematically on exposure to stimuli feared during penetration, while simultaneously reducing avoidant behavior by intensive therapist guidance appears to be an effective treatment for women with vaginismus. Furthermore, the efficacy of CBT seems to differ depending on the specific sexual dysfunction to be treated; HSDD, OD, and vaginismus seem to have a better prognosis than dyspareunia. Little is known about which treatment components are most effective.[14] However, component control studies are generally rare, even in much better researched areas as CBT for depression or anxiety. In conclusion, despite their widespread acceptance in clinical practice, few CBT treatments for women's sexual dysfunction have yet been empirically investigated in a methodologically sound way and little is known about which of the treatment components are most effective.

REFERENCES

1. American Psychiatric Association. Diagnostic and statistical manual of mental disorders. 4th edition and text revision . Washington, DC: American Psychiatric Association; 2000.
2. Basson R, Leiblum S, Brotto L, et al. Definitions of women's sexual dysfunction reconsidered: advocating expansion and revision. J Psychosom Obstet Gynaecol 2003;24(4):221–9.
3. Basson R, Wierman ME, Van Lankveld J, et al. Summary of the recommendations on sexual dysfunctions in women. J Sex Med 2010;7(1):314–26.
4. Chambless DL, Hollon SD. Defining empirically supported treatments. J Consult Clin Psychol 1998;66:7–18.
5. Bancroft J, Loftus J, Long JS. Distress about sex: a national survey of women in heterosexual relationships. Arch Sex Behav 2003;32(3):193–208.
6. Laan E, van Driel EM, van Lunsen RH. Genital responsiveness in healthy women with and without sexual arousal disorder. J Sex Med 2008;5(6):1424–35.
7. Laan E, Everaerd W, Both S. Female sexual arousal disorders. In: Balon R, Segraves RT, editors. Handbook of sexual dysfunctions. New York: Marcel Dekker Inc; 2005. p. 123–54.
8. Brotto LA, Bitzer J, Laan E, et al. Women's sexual desire and arousal disorders. J Sex Med 2010;7(1):586–614.
9. Segraves KB, Segraves RT. Hypoactive sexual desire disorder: prevalence and comorbidity in 906 subjects. J Sex Marital Ther 1991;17(1):55–8.
10. Laurent SM, Simons AD. Sexual dysfunction in depression and anxiety: conceptualizing sexual dysfunction as part of an internalizing dimension. Clin Psychol Rev 2009;29(7):573–85.
11. Hoyer J, Uhmann S, Rambow J, et al. Reduction of sexual dysfunction: byproduct of cognitive-behavioural therapy for psychological disorders? Sex Rel Ther 2009;24(1):64–73.
12. Leonard LM, Follette VM. Sexual functioning in women reporting a history of child abuse. Review of the empirical literature and clinical implications. Annu Rev Sex Res 2002;13:375–87.
13. Mchichi A, Kadri N. Moroccan women with a history of child sexual abuse and its long-term repercussions: a population-based epidemiological study. Arch Womens Ment Health 2004;7(4):237–42.
14. Meston CM, Bradford A. Sexual dysfunctions in women. Annu Rev Clin Psychol 2007;3:233–56.
15. Kaplan HS. Disorders of sexual desire. New York: Brunner/Mazel; 1977.
16. Masters WH, Johnson VE. Human sexual response. Boston: Little Brown; 1966.
17. Basson R. The female sexual response: a different model. J Sex Marital Ther 2000;26(1):51–65.
18. Both S, Everaerd W, Laan E. Desire emerges from excitement: a psychophysiological perspective on sexual motivation. In: Janssen E, editor. The psychophysiology of sex. Bloomington (IN): Indiana University Press; 2007. p. 327–39.
19. Meston CM, Buss DM. Why humans have sex. Arch Sex Behav 2007;36(4):477–507.
20. Barlow DH. Causes of sexual dysfunction: the role of anxiety and cognitive interference. J Consult Clin Psychol 1986;54(2):140–8.

21. van den Hout M, Barlow D. Attention, arousal and expectancies in anxiety and sexual disorders. J Affect Disord 2000;61(3):241–56.
22. Bach AK, Brown TA, Barlow DH. The effects of false negative feedback on efficacy expectancies and sexual arousal in sexually functional males. Behav Ther 1999;30(1):79–95.
23. Meston CM. The effects of state and trait self-focused attention on sexual arousal in sexually functional and dysfunctional women. Behav Res Ther 2006;44(4): 515–32.
24. Elliott AN, O'Donohue WT. The effects of anxiety and distraction on sexual arousal in a nonclinical sample of heterosexual women. Arch Sex Behav 1997;26(6): 607–24.
25. Salemink E, van Lankveld JJ. The effects of increasing neutral distraction on sexual responding of women with and without sexual problems. Arch Sex Behav 2006;35(2):179–90.
26. Bancroft J, Janssen E. The dual control model of male sexual response: a theoretical approach to centrally mediated erectile dysfunction. Neurosci Biobehav Rev 2000;24(5):571–9.
27. Brotto LA. The DSM diagnostic criteria for hypoactive sexual desire disorder in women. Arch Sex Behav 2010;39(2):221–39.
28. Graham CA. The DSM diagnostic criteria for female sexual arousal disorder. Arch Sex Behav 2010;39(2):240–55.
29. Masters WH, Johnson VE. Human sexual inadequacy. Boston: Little Brown; 1970.
30. Trudel G, Marchand A, Ravart M, et al. The effect of a cognitive behavioral group treatment on hypoactive sexual desire in women. Sex Rel Ther 2001;16:145–64.
31. Hurlbert DF. A comparative study using orgasm consistency training in the treatment of women reporting hypoactive sexual desire. J Sex Marital Ther 1993; 19(1):41–55.
32. Hurlbert DF, White LC, Powell RD, et al. Orgasm consistency training in the treatment of women reporting hypoactive sexual desire: an outcome comparison of women-only groups and couples-only groups. J Behav Ther Exp Psychiatry 1993;24(1):3–13.
33. van Lankveld JJDM, Everaerd W, Grotjohann Y. Cognitive-behavioral bibliotherapy for sexual dysfunctions in heterosexual couples: a randomized waiting-list controlled clinical trial in the Netherlands. J Sex Res 2001;38(1):51–67.
34. Cohen J. Statistical power analysis for the behavioral sciences. Revised edition. New York: Academic Press; 1977.
35. Meston CM, Hull E, Levin RJ, et al. Disorders of orgasm in women. J Sex Med 2004;1(1):66–8.
36. Derogatis LR, Conklin-Powers B. Psychological assessment measures of female sexual functioning in clinical trials. Int J Impot Res 1998;10(Suppl 2):S111–6.
37. Simons JS, Carey MP. Prevalence of sexual dysfunctions: results from a decade of research. Arch Sex Behav 2001;30(2):177–219.
38. Laumann EO, Paik A, Rosen RC. Sexual dysfunction in the United States: prevalence and predictors. JAMA 1999;281(6):537–44.
39. Sipski M. SCI women do have orgasms! Spinal Cord 1998;36(8):596.
40. LoPiccolo J, Lobitz WC. The role of masturbation in the treatment of orgasmic dysfunction. Arch Sex Behav 1972;2(2):163–71.
41. Barbach LG. Group treatment of preorgasmic women. J Sex Marital Ther 1974; 1(2):139–45.
42. Kegel AH. Sexual functions of the pubococcygeus muscle. West J Surg Obstet Gynecol 1952;60(10):521–4.

43. Heiman JR, LoPicolo J. Becoming orgasmic: a sexual and personal growth program for women. New York: Simon & Schuster; 1988.
44. Heiman JR, Meston CM. Empirically validated treatment for sexual dysfunction. Annu Rev Sex Res 1997;8:148–94.
45. Meston CM, Levin RJ, Sipski ML, et al. Women's orgasm. Annu Rev Sex Res 2004;15:173–257.
46. McMullen S, Rosen RC. Self-administered masturbation training in the treatment of primary orgasmic dysfunction. J Consult Clin Psychol 1979;47(5):912–8.
47. Hurlbert DF, Apt C. The coital alignment technique and directed masturbation: a comparative study on female orgasm. J Sex Marital Ther 1995;21(1):21–9.
48. Andersen BL. A comparison of systematic desensitization and directed masturbation in the treatment of primary orgasmic dysfunction in females. J Consult Clin Psychol 1981;49(4):568–70.
49. Riley AJ, Riley EJ. A controlled study to evaluate directed masturbation in the management of primary orgasmic failure in women. Br J Psychiatry 1978;133:404–9.
50. Roughan PA, Kunst L. Do pelvic floor exercises really improve orgasmic potential? J Sex Marital Ther 1981;7(3):223–9.
51. Friedrich EG. Vulvar vestibulitis syndrome. J Reprod Med 1987;32(2):110–4.
52. Moyal-Barracco M, Lynch PJ. 2003 ISSVD terminology and classification vulvodynia: a historical perspective. J Reprod Med 2004;49(10):772–7.
53. Harlow BL, Wise LA, Stewart EG. Prevalence and predictors of chronic lower genital tract discomfort. Am J Obstet Gynecol 2001;185(3):545–50.
54. Van Lankveld JJ, Granot M, Weijmar SW, et al. Women's sexual pain disorders. J Sex Med 2010;7(1):615–31.
55. Spano L, Lamont JA. Dyspareunia: a symptom of female sexual dysfunction. Cancer Nurs 1975;71(8):22–5.
56. ter Kuile MM, Weijenborg PT. A cognitive-behavioral group program for women with vulvar vestibulitis syndrome (VVS): factors associated with treatment success. J Sex Marital Ther 2006;32(3):199–213.
57. van der Velde J, Laan E, Everaerd W. Vaginismus, a component of a general defensive reaction. An investigation of pelvic floor muscle activity during exposure to emotion-inducing film excerpts in women with and without vaginismus. Int Urogynecol J Pelvic Floor Dysfunct 2001;12(5):328–31.
58. van der Velde J, Everaerd W. The relationship between involuntary pelvic floor muscle activity, muscle awareness and experienced threat in women with and without vaginismus. Behav Res Ther 2001;39(4):395–408.
59. Reissing ED, Binik YM, Khalife S, et al. Vaginal spasm, pain, and behavior: an empirical investigation of the diagnosis of vaginismus. Arch Sex Behav 2004; 33(1):5–17.
60. Reissing ED, Binik YM, Khalife S, et al. Etiological correlates of vaginismus: sexual and physical abuse, sexual knowledge, sexual self-schema, and relationship adjustment. J Sex Marital Ther 2003;29(1):47–59.
61. Pukall CF, Binik YM, Khalife S, et al. Vestibular tactile and pain thresholds in women with vulvar vestibulitis syndrome. Pain 2002;96(1-2):163–75.
62. Pukall CF, Baron M, Amsel R, et al. Tender point examination in women with vulvar vestibulitis syndrome. Clin J Pain 2006;22(7):601–9.
63. Payne KA, Binik YM, Amsel R, et al. When sex hurts, anxiety and fear orient attention towards pain. Eur J Pain 2005;9(4):427–36.
64. Payne KA, Binik YM, Pukall CF, et al. Effects of sexual arousal on genital and nongenital sensation: a comparison of women with vulvar vestibulitis syndrome and healthy controls. Arch Sex Behav 2007;36(2):289–300.

65. Brauer M, ter Kuile MM, Janssen SA, et al. The effect of pain-related fear on sexual arousal in women with superficial dyspareuma. Eur J Pain 2007;11(7): 788–98.
66. Brauer M, ter Kuile MM, Laan E. Effects of appraisal of sexual stimuli on sexual arousal in women with and without superficial dyspareunia. Arch Sex Behav 2009;38(4):476–85.
67. Brauer M, ter Kuile MM, Laan E, et al. Cognitive-affective correlates and predictors of superficial dyspareunia. J Sex Marital Ther 2009;35(1):1–24.
68. Desrochers G, Bergeron S, Khalife S, et al. Fear avoidance and self-efficacy in relation to pain and sexual impairment in women with provoked vestibulodynia. Clin J Pain 2009;25(6):520–7.
69. Desrochers G, Bergeron S, Khalife S, et al. Provoked vestibulodynia: psychological predictors of topical and cognitive-behavioral treatment outcome. Behav Res Ther 2010;48:106–15.
70. Klaassen M, ter Kuile MM. Development and initial validation of the Vaginal Penetration Cognition Questionnaire (VPCQ) in a sample of women with vaginismus and dyspareunia. J Sex Med 2009;6(6):1617–27.
71. Landry T, Bergeron S, Dupuis MJ, et al. The treatment of provoked vestibulodynia—a critical review. Clin J Pain 2008;24(2):155–71.
72. Bergeron S, Binik YM, Khalife S, et al. A randomized comparison of group cognitive-behavioral therapy, surface electromyographic biofeedback, and vestibulectomy in the treatment of dyspareunia resulting from vulvar vestibulitis. Pain 2001;91(3):297–306.
73. Bornstein J, Livnat G, Stolar Z, et al. Pure versus complicated vulvar vestibulitis: a randomized trial of fluconazole treatment. Gynecol Obstet Invest 2000;50(3): 194–7.
74. Nyirjesy P, Sobel JD, Weitz MV, et al. Cromolyn cream for recalcitrant idiopathic vulvar vestibulitis: results of a placebo controlled study. Sex Transm Infect 2001;77(1):53–7.
75. Danielsson I, Torstensson T, Brodda-Jansen G, et al. EMG biofeedback versus topical lidocaine gel: a randomized study for the treatment of women with vulvar vestibulitis. Acta Obstet Gynecol Scand 2006;85(11):1360–7.
76. Bergeron S, Khalife S, Dupuis MJ. A randomized comparison of cognitive-behavioral therapy and medical management. In: Paper presented as part of a symposium at the annual meeting of the International Society for the Study of Women's Sexual Health. San Diego (CA); 2008.
77. Murina F, Bianco V, Radici G, et al. Transcutaneous electrical nerve stimulation to treat vestibulodynia: a randomised controlled trial. Br J Obstet Gynaecol 2008; 115(9):1165–70.
78. Petersen CD, Giraldi A, Lundvall L, et al. Botulinum toxin type A—a novel treatment for provoked vestibulodynia? Results from a randomized, placebo controlled, double blinded study. J Sex Med 2009;6(9):2523–37.
79. Masheb RM, Kerns RD, Lozano C, et al. A randomized clinical trial for women with vulvodynia: cognitive-behavioral therapy vs. supportive psychotherapy. Pain 2009;141(1–2):31–40.
80. Brown CS, Wan J, Bachmann G, et al. Self-management, amitriptyline, and amitriptyline plus triamcinolone in the management of vulvodynia. J Womens Health 2009;18(2):163–9.
81. Glazer HI, Rodke G, Swencionis C, et al. Treatment of vulvar vestibulitis syndrome with electromyographic biofeedback of pelvic floor musculature. J Reprod Med 1995;40(4):283–90.

82. Bergeron S, Khalife S, Glazer HI, et al. Surgical and behavioral treatments for ves-tibulodynia - two-and-one-half-year follow-up and predictors of outcome. Obstet Gynecol 2008;111(1):159–66.
83. Binik YM. The DSM diagnostic criteria for dyspareunia. Arch Sex Behav 2010; 39(2):292–303.
84. Binik YM. The DSM diagnostic criteria for vaginismus. Arch Sex Behav 2010; 39(2):278–91.
85. Lewis RW, Fugl-Meyer KS, Bosch R, et al. Epidemiology/risk factors of sexual dysfunction. J Sex Med 2004;1(1):35–9.
86. Vlaeyen JWS, Linton SJ. Fear-avoidance and its consequences in chronic muscu-loskeletal pain: a state of the art. Pain 2000;85(3):317–32.
87. Reissing ED. Vaginismus: evaluation and management. In: Goldstein AT, Pukall CF, Goldstein I, editors. Female sexual pain disorders: evaluation and management. Oxford (UK): Wiley-Blackwell; 2009. p. 229–34.
88. ter Kuile MM, van Lankveld JJ, de Groot HE, et al. Cognitive behavioural therapy for women with lifelong vaginismus: process and prognostic factors. Behav Res Ther 2007;45:359–73.
89. Leiblum SR. Vaginismus. A most perplexing problem. In: Leiblum SR, Rosen RC, editors. Principles and practice of sex therapy. 3rd edition. New York: Guilford Press; 2000. p. 181–202.
90. ter Kuile MM, Bulte I, Weijenborg PT, et al. Therapist-aided exposure for women with lifelong vaginismus: a replicated single-case design. J Consult Clin Psychol 2009;77(1):149–59.
91. McGuire H, Hawton KKE. Interventions for vaginismus. Cochrane Database Syst Rev 2001;2:CD001760.
92. Reissing ED, Binik YM, Khalife S. Does vaginismus exist? A critical review of the literature. J Nerv Ment Dis 1999;187(5):261–74.
93. Schnyder U, Schnyder-Luthi C, Ballinari P, et al. Therapy for vaginismus: in vivo versus in vitro desensitization. Can J Psychiatry 1998;43(9):941–4.
94. van Lankveld JJ, ter Kuile MM, de Groot HE, et al. Cognitive-behavioral therapy for women with lifelong vaginismus: a randomized waiting-list controlled trial of efficacy. J Consult Clin Psychol 2006;74:168–78.
95. ter Kuile MM, Melles R, Groot HE, et al. Therapist-aided exposure for women with lifelong vaginismus: a randomized waiting-list controlled trial of efficacy. Submitted for publication.

Cognitive Behavioral Therapy for Eating Disorders

Rebecca Murphy, DClinPsych*,
Suzanne Straebler, APRN - Psychiatry, MSN, Zafra Cooper, DPhil, DipPsych,
Christopher G. Fairburn, DM, FMedSci, FRCPsych

KEYWORDS

- Cognitive behavioral therapy • Eating disorders
- Anorexia nervosa • Bulimia nervosa

The eating disorders provide one of the strongest indications for cognitive behavioral therapy (CBT). Two considerations support this claim. First, the core psychopathology of eating disorders, the overevaluation of shape and weight, is cognitive in nature. Second, it is widely accepted that CBT is the treatment of choice for bulimia nervosa[1] and there is evidence that it is as effective with cases of "eating disorder not otherwise specified" (eating disorder NOS),[2] the most common eating disorder diagnosis. This article starts with a description of the clinical features of eating disorders and then reviews the evidence supporting cognitive behavioral treatment. Next, the cognitive behavioral account of eating disorders is presented and, last, the new "transdiagnostic" form of CBT is described.

EATING DISORDERS AND THEIR CLINICAL FEATURES
Classification and Diagnosis

Eating disorders are characterized by a severe and persistent disturbance in eating behavior that causes psychosocial and, sometimes, physical impairment. The DSM-IV classification scheme for eating disorders recognizes 2 specific diagnoses, anorexia nervosa (AN) and bulimia nervosa (BN), and a residual category termed eating disorder NOS.[3]

The diagnosis of anorexia nervosa is made in the presence of the following features:

1. The overevaluation of shape and weight; that is, judging self-worth largely, or even exclusively, in terms of shape and weight. This has been described in various ways and is often expressed as strong desire to be thin combined with an intense fear of weight gain and fatness.

C.G.F. is supported by a Principal Research Fellowship from the Wellcome Trust (046386). R.M., S.S., and Z.C. are supported by a program grant from the Wellcome Trust (046386).
Department of Psychiatry, Warneford Hospital, Warneford Lane, Oxford University, Oxford OX3 7JX, UK
* Corresponding author.
E-mail address: Rebecca.Murphy@psych.ox.ac.uk

Psychiatr Clin N Am 33 (2010) 611–627
doi:10.1016/j.psc.2010.04.004
0193-953X/10/$ – see front matter © 2010 Elsevier Inc. All rights reserved.

2. The active maintenance of an unduly low body weight. This is commonly defined as maintaining a body weight less than 85% of that expected or a body mass index (BMI; weight kg/height m^2 or weight lb/[height in]^2 × 703) of 17.5 or less.
3. Amenorrhea, in postpubertal females not taking an oral contraceptive.

The unduly low weight is pursued in a variety of ways with strict dieting and excessive exercise being particularly prominent. A subgroup also engages in episodes of binge eating and/or "purging" through self-induced vomiting or laxative misuse.

For a diagnosis of bulimia nervosa 3 features need to be present:

1. Overevaluation of shape and weight, as in anorexia nervosa.
2. Recurrent binge eating. A "binge" is an episode of eating during which an objectively large amount of food is eaten for the circumstances and there is an accompanying sense of loss of control.
3. Extreme weight-control behavior, such as recurrent self-induced vomiting, regular laxative misuse, or marked dietary restriction.

In addition, the diagnostic criteria for anorexia nervosa should not be met. This "trumping rule" ensures that patients do not receive both diagnoses at one time.

There are no positive criteria for the diagnosis of eating disorder NOS. Instead, this diagnosis is reserved for eating disorders of clinical severity that do not meet the diagnostic criteria of AN or BN. Eating disorder NOS is the most common eating disorder encountered in clinical settings constituting about half of adult outpatient eating-disordered samples, with patients with bulimia nervosa constituting about a third, and the rest being cases of anorexia nervosa.[4] In inpatient settings the great majority of cases are either underweight forms of eating disorder NOS or anorexia nervosa.[5]

In addition, DSM-IV recognizes "binge eating disorder" (BED) as a provisional diagnosis in need of further study. The criteria for BED are recurrent episodes of binge eating in the absence of extreme weight-control behavior. It is proposed that BED be recognized as a specific eating disorder in DSM-V.[6]

Clinical Features

Anorexia nervosa, bulimia nervosa, and most cases of eating disorder NOS share a core psychopathology: the overevaluation of the importance of shape and weight and their control. Whereas most people judge themselves on the basis of their perceived performance in a variety of domains of life (such as the quality of their relationships, their work performance, their sporting prowess), for people with eating disorders self-worth is dependent largely, or even exclusively, on their shape and weight and their ability to control them. This psychopathology is peculiar to the eating disorders (and to body dysmorphic disorder).

In anorexia nervosa, patients become underweight largely as a result of persistent and severe restriction of both the amount and the type of food that they eat. In addition to strict dietary rules, some patients engage in a driven form of exercising, which further contributes to their low body weight. Patients with anorexia nervosa typically value the sense of control that they derive from undereating. Some practice self-induced vomiting, laxative and/or diuretic misuse, especially (but not exclusively) those who experience episodes of loss of control over eating. The amount of food eaten during these "binges" is often not objectively large; hence, they are described as "subjective binges." Many other psychopathological features tend to be present, some as a result of the semistarvation. These include depressed and labile mood, anxiety features, irritability, impaired concentration, loss of libido, heightened obsessionality and sometimes frank obsessional features, and social withdrawal. There are also a multitude of physical features, most of which are secondary to being under-weight. These include poor sleep, sensitivity to the cold, heightened fullness, and decreased energy.

Patients with bulimia nervosa resemble those with anorexia nervosa both in terms of their eating habits and methods of weight control. The main feature distinguishing these 2 groups is that in patients with bulimia nervosa attempts to restrict food intake are regularly disrupted by episodes of (objective) binge eating. These episodes are often followed by compensatory self-induced vomiting or laxative misuse, although there is also a subgroup of patients who do not purge (nonpurging bulimia nervosa). As a result of the combination of undereating and overeating the weight of most patients with bulimia nervosa tends to be unremarkable and is within the healthy range, BMI = 20–25. Features of depression and anxiety are prominent in these patients. Certain of these patients engage in self-harm and/or substance and alcohol misuse and may attract the diagnosis of borderline personality disorder. Most have few physical complaints, although electrolyte disturbance may occur in those who vomit or take laxatives or diuretics frequently.

The clinical features of patients with eating disorder NOS closely resemble those seen in anorexia nervosa and bulimia nervosa and are of comparable duration and severity.[7] Within this diagnostic grouping 3 subgroups may be distinguished, although there are no sharp boundaries among them. The first group consists of cases that closely resemble anorexia nervosa or bulimia nervosa but just fail to meet the threshold set by the diagnostic criteria (eg, binge eating may not be frequent enough to meet criteria for BN or weight may be just above the threshold in AN); the second and largest subgroup comprises cases in which the features of AN and BN occur in different combinations from that seen in the prototypic disorders—these states may be best viewed as "mixed" in character—and the third subgroup comprises those with binge-eating disorder. Most patients with binge-eating disorder are overweight (BMI = 25–30) or meet criteria for obesity (BMI ≥ 30).

THE EMPIRICAL STATUS OF COGNITIVE BEHAVIORAL THERAPY FOR EATING DISORDERS

Consistent with the current way of classifying eating disorders, the research on their treatment has focused on the particular disorders in isolation. Wilson and colleagues[8] have provided a narrative review of the studies of the treatment of the 2 specific eating disorders as well as eating disorder NOS, and an authoritative meta-analysis has been conducted by the UK National Institute for Health and Clinical Excellence (NICE).[1] This systematic review is particularly rigorous and, as with all NICE reviews, it forms the basis for evidence-based guidelines for clinical management.

The conclusion from the NICE review, and 2 other recent systematic reviews,[9,10] is that cognitive behavioral therapy (CBT-BN) is the clear leading treatment for bulimia nervosa in adults. However, this is not to imply that CBT-BN is a panacea, as the orig-inal version of the treatment resulted in only fewer than half of the patients who completed treatment making a full and lasting recovery.[8] The new "enhanced" version of the treatment (CBT-E) appears to be more effective.[2]

Interpersonal psychotherapy (IPT) is a potential evidence-based alternative to CBT-BN in patients with bulimia nervosa and it involves a similar amount of thera-peutic contact, but there have been fewer studies of it.[11,12] IPT takes 8 to 12 months longer than CBT-BN to achieve a comparable effect. Antidepressant medication (eg, fluoxetine at a dose of 60 mg daily) has also been found to have a beneficial effect on binge eating in bulimia nervosa but not as great as that obtained with CBT-BN and the long-term effects remain largely untested.[13] Combining CBT-BN with antidepressant medication does not appear to offer any clear advantage over CBT-BN alone.[13] The treatment of adolescents with bulimia nervosa has received relatively little research attention to date.

There has been much less research on the treatment of anorexia nervosa. Most of the studies suffer from small sample sizes and some from high rates of attrition. As a result, there is little evidence to support any psychological treatment, at least in adults. In adolescents the research has focused mainly on family therapy, with the result that the status of CBT in younger patients is unclear.

Preliminary findings have been reported from a 3-site study of the use of the enhanced form of CBT (CBT-E) to treat outpatients with anorexia nervosa.[14] This is the largest study of the treatment of anorexia nervosa to date. In brief, it appears that the treatment can be used to treat about 60% of outpatients with the disorder (BMI 15.0 to 17.5) and that in these patients about 60% have a good outcome. Interestingly and importantly the relapse rate appears low.

There is a growing body of research on the treatment of binge-eating disorder. This research has been the subject of a recent narrative review[15] and several systematic reviews.[1,16,17] The strongest support is for a form of CBT similar to that used to treat BN (CBT-BED). This treatment has been found to have a sustained and marked effect on binge eating, but it has little effect on body weight, which is typically raised in these patients. Arguably the leading first-line treatment is a form of guided cognitive behavioral self-help as it is relatively simple to administer and reasonably effective.[18]

Until recently, there had been almost no research on the treatment of forms of eating disorder NOS other than binge-eating disorder despite their severity and prevalence.[7] However, recently the first randomized controlled trial of the enhanced form of CBT found that CBT-E was as effective for patients with eating disorder NOS (who were not significantly underweight; BMI >17.5) as it was for patients with bulimia nervosa with two-thirds of those who completed treatment having a good outcome.[2]

In summary, CBT is the treatment of choice for bulimia nervosa and for binge-eating disorder with the best results being obtained with the new "enhanced" form of the treatment. Recent research provides support for the use of this treatment with patients with eating disorder NOS and those with anorexia nervosa.

The remainder of this article provides a description of this transdiagnostic form of CBT.

THE COGNITIVE BEHAVIORAL ACCOUNT OF EATING DISORDERS

Although the DSM-IV classification of eating disorders encourages the view that they are distinct conditions, each requiring their own form of treatment, there are reasons to question this view. Indeed, it has recently been pointed out that what is most striking about the eating disorders is not what distinguishes them but how much they have in common.[19] As noted earlier, they share many clinical features, including the characteristic core psychopathology of eating disorders: the overevaluation of the importance of shape and weight. In addition, longitudinal studies indicate that most patients migrate among diagnoses over time.[20] This temporal movement among diagnostic categories, together with the shared psychopathology, has led to the proposal that there may be limited utility in distinguishing among the disorders[19] and furthermore that common "transdiagnostic" mechanisms may be involved in their maintenance.

The transdiagnostic cognitive behavioral account of the eating disorders[19] extends the original theory of bulimia nervosa[21] to all eating disorders. According to this theory, the overevaluation of shape and weight and their control is central to the maintenance of all eating disorders. Most of the other clinical features can be understood as result-ing directly from this psychopathology. It results in dietary restraint and restriction; preoccupation with thoughts about food and eating, weight and shape; the repeated checking of body shape and weight or its avoidance; and the engaging in extreme methods of weight control. The one feature that is not a direct expression of the core psychopathology is binge eating. This occurs in all cases of bulimia nervosa, many cases of eating disorder NOS, and some cases of anorexia nervosa. The cogni-tive behavioral account proposes that such episodes are largely the result of attempts to adhere to multiple extreme, and highly specific, dietary rules. The repeated breaking of these rules is almost inevitable and patients tend to react negatively to such dietary slips, generally viewing them as evidence of their poor self-control. They typically respond by temporarily abandoning their efforts to restrict their eating with binge eating being the result. This in turn maintains the core psychopathology by intensifying patients' concerns about their ability to control their eating, shape, and weight. It also encourages more dietary restraint, thereby increasing the risk of further binge eating.

Three further processes may also maintain binge eating. First, difficulties in the patient's life and associated mood changes make it difficult to maintain dietary restraint. Second, as binge eating temporarily alleviates negative mood states and distracts patients from their difficulties, it can become a way of coping with such prob-lems. Third, in patients who engage in compensatory purging, the mistaken belief in the effectiveness of vomiting and laxative misuse as a means of weight control results in a major deterrent against binge eating being removed.

In patients who are underweight, the physiological and psychological conse-quences may also contribute to the maintenance of the eating disorder. For example, delayed gastric emptying leads to feelings of fullness even after patients have eaten only modest amounts of food. In addition, the social withdrawal and loss of previous interests prevent patients from being exposed to experiences that might diminish the importance they place on shape and weight.

The composite "transdiagnostic" formulation is shown in **Fig. 1**. This illustrates the core processes that are hypothesized to maintain the full range of eating disorders.

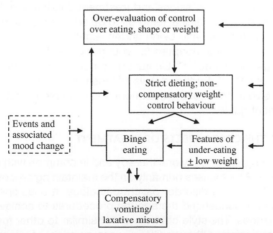

Fig. 1. The composite "transdiagnostic" cognitive behavioral formulation. (Fairburn CG. Eating disorders: the transdiagnostic view and the cognitive behavioral theory. In: Fair-burn CG. Cognitive behavior therapy and eating disorders. New York: Guilford Press; 2008. p. 7–22).

When applied to individual patients, its precise form will depend on the psychopathology present. In some patients, most of the processes are in operation (for example, in cases of anorexia nervosa binge-purge subtype) but in others only a few are active (for example, in binge-eating disorder). Thus, for each patient the formulation is driven by their individual psychopathology rather than their DSM diagnosis. As such, the formulation provides a guide to those processes that need to be addressed in treatment.

ENHANCED COGNITIVE BEHAVIORAL THERAPY

"Enhanced" cognitive behavioral therapy (CBT-E) is based on the transdiagnostic theory outlined earlier and was derived from CBT-BN. It is designed to treat eating disorder psychopathology rather than an eating disorder diagnosis, with its exact form in any particular case depending on an individualized formulation of the processes maintaining the disorder. CBT-E is designed to be delivered on an individual basis to adult patients with any eating disorder of clinical severity who are appropriate to treat on an outpatient basis. It is described as "enhanced" because it uses a variety of new strategies and procedures to improve outcome and because it includes modules to address certain obstacles to change that are "external" to the core eating disorder, namely clinical perfectionism, low self-esteem, and interpersonal difficulties.

There are 2 forms of CBT-E. The first is the "focused" form (CBT-Ef) that exclusively addresses eating disorder psychopathology. Current evidence suggests that this form should be viewed as the "default" version, as it is optimal for most patients with eating disorders.[2] The second, a broad form of the treatment (CBT-Eb), addresses external obstacles to change, in addition to the core eating disorder psychopathology. Preliminary evidence suggests that this more complex form of CBT-E should be reserved for patients in whom clinical perfectionism, core low self-esteem, or interpersonal difficulties are pronounced and maintaining the eating disorder.[2]

There are also 2 intensities of CBT-E. With patients who are not significantly underweight (BMI above 17.5), it consists of 20 sessions over 20 weeks. This version is suitable for the great majority of adult outpatients. For patients who have a BMI below 17.5, a commonly used threshold for anorexia nervosa, treatment involves 40 sessions over 40 weeks. The additional sessions and treatment duration are designed to allow sufficient time for 3 additional clinical features to be addressed, namely, limited motivation to change, undereating, and being underweight.

In addition CBT-E has been adapted for younger patients[22] and for inpatient and day patient settings treatment.[23,24] Limitations on space preclude a description of these other forms of CBT-E. Further details of these adaptations of CBT-E, together with a comprehensive account of the treatment and its implementation, can be found in the main treatment guide.[25]

AN OVERVIEW OF THE CORE ASPECTS OF TREATMENT

CBT-E is a form of cognitive behavioral therapy and in common with other empirically supported forms of CBT it focuses primarily on the maintaining processes, in this case those maintaining the eating disorder psychopathology. It uses specified strategies and a flexible series of sequenced therapeutic procedures to achieve both cognitive and behavioral changes. The style of treatment is similar to other forms of CBT, that of collaborative empiricism. Although CBT-E uses a variety of generic cognitive and behavioral interventions (such as addressing cognitive biases), unlike some forms of CBT, it favors the use of strategic changes in behavior to modify thinking rather than direct cognitive restructuring. The eating disorder psychopathology may be likened to a house of cards with the strategy being to identify and remove the key cards that are supporting the eating disorder, thereby bringing down the entire house. Following, we summarize the core features of the focused and broad versions of CBT-E, including adaptations that need to be made for patients who are underweight. The treatment has 4 defined stages.

PREPARATION FOR TREATMENT AND CHANGE

An evaluation interview assessing the nature and extent of the patient's psychiatric problems is conducted before starting treatment.[26] This interview usually takes place over 2 or more appointments. The assessment process is collaborative and designed to put the patient at ease and begin to engage the patient in treatment and in change. Information from the assessment informs how best to proceed and, in particular, whether CBT-E is appropriate. If CBT-E is deemed to be appropriate, the main aspects of the therapy are described and patients are encouraged to make the most of the opportunity to overcome their eating disorder.

It is important that from the outset of CBT-E the patient is in a position to make optimum use of treatment. For this reason any potential barriers to benefiting from CBT-E should be explored. Important contraindications to beginning treatment immediately are physical features of concern, the presence of severe clinical depression, significant substance abuse, major distracting life events or crises, and competing commitments. Such factors should be addressed first before embarking on treatment.

STAGE ONE

It is crucial that treatment starts well. This is consistent with evidence that the magnitude of change achieved early in treatment is a good predictor of treatment outcome.[27,28] This initial intensive stage, designed to achieve initial therapeutic momentum, involves approximately 8 sessions held twice weekly over 4 weeks. The aims of this first stage are to engage the patient in treatment and change, to derive a personalized formulation (case conceptualization) with the patient, to provide education about treatment and the disorder, and to introduce and implement 2 important procedures: collaborative "weekly weighing" and "regular eating." The changes made in this first stage of treatment form the foundation on which other changes are built.

Engaging the Patient in Treatment and Change

Many patients with eating disorders are ambivalent about treatment and change. Getting patients "on board" with treatment is a necessary first step. Engagement can be enhanced by conducting the assessment of the eating disorder in a way that helps the patient to become involved in, and hopeful about, the possibility of change and encourages the patient to take "ownership" of treatment.

Jointly Creating the Formulation

This is usually done in the first treatment session and is a personalized visual representation of the processes that appear to be maintaining the eating problem. The therapist draws out the relevant sections of **Fig. 1** in collaboration with the patient, incorporating the patient's own experiences and words. It is usually best to start with something the patient wishes to change (eg, binge eating). The formulation helps patients to realize both that their behavior is comprehensible and that it is maintained by a series of interacting self-perpetuating mechanisms that are open to change. It is explained that "the diagram" provides a guide to what needs to be targeted in treatment if patients are to achieve a full and lasting recovery. At this early stage in treatment the therapist should explain that it is provisional and may need to be modified as treatment progresses and understanding of the patient's eating problem increases.

Establishing Real-time Self-monitoring

This is the ongoing "in-the-moment" recording of eating and other relevant behavior, thoughts, feelings, and events (**Fig. 2** is an example of a monitoring record). Self-monitoring is introduced in the initial session and continues to occupy an essential and central role throughout most of treatment. Therapists should clearly explain the reasons for self-monitoring. First, that it enables further understanding of the eating problem and it identifies progress. Second, and more importantly, it helps patients

Day ...... **Monday** ....   Date ...... **March 19** ....

Time	Food and drink consumed	Place	*	v/l	Context and comments
6.30	Glass water	Kitchen			Feeling good this morning
7:10	Banana Bowl cheerios Skim milk Black coffee	Cafe			Normal breakfast
10:00	Apple Cereal bar	Desk at work			Didn't want to have this as having big lunch, but wanted to stick to plan.
1:00	Greek salad with feta cheese and dressing Roll water	Cafe			Decided that I would eat 3/4 of salad beforehand. Was pretty nervous the whole time, but was able to eat it and keep it down!
3:00	Yogurt	Desk at work			Thought about not eating this, but didn't want a huge gap.
6:30	Salmon (small piece) Rice (1/2 cup) spinach	Kitchen			Feeling ok.
9:30	Ice cream cone with hot fudge	Ice cream parlor with friends			Planned to have 2 scoops and was fine! Really enjoyed getting this with my friends as I usually don't go.

Fig. 2. An example monitoring record. (Fairburn CG, Cooper Z, Shafran R, et al. Enhanced cognitive behavior therapy for eating disorders: the core protocol. In: Fairburn CG. Cognitive behavior therapy and eating disorders. New York: Guilford Press; 2008. p. 47–193.)

to be more aware of what is happening *in the moment* so that they can begin to make changes to behavior that may have seemed automatic or beyond their control. Fundamental to establishing accurate recording is jointly reviewing the patient's records each session and discussing the process of recording and any difficulties with this. The records also help inform the agenda for the session: it is best to save any problems identified in the records for the main part of the session.

Establishing Collaborative "Weekly Weighing"

The patient and therapist check the patient's weight once a week and plot it on an individualized weight graph. Patients are strongly encouraged not to weigh themselves at other times. Weekly in-session weighing has several purposes. First, it provides an opportunity for the therapist to educate patients about body weight and help patients to interpret the numbers on the scale, which otherwise they are prone to misinterpret. Second, it provides patients with accurate data about their weight at a time when their eating habits are changing. Third, and most importantly, it addresses the maintaining processes of excessive body weight checking or its avoidance.

Providing Education

From session 1 onward, an important element of treatment is education about weight and eating, as many patients have misconceptions that maintain their eating disorder. Some of the main topics to cover are as follows:

- The characteristic features of eating disorders including their associated physical and psychosocial effects
- Body weight and its regulation: the body mass index and its interpretation; natural weight fluctuations; and the effects of treatment on weight
- Ineffectiveness of vomiting, laxatives, and diuretics as a means of weight control
- Adverse effects of dieting: the types of dieting that promote binge eating; dietary rules versus dietary guidelines.

To provide reliable information on these topics, patients are asked to read relevant sections from one of the authoritative books on eating disorders[29,30] and their reading is discussed in subsequent treatment sessions.

Establishing "Regular Eating"

Establishing a pattern of regular eating is fundamental to successful treatment whatever the form of the eating disorder. It addresses an important type of dieting ("delayed eating"); it displaces most episodes of binge eating; it structures people's days and, for underweight patients, it introduces meals and snacks that can be subsequently increased in size. Early in treatment (usually by the third session) patients are asked to eat 3 planned meals each day plus 2 or 3 planned snacks so that there is rarely more than a 4-hour interval between them. Patients are also asked to confine their eating to these meals and snacks. They should choose what they eat with the only condition being that the meals and snacks are not followed by any compensatory behavior (eg, self-induced vomiting or laxative misuse). The new eating pattern should take precedence over other activities but should not be so inflexible as to preclude the possibility of adjusting timings to suit the patients' commitments each day.

Patients should be helped to adhere to their regular eating plan and to resist eating between the planned meals and snacks. Two rather different strategies may be used to achieve the latter goals. The first involves helping patients to identify activities that are incompatible with eating and likely to distract them from the urge to binge eat (eg, taking a brisk walk) and strategies that make binge eating less likely (eg, leaving the kitchen). The second is to help patients to recognize that the urge to binge eat is a temporary phenomenon that can be "surfed." Some "residual binges" are likely to persist, however, and these are addressed later.

Involving Significant Others

The treatment is primarily an individual treatment for adults. Despite this, "significant others" are seen if this is likely to facilitate treatment and the patient is willing for this to happen. There are 2 reasons for seeing others: if they could help the patient in making changes or if others are making it difficult for the patient to change, for example, by commenting adversely on eating or appearance.

STAGE TWO

Stage two is a brief, but essential, transitional stage that generally comprises 2 appointments, a week apart. While continuing with the procedures introduced in Stage one, the therapist and patient take stock and conduct a joint review of progress, the goal being to identify problems still to be addressed and any emerging barriers to change, to revise the formulation if necessary, and to design Stage three. The review serves several purposes. If patients are making good progress they should be praised for their efforts and helpful changes reinforced. If patients are not doing well, the explanation needs to be understood and addressed. If clinical perfectionism, core low self-esteem or relationship difficulties appear to be responsible, this would be an indication for implementing the broad version of the treatment.

STAGE THREE

This is the main body of treatment. Its aim is to address the key processes that are maintaining the patient's eating disorder. The mechanisms addressed, and the order in which these are tackled, depend upon their role and relative importance in maintaining the patient's psychopathology. There are generally 8 weekly appointments.

Addressing the Overevaluation of Shape and Weight

Identifying the overevaluation and its consequences

The first step involves explaining the concept of self-evaluation and helping patients identify how they evaluate themselves. The relative importance of the various domains that are relevant may be represented as a pie chart (**Fig. 3** is an example of a pie chart with extended formulation), which for most patients is dominated by a large slice representing shape and weight and controlling eating.

The patient and therapist then identify the problems inherent in this scheme for self-evaluation. Briefly there are 3 related problems: first, self-evaluation is overly dependent on performance in one area of life with the result that domains other than shape and weight are marginalized; second, the area of controlling shape and weight is one in which success is elusive, thus undermining self-esteem; and third, the overevaluation is responsible for the behavior that characterizes the eating disorder (dieting, binge eating, and so forth).[31]

The final step in the consideration of self-evaluation is the creation of an "extended formulation" depicting the main expressions of the overevaluation of shape and weight: dieting, body checking and body avoidance, feeling fat, and marginalization of other areas of life. The therapist uses this extended formulation to explain how these

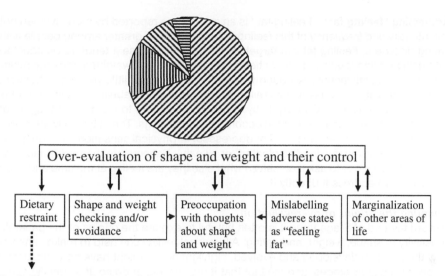

Fig. 3. The overevaluation of shape and weight and their control: an extended formulation. (Fairburn CG, Cooper Z, Shafran R, et al. Enhanced cognitive behavior therapy for eating disorders: the core protocol. In: Fairburn CG. Cognitive behavior therapy and eating disorders. New York: Guilford Press; 2008. p. 47–193.)

behaviors and experiences serve to maintain and magnify the patient's concerns about shape and weight and thus they need to be addressed in treatment.

Enhancing the importance of other domains for self-evaluation
An indirect, yet powerful, means of diminishing the overevaluation of shape and weight is helping patients increase the number and significance of other domains for self-evaluation. Engaging in other aspects of their life that may have been pushed aside by the eating disorder results in these other areas becoming more important in the patient's self-evaluation. Briefly, this involves identifying activities or areas of life that the patient would like to engage in and helping them do so.

A second, direct, strategy is to target the behavioral expressions of the overevaluation of shape and weight. This is done at the same time as enhancing the other domains for self-evaluation and it involves tackling body checking, body avoidance, and feeling fat.

Addressing body checking and avoidance Patients are often not aware that they are engaging in body checking and that it is maintaining their body dissatisfaction. The first step is therefore to obtain detailed information about their checking behavior by asking patients to monitor it. Patients are then educated about the adverse effects of repeated body checking as the way in which they check tends to provide biased information that leads them to feel dissatisfied. For example, scrutinizing parts of one's body magnifies apparent defects, and only comparing oneself to thin and attractive people leads one to draw the conclusion that one is unattractive. Most patients need substantial and detailed help to curb their repeated body checking and invariably attention needs to be devoted to their mirror use.

Patients who avoid seeing their bodies also need considerable help. They should be encouraged to progressively get used to the sight and feel of their body. This may take many successive sessions.

Addressing "feeling fat" "Feeling fat" is an experience reported by many women but the intensity and frequency of this feeling appears to be far greater among people with eating disorders. Feeling fat is a target for treatment because it tends to be equated with being fat (irrespective of the patient's actual shape and weight) and hence maintains body dissatisfaction. Although this topic has received little research attention, clinical observation suggests that feeling fat is a result of mislabeling certain emotions and bodily experiences. Consequently, patients are helped to identify the triggers of their feeling fat experiences and the accompanying feelings. These typically are negative mood states (eg, feeling bored or depressed) or physical sensations that heighten body awareness (eg, feeling full, bloated, or sweaty). Patients are then helped to view "feeling fat" as a cue to ask themselves what else they are feeling at the time and once recognized to address it directly.

Exploring the origins of overevaluation

Toward the end of Stage three it is often helpful to explore the origins of the patient's sensitivity to shape, weight, and eating. A historical review can help to make sense of how the problem developed and evolved, highlight how it might have served a useful function in its early stages, and the fact that it may no longer do so. If a specific event appears to have played a critical role in the development of the eating problem, the patient should be helped to reappraise this from the vantage point of the present. This review helps patients distance themselves further from the eating disorder frame of mind or "mindset."

Addressing Dietary Rules

Patients are helped to recognize that their multiple extreme and rigid dietary rules impair their quality of life and are a central feature of the eating disorder. A major goal of treatment is therefore to reduce, if not eliminate altogether, dieting. The first step in doing so is to identify the patient's various dietary rules together with the beliefs that underlie them. The patient is then helped to break these rules to test the beliefs in question and to learn that the feared consequences that maintain the dietary rule (typically weight gain or binge eating) are not an inevitable result. With patients who binge eat, it is important to pay particular attention to "food avoidance" (the avoidance of specific foods) as this is a major contributory factor. These patients need to systematically re-introduce the avoided food into their diet.

Addressing Event-related Changes in Eating

Among many patients with eating disorders, eating habits change in response to outside events and changes in their mood. The change may involve eating less, stopping eating altogether, overeating, or binge eating. If these changes are prominent, patients need help to deal directly with the triggers. Generally this may be achieved by training them in "proactive" problem solving coupled with the use of functional means of modulating mood.

Addressing Clinical Perfectionism, Low Self-esteem, and Interpersonal Problems

As noted earlier, there are 2 main forms of CBT-E. The components of the focused version are described previously. The "broad" version also includes these strategies and procedures but, in addition, addresses one or more "external" (to the core eating disorder) processes that may be maintaining the eating disorder. It is designed for patients in whom clinical perfectionism, core low self-esteem, or marked interpersonal problems are pronounced and appear to be contributing to the eating disorder. If the therapist decides, in the review of progress (Stage two), to use one or more of these modules, they should become a major component of all subsequent sessions. In the original version of the broad form of CBT-E a fourth module, "mood intolerance," was included but this has since been integrated in to the standard, focused, form of the treatment as part of addressing events and moods. A description of the main elements of the 3 modules follows. A more detailed account is available in the main treatment guide.[32]

Addressing clinical perfectionism

The psychopathology of clinical perfectionism is similar to that of an eating disorder.[33] Its core is the overevaluation of striving to achieve and achievement itself. People with clinical perfectionism judge themselves largely, or exclusively, in terms of working hard toward, and meeting, personally demanding standards in areas of life that they value. If they have a coexisting eating disorder such extreme standards are applied to their eating, weight, and shape. This intensifies key aspects of the eating disorder including dietary restraint, exercise, and shape checking. It is usually evident from the patient's behavior and it can interfere with important aspects of treatment, leading to, for example, overly detailed recording and a strong resistance to relaxing dietary restraint.

The strategy for addressing clinical perfectionism mirrors that used to address the overevaluation of shape and weight and the two can be addressed more or less at the same time. The first step is to add perfectionism to the patient's formulation and to consider the consequences of this for the patient and his or her life, including the self-evaluation pie-chart. Patients are then encouraged to take steps to enhance the importance of other, nonperformance related, domains for self-evaluation.

It is helpful to consider collaboratively patients' goals in areas of life that they value, which are usually multiple, rigid, and extreme, and whether these goals are in fact counterproductive and impairing their actual performance. Performance checking is addressed similarly to shape checking, beginning by first asking patients to record times when they are checking their performance. Then the therapist helps them appreciate that the data they obtain is likely to be skewed as a result of using biased assessment processes, such as selective attention to failure. Avoidance and procrastination also need to be addressed, as they interfere with patients being able to assess their true ability with the result that their fears of failure are maintained.

Addressing core low self-esteem

People with core low self-esteem (CLSE) have a longstanding and pervasive negative view of themselves. It is largely independent of the person's actual performance in life (ie, it is unconditional) and is not secondary to the presence of the eating disorder. The presence of CLSE results in the individual striving especially hard to control eating, weight, and shape to retain some sense of self-worth. It is generally a barrier to engaging in treatment as patients do not feel they deserve treatment nor do they believe that they can benefit from it.

If it is to be directly addressed in treatment, it is added to the patient's formulation in Stage two and tackled alongside, although slightly later than, the steps addressing the overevaluation of shape and weight. This involves educating patients about the role of CLSE in maintaining the eating disorder and contributing to other difficulties in their life. Patients are helped to identify and modify the main cognitive maintaining processes, including discounting positive qualities and the overgeneralization of apparent failures. Previous views of the self are reappraised, using both cognitive restructuring and behavioral experiments, to help patients to reach a more balanced view of their self-worth.

Addressing interpersonal problems

Interpersonal problems are common among patients with eating disorders, although they generally improve as the eating disorder resolves. Such problems may include conflict with others and difficulties developing close relationships. If these problems, and the resulting effects on mood, directly influence the patient's eating, they may be addressed through the use of proactive problem solving and functional mood modulation and acceptance (as described earlier). However, in some cases interpersonal problems powerfully maintain the eating disorder through a variety of direct and indirect processes or they interfere with treatment itself. Under these circumstances, they need to become a focus of treatment in their own right.

The strategy used in CBT-E is to use a different psychological treatment to achieve interpersonal change, namely Interpersonal Psychotherapy (IPT). This is an evidence-based treatment that helps patients identify and address current interpersonal problems. In style and content IPT is very different from CBT-E. For this reason it is not "integrated" with CBT-E as such: rather, each session has a CBT-E component and an IPT one. More detailed information about IPT and its use with patients with eating disorders is available in a recent book chapter.[34]

STAGE FOUR

Stage four, the final stage in treatment, is concerned with ending treatment well. The focus is on maintaining the progress that has already been made and reducing the risk of relapse. Typically there are 3 appointments about 2 weeks apart. During this stage, as part of their preparation for the ending of treatment, patients discontinue self-monitoring and begin weekly weighing at home.

To maximize the chances that progress is maintained, the therapist and patient jointly devise a personalized plan for the following few months until a posttreatment review appointment (usually about 20 weeks later). Typically this includes further work on body checking, food avoidance, and perhaps further practice at problem solving. In addition, patients are encouraged to continue their efforts to develop new interests and activities.

There are 2 elements to minimizing the risk of relapse. First, patients need to have realistic expectations regarding the future. Expecting never to experience any eating difficulties again makes patients vulnerable to relapse because it encourages a negative reaction to even minor setbacks. Instead, patients should view their eating problem as an Achilles heel. The goal is that patients identify setbacks as early as possible, view them as a "lapse" rather than a "relapse," and actively address them using strategies that they learned during treatment.

UNDERWEIGHT PATIENTS

The strategies and procedures described so far are also relevant to patients who are underweight (mostly cases of anorexia nervosa but some cases of eating disorder NOS). However, CBT-E has to be modified to address certain characteristics of these patients.

The first priority is to address motivation, as often these patients do not view undereating or being underweight as a problem. This may be done in several ways and relies on a good therapeutic alliance. The patient is provided with a personalized education about the psychological and physical effects of being underweight. This helps them to understand that some of the things that they find difficult (eg, being obsessive and indecisive, being unable to be spontaneous, being socially avoidant, lacking sexual appetite) are a direct consequence of being a low weight rather than being a reflection of their true personality. The patient is helped to think through the advantages and disadvantages of change, including a consideration of how things are likely to be in the future if they choose not to change and how this would fit with their aspirations. The therapist shows intense interest in the patient as a person, beyond the eating disorder, and helps them to reflect on the state of all aspects of their life, including their relationships, their physical and psychological well-being, their work, and their personal values. The patient is encouraged to experiment with making changes to learn more about the pros and cons of their current behavior. The goal is for patients themselves to decide to regain weight rather than this decision being imposed by the therapist. If this is successful, it greatly assists subsequent weight regain.

Second, the undereating and the consequent state of starvation must be addressed. It is important to help patients to realize that undereating, and being underweight maintain the eating disorder and this is illustrated in a personalized formulation. Once the patient has agreed to regain weight it is explained that weight regain should be gradual and steady and that they should aim to maintain an average energy surplus of 500 calories each day to regain an average of 0.5 kg (1.1 lb) per week. The therapist helps the patient to devise and implement a daily plan of eating (which may be supplemented by energy-rich drinks) that meets this target.

Treatment needs to be extended from the typical 20 weeks to about 40 weeks to allow sufficient time for patients to decide to change, to reach a healthy weight, and then practice maintaining it. It can be helpful to involve others in the weight-gain process to facilitate the patient's own efforts. This is especially so with young patients who are living at home with their parents.

FINAL COMMENTS

Hopefully it will be clear from this brief account of CBT for eating disorders that major advances have been made and are continuing to be made. Perhaps most prominent among these is the adoption of a transdiagnostic approach to treatment whereby treatment is no longer for a specific eating disorder (eg, bulimia nervosa) but is directed at eating disorder psychopathology and the processes that maintains it. As a result, an empirically supported treatment approach has evolved that is suitable for all forms of eating disorder and one that is highly individualized.

Many challenges remain. First and foremost, treatment outcome needs to be further improved, especially in the case of patients who are substantially underweight. Second, understanding more about the way in which treatment works, and the active ingredients of treatment, could inform the design of a more potent version. Doubtless some elements could be discarded whereas others may need to be enhanced.[35] We need treatments that are effective and efficient. Last, we need to facilitate the dissemination of evidence-based practice. Many patients receive suboptimal treatment. There are several possible reasons for this but prominent among them is the fact that few therapists have received the necessary training.

REFERENCES

1. National Institute for Clinical Excellence (NICE). Eating disorders—core interventions in the treatment and management of anorexia nervosa, bulimia nervosa and related eating disorders. London: NICE; 2004. Available at: http://www.nice.org. uk. Accessed October 2009. NICE Clinical Guidance No. 9.
2. Fairburn CG, Cooper Z, Doll HA, et al. Transdiagnostic cognitive behavioral therapy for patients with eating disorders: a two-site trial with 60-week follow-up. Am J Psychiatry 2009;166:311–9.

3. American Psychiatric Association. Diagnostic and statistical manual of mental disorders. 4th edition. Washington, DC: American Psychiatric Association; 1994.

4. Fairburn CG, Bohn K. Eating disorder NOS (EDNOS): an example of the troublesome "not otherwise specified" (NOS) category in DSM-IV. Behav Res Ther 2005; 43:691–701.

5. Dalle Grave R, Calugi S. Eating disorder not otherwise specified on an inpatient unit. Eur Eat Disord Rev 2007;15:340–9.

6. Miller G, Holden C. Proposed revisions to psychiatry's canon unveiled. Science 2010;327(5967):770–1.

7. Fairburn CG, Cooper Z, Bohn K, et al. The severity and status of eating disorder NOS: implications for DSM-V. Behav Res Ther 2007;45(8):1705–15.

8. Wilson GT, Grilo CM, Vitousek KM. Psychological treatment of eating disorders. Am Psychol 2007;62(3):199–216.

9. Shapiro JR, Berkamn ND, Brownley KA, et al. Bulimia nervosa treatment: a systematic review of randomized controlled trials. Int J Eat Disord 2007;40(4):321–36.

10. Hay PPJ, Bacaltchuk J, Stefano S, et al. Psychological treatments for bulimia nervosa and binging. Cochrane Database Syst Rev 2009;4:CD000562.

11. Fairburn CG, Jones R, Peveler RC, et al. Psychotherapy and bulimia nervosa: the longer-term effects of interpersonal psychotherapy, behaviour therapy and cognitive behaviour therapy. Arch Gen Psychiatry 1993;50:419–28.

12. Agras WS, Walsh BT, Fairburn CG, et al. A multicenter comparison of cognitive behavioral therapy and interpersonal psychotherapy for bulimia nervosa. Arch Gen Psychiatry 2000;57:459–66.

13. Wilson GT, Fairburn CG. Treatments for eating disorders. In: Nathan PE, Gorman JM, editors. A guide to treatments that work. 3rd edition. New York: Oxford University Press; 2007. p. 581–3.

14. Fairburn CG. Transdiagnostic CBT for eating disorders "CBT-E", presented at association for behavioral and cognitive therapy. New York; 2009.

15. Mitchell J, Devlin M, de Zwaan M, et al. Binge eating disorder. Clinical foundations and treatment. New York: Guilford; 2008. p. 65–9.

16. Brownley KA, Berkman ND, Sedway JA, et al. Binge eating disorder treatment: a systematic review of randomized controlled trials. Int J Eat Disord 2007;40: 337–48.

17. Sysko R, Walsh T. A critical evaluation of the efficacy of self-help interventions for the treatment of bulimia nervosa and binge-eating disorder. Int J Eat Disord 2008; 41:97–112.

18. Wilson GT, Wilfley DE, Agras WS, et al. Psychological treatments of binge eating disorder. Arch Gen Psychiatry 2010;67(1):94–101.

19. Fairburn CG, Cooper Z, Shafran R. Cognitive behaviour therapy for eating disorders: a "transdiagnostic" theory and treatment. Behav Res Ther 2003;41:509–28.

20. Fairburn CG, Harrison PJ. Eating disorders. Lancet 2003;361:407–16.

21. Fairburn CG, Cooper Z, Cooper P. The clinical features and maintenance of bulimia nervosa. In: Brownwell KD, Foreyt JP, editors. Physiology, psychology and treatment of eating disorders. New York: Basic Books; 1986. p. 389–404.

22. Cooper Z, Stewart A. CBT-E and the younger patient. In: Fairburn CG, editor. Cognitive behavior therapy and eating disorders. New York: Guilford Press; 2008. p. 221–30.

23. Dalle Grave R, Bohn K, Hawker D, et al. Inpatient, day patient, and two forms of outpatient CBT-E. In: Fairburn CG, editor. Cognitive behavior therapy and eating disorders. New York: Guilford Press; 2008. p. 231–44.

24. Dalle Grave R, Fairburn CG. Intensive CBT for eating disorders. New York: Guilford Press, in press.
25. Fairburn CG. Cognitive behavior therapy and eating disorders. New York: Guilford Press; 2008.
26. Fairburn CG, Cooper Z, Waller D. The patients: their assessment, preparation for treatment and medical management. In: Fairburn CG, editor. Cognitive behavior therapy and eating disorders. New York: Guilford Press; 2008. p. 35–40.
27. Fairburn CG, Agras WS, Walsh BT, et al. Prediction of outcome in bulimia nervosa by early change in treatment. Am J Psychiatry 2004;161:2322–4.
28. Agras WS, Crow SJ, Halmi KA, et al. Outcome predictors for the cognitive-behavioral treatment of bulimia nervosa: data from a multisite study. Am J Psychiatry 2000;157:1302–8.
29. Fairburn CG. Overcoming binge eating. New York: Guilford Press; 1995.
30. Schmidt U, Treasure J. Getting better bit(e) by bit(e). A survival guide for sufferers of bulimia nervosa and binge eating disorders. Hove (UK): Psychology Press; 1993.
31. Fairburn CG, Cooper Z, Shafran R, et al. Enhanced cognitive behavior therapy for eating disorders: the core protocol. In: Fairburn CG, editor. Cognitive behavior therapy and eating disorders. New York: Guilford Press; 2008. p. 47–193.
32. Fairburn CG, Cooper Z, Shafran R, et al. Clinical perfectionism, core low self-esteem and interpersonal problems. In: Fairburn CG, editor. Cognitive behavior therapy and eating disorders. New York: Guilford Press; 2008. p. 47–123.
33. Shafran R, Cooper Z, Fairburn CG. Clinical perfectionism: a cognitive-behavioural analysis. Behav Res Ther 2002;40:773–91.
34. Murphy R, Straebler S, Cooper Z, et al. Interpersonal psychotherapy (IPT) for eating disorders. In: Dancyger IF, Fornari VM, editors. Evidence based treatments for eating disorders. New York: Nova Science Publishers; 2009. p. 257–74.
35. Kazdin AE, Nock MK. Delineating mechanisms of change in child and adolescent therapy: methodological issues and research recommendations. J Child Psychol Psychiatry 2003;44:1116–29.

Cognitive Behavioral Therapy for Sleep Disorders

Kimberly A. Babson, MA*, Matthew T. Feldner, PhD,
Christal L. Badour, BA

KEYWORDS

- Primary insomnia • Cognitive behavioral therapy
- Sleep disorders • Outcomes research

Primary sleep disorders are defined as sleep disorders in which the etiology is not due to another mental disorder, medical condition, or substance use. Instead, the cause of primary sleep disorders is thought to arise from organic complications in the sleep-wake cycle.[1] Primary sleep disorders can be divided into two subgroups. First, dyssomnias (complications in the amount, quality, or timing of sleep) include primary insomnia, primary hypersomnia, narcolepsy, breathing-related sleep disorder, circadian-rhythm sleep disorder, and dyssomnia not otherwise specified. Second, parasomnias (abnormal behavioral or physiological events occurring during sleep, specific sleep stages, or sleep-wake transitions) include nightmare disorder, sleep terror disorder, sleepwalking disorder, and parasomnia not otherwise specified.[1] Of these sleep disorders, dyssomnias are the most common primary forms. Primary insomnia (PI), defined as difficulty initiating or maintaining sleep or nonrestorative sleep that persists for at least 1 month and is accompanied by significant distress or functional impairment,[1] is the most common form of dyssomnia. Over 70 million people within the United States experience PI at some point in their life, resulting in an estimated $65 billion in health care costs and lost productivity; this makes PI one of the most common health care problems in the United States.[2] Worldwide, PI accounts for 3.6 million years of productive life lost.[3] To mollify the negative effects of PI, scholars have sought to evaluate and improve treatments for this costly health care problem.

Early cognitive behavioral approaches for PI incorporated behavioral techniques including relaxation, stimulus control, sleep restriction, and sleep hygiene. Relaxation therapy includes techniques such as progressive muscle relaxation, breathing retraining, guided imagery, autogenic training, meditation, and biofeedback. Relaxation therapies target reductions in cognitive and/or physiological arousal. When relaxation

Department of Psychology, University of Arkansas, 216 Memorial Hall, Fayetteville, AR 72701, USA
* Corresponding author.
E-mail address: kbabson@uark.edu

Psychiatr Clin N Am 33 (2010) 629–640
doi:10.1016/j.psc.2010.04.011
0193-953X/10/$ – see front matter © 2010 Elsevier Inc. All rights reserved.

strategies are employed in the sleep environment, the environment can become conditioned to initiate relaxation instead of arousal. Stimulus control therapy (SCT) is a second behavioral treatment for PI. SCT aims to recondition the sleep environment for successful sleep. To do this, individuals are instructed: (1) go to bed only when tired; (2) wake up at the same time every day; (3) get out of bed when unable to sleep; (4) avoid other activities in bed, such as reading, eating, and working; and (5) eliminate napping. A third behavioral technique is sleep restriction therapy (SRT). SRT begins by calculating average total sleep time, which is accomplished by completing sleep logs that record amount of time in bed and total amount of time spent sleeping. Total time in bed is then restricted to the average total sleep time. This regime functions to consolidate sleep such that time passed in bed is spent sleeping rather than awake. Following successful sleep consolidation, total time in bed is then increased by 15 to 30 minutes. A final common behavioral component of PI is sleep hygiene. Sleep hygiene is primarily psychoeducational in nature. Clients are provided information about healthy sleep habits. Topics include recommendations to create a restful and calm sleep environment, incorporate daily exercise not too close to bed time, and limiting substance use (including primarily nicotine, alcohol, and caffeine).

SCT and SRT have been shown to be the most efficacious behavioral techniques for PI.[4] However, current conceptualizations of the etiology of PI suggest these behavioral techniques in isolation do not target all of the mechanisms implicated in the maintenance of insomnia. Current theory[5,6] suggests cognitions and behaviors interact to initiate and maintain a cycle of insomnia. For example, cognitive arousal (eg, worry about the consequences of sleep loss) may lead to disruptive sleep behavior (eg, excessive wakeful time in bed). This time spent awake and worrying in bed can result in conditioned behavioral and emotional responses to sleep and sleep cues (eg, bed) culminating in environmental (conditioned response to a bed of wakefulness instead of sleepiness) and physiological (disruption of circadian rhythms) inhibitors of sleep that can initiate and maintain a cycle of insomnia. Based on the theoretical model of insomnia, a combination of techniques has been melded to create current approaches to cognitive behavioral therapy (CBT), which is now the most common nonpharmacological treatment for PI. CBT for PI employs sleep hygiene for psychoeducation, a combination of SCT and SRT to modify behavioral conditioning, and cognitive restructuring of maladaptive beliefs and thoughts. The combination of these components has led to the development of a comprehensive treatment that targets the underlying mechanisms thought to maintain primary insomnia. Of note, terms for the techniques employed during CBT for insomnia are often used interchangeably and may fall into more than one broad category. For example, individuals are instructed to limit the amount of time spent awake in bed; this is a component of both sleep hygiene and stimulus control. For ease of presentation, here the authors use the terminology and definitions as outlined above.

CBT OUTCOME RESEARCH

There has been a wealth of studies conducted to examine whether CBT for PI can work (ie, efficacy studies) as well as whether CBT for PI does work in applied settings (ie, effectiveness studies). These studies examine whether CBT for PI impacts multiple different measures of sleep (ie, sleep parameters). While a range of sleep parameters has been employed, the majority of efficacy and effectiveness research implements 6 main parameters: subjective sleep quality (self-reported quality of sleep), wake after sleep onset (amount of time awake after initially falling asleep), sleep efficiency (ratio between total time asleep and the amount of time spent in bed), total sleep time (total amount of time spent asleep), sleep onset latency (amount of time it takes to fall asleep), and number of awakenings (number of times an individual wakes during the night). An overview of research in this domain now follows.

Efficacy Studies

Treatment efficacy research tests whether treatments can work under controlled conditions, such as when delivered by highly trained clinicians or with specific types of clients. More than 50 randomized clinical trials (RCTs) have demonstrated that CBT for primary insomnia results in reliable and robust improvements across several sleep parameters (including both subjective and objective measures used to index sleep disturbance).[6] For example, 75 adults in a placebo-controlled RCT were assigned to one of the following groups: (1) CBT; (2) progressive muscle relaxation training (RT); or (3) quasi-desensitization (placebo) group. Treatment was conducted in 6 weekly individual sessions led by a beginning-level clinician. In addition, a 6-month follow-up assessment gauged the maintenance of treatment gains. Findings suggested that CBT resulted in greater improvements in subjective sleep problems (sleep quality, wake after sleep onset, and sleep efficiency) and objective sleep problems measured via polysomnograph (total sleep time, wake after sleep onset, and sleep efficiency) compared with both control groups. Furthermore, results were maintained at the 6-month follow-up. In addition, results indicated a nonsignificant difference between the relaxation and placebo groups. Specifically, there was an average of 16% reduction in sleep problems in the relaxation group, whereas a 12% reduction in sleep problems was observed in the placebo condition.[7] In fact, over the past 15 years a series of systematic qualitative and quantitative reviews provide cumulative support for the efficacy of CBT for PI.[4-6,8-15]

Meta-analyses have provided quantitative reviews of the treatment outcome research in this area, yielding estimates of the magnitude of treatment effects resulting from CBT for PI. The most commonly employed index of effect size is Cohen's d statistic, where $d \leq .20$ is considered a small effect and $d \geq .80$ is considered a large effect.[16] A review of 59 studies concluded that CBT for insomnia led to a decrease in sleep onset latency of 27.7 minutes ($d = .88$) and a 32.7-minute improvement in wake after sleep onset ($d = .65$) relative to waitlist and placebo control groups.[4] A second meta-analysis conducted by Murtagh and Greenwood[17] including 66 studies concluded that CBT, compared with a placebo control, led to a 24-minute decrease in sleep onset latency ($d = .88$), 1.2 fewer number of awakenings during the night ($d = .63$), and 32 more minutes of total sleep time ($d = .49$). Of note, treatment gains appeared to be maintained through 8 months.

The efficacy of CBT for PI has also been demonstrated among children and elderly populations. A series of controlled studies and clinical case reports have demonstrated that CBT is an efficacious treatment for childhood sleep disorders.[18] Most research in this area has focused on parent-directed CBT for sleep problems among infants and toddlers.[18] Further research is now needed to extend our knowledge of the efficacy of CBT for treating sleep problems among older children and adolescents. The efficacy of CBT for insomnia has also been investigated among the elderly, in whom sleep problems are experienced at a greater frequency and severity than any other age group.[19] In a meta-analysis of 23 RCTs on CBT for insomnia conducted with elderly samples [2 age cohorts were created: (1) young elderly, with a mean age of 55 and (2) elderly, in which participants were 55 years or older], results indicated significant improvements in sleep quality ($d = .76$), sleep onset latency ($d = .52$), and wake after sleep onset ($d = .64$) across both cohorts (no differences between age cohorts were observed).[20] These results are similar to those demonstrated among young and middle-aged adults.

Overall, meta-analyses of clinical trials have demonstrated that CBT for insomnia is associated with improvements in sleep onset latency, number of awakenings during the night, duration of awakenings during the night, total sleep time, and subjective sleep quality, with effect sizes ranging from moderate to large across multiple age ranges. These statistically significant improvements are further bolstered by the clinical significance of these findings. Clinically meaningful markers have been identified indicating that gains observed in a study are clinically significant, in addition to statistically significant. Markers of clinical significance include: (1) the proportion of individuals who reach 50% or greater improvement on target symptoms, (2) the number of symptoms that fall below the 30-minute cut-off criterion for clinical levels of insomnia (eg, sleep onset latency or wake after sleep onset decreases below 30 minutes), (3) the proportion of people that reach a sleep efficiency of 80%, and (4) the number of people that discontinue use of sleep medications.[15] Based on these markers, meta-analyses have also indicated clinically significant improvements resulting from CBT for PI. For example, Morin and colleagues[4] concluded that 50% of individuals with insomnia reached a 50% or greater level of improvement on target symptoms while 38% of individuals reached 80% or greater improvement in sleep efficiency.

Effectiveness Studies

Extending the efficacy studies summarized above, researchers have investigated if CBT for PI works under less controlled conditions. This type of "real-world" research, referred to here as effectiveness research, has further supported the use of CBT for PI. Effectiveness studies have tested CBT for PI within primary care settings, when used with relatively diverse populations, and when administered by a range of health professionals.

First, the clinical effectiveness of administering CBT within small clinical sleep treatment settings has been examined. Here, patients were referred to the sleep clinics by physicians for the treatment of insomnia. CBT was administered by doctoral level clinical psychologists over 6 sessions. Findings indicated that CBT resulted in decreases in both wake time during the night and sleep onset latency.[21] In a similar study, individuals with insomnia reported decreased sleep onset latency and awakenings after sleep onset as well as increased sleep efficiency 1 month after CBT.[22] These studies combine to suggest that CBT can be effectively administered in small sleep clinic settings for individuals referred with chronic insomnia.

Second, studies have examined the effectiveness of CBT for PI when administered within a primary care setting by nurses trained in the administration of CBT. Treatment consisted of 6 group sessions of CBT. Here, CBT resulted in improvements in both sleep onset latency and awakenings during the night compared with a self-monitoring control group. In addition, treatment outcomes were maintained at a 1-year follow-up and 84% of patients discontinued use of hypnotic sleep medications.[23] The relative impact of individual components of CBT also was investigated during the 1-year follow-up of this study. Results suggested that home use of stimulus control and sleep restriction techniques resulted in the most improvement in sleep onset latency and nighttime awakenings, whereas cognitive restructuring led to a decrease in the amount of time awake during the night; relaxation did not predict improvement in any sleep parameter.[24] These results combine to indicate that CBT administered in a primary care setting by a nurse practitioner trained in CBT administration resulted in both short- and long-term improvement. Of note, continued home use of stimulus control and sleep restriction predicted the best global outcome 1 year post treatment.[23,24]

The effectiveness of group-format CBT for PI also has been investigated. For example, veterans with insomnia and both comorbid psychiatric and physiological conditions in a Veterans' Affairs setting completed CBT in groups of 4 individuals. Treatment was administered by 2 clinical psychologists and was conducted over 8 to 10 weeks. Results indicated improvements in wake after sleep onset, total sleep time, and sleep efficiency among the veterans. In addition, hypnotic sleep medication use was decreased by 50%.[25] While this study investigated the short-term effectiveness of group CBT, a separate study investigated the long-term effects of a brief (4 sessions) group CBT for PI administered by clinical psychologists. Results indicated that brief group CBT was effective for patients with chronic PI. Improvements were noted in total sleep time and sleep efficiency, as well as mood, including a decrease in negative cognitions and depression. Of note, these treatment gains were maintained through a 3-year follow-up.[26] Overall, these findings suggest that group CBT is effective (in as few as 4 sessions) in improving several sleep parameters (ie, total sleep time, sleep efficiency, number of awakenings, amount of time awake after sleep onset, and sleep onset latency) and mood (ie, depression and negative cognitions) in the short term as well as long term. Moreover, these studies suggest group treatment for insomnia is an effective therapy for individuals with comorbid physical and mental health conditions.

The efficacy and effectiveness research summarized here can be used to index the overall empirical support for CBT for PI. According to criteria defined by the American Psychological Association's Division 12 Task Force, a treatment is deemed well established if at least 2 between-group design experiments have demonstrated efficacy by evidencing either superiority over a placebo or other treatment, or equivalence to an already well-established treatment.[27] According to these guidelines, and based on the research highlighted here, CBT may be considered a well-established treatment for PI.

PRACTITIONER CONSIDERATIONS: FACTORS THAT MAY AFFECT CBT

A wealth of research has combined to suggest that CBT is an effective treatment for PI. However, there are underlying factors that may affect the outcome of CBT. The authors now discuss several issues that practitioners may take into consideration when implementing CBT for PI.

Pharmacotherapy

Pharmacotherapy and CBT for insomnia are the only two treatment modalities that have sufficient support to be considered efficacious and effective treatments for insomnia.[28] Sedative-hypnotics are the most frequently prescribed medication for the treatment of insomnia, and the negative side effects may potentially outweigh the benefits. Sedative-hypnotics can result in tolerance, dependency, daytime sedation, impairments in psychomotor and cognitive processes, iatrogenic sleep disturbance, rebound insomnia, and rapid eye movement sleep rebound.[29-31] More recently, nonbenzodiazepine γ-aminobutyric acid agonists (ie, zolpidem, eszopiclone) as well as a melatonin agonist (ramelteon) have been introduced to limit negative effects. Recent RCTs have been conducted to compare CBT with pharmacotherapy to better understand the efficacy of these treatments singly and in combination. First, results from an RCT comparing CBT (delivered by 2 clinical psychologists across 6 weeks), zopiclone (a nonbenzodiazapine hypnotic), and a placebo control indicated CBT had greater short- and long-term outcomes on sleep parameters including total wake time, sleep efficiency, and slow-wave sleep as indicated by polysomnography immediately posttreatment as well as 6 months later.[32] Total sleep time was the only parameter in which no group differences emerged.[32] Research combines to suggest that CBT alone compared with both medication alone and a placebo leads to short-term improvement across multiple sleep parameters.[32–34] Whereas evidence suggests CBT alone results in greater improvements than placebos and medications,[32] the combination of pharmacotherapy and CBT has been shown to lead to greater improvements compared with either intervention alone in one sleep parameter (ie, increases in total time asleep).[34] Treatment gains from CBT also appear to be maintained while gains from pharmacotherapy decline across time.[33,34] In fact, a recent RCT suggests the best long-term outcomes are experienced by individuals who discontinue medication and use CBT as a maintenance therapy.[34] Overall, these lines of research converge to suggest pharmacotherapy may be an efficacious short-term, fast-acting approach to increasing total time asleep. However, CBT has been shown to have greater short- and long-term effects on several critical sleep parameters. For individuals with persistent insomnia, optimal treatment outcomes may result from initially combining CBT and medication. However, to obtain the best long-term outcomes medication should be tapered to discontinuation as CBT treatment progresses.

Treatment Format: Group Versus Individual

Although a majority of past research on CBT for PI has examined individual treatment, there has been a recent surge of research that has investigated the efficacy of group CBT for PI. For example, in a recent RCT patients seeking treatment for insomnia were randomized into a self-help control group or a group-format CBT. A therapist trained in CBT delivered weekly 2-hour sessions for 6 weeks. Results indicated that compared with the control condition, CBT reduced dysfunctional beliefs and attitudes about sleep and negative daytime symptoms. Furthermore, CBT improved sleep latency, time awake after sleep onset, total sleep time, sleep quality, and sleep efficiency compared with the control group.[35] Researchers have also compared group versus individual format CBT for PI. Individuals with primary or secondary insomnia (as a result of psychopathology) were assigned to either group or individual CBT. Both formats consisted of the same material and were administered by a clinical psychologist weekly for 6 weeks. Results indicated that both individual and group CBT led to significant improvements in subjective sleep quality, quality of life, and attitudes about sleep at posttreatment and during a 9-month follow-up, but the individual and group formats did not differ in efficacy.[36] Overall, these results combine to suggest group CBT outperforms a control group and appears to perform as well as individual treatment for PI. Furthermore, group treatment has the added benefit of providing social support, and this format likely is more cost effective, with the average group size ranging from 6 to 8 people.

Predictors of Treatment Dropout

While CBT for insomnia has been deemed the standard treatment for chronic insomnia by the American Academy of Sleep Medicine,[37] effectiveness studies within clinical outpatient settings have indicated attrition rates ranging from 13.7% to 34%.[23,38] Recent research has focused on improving understanding of factors that affect treatment dropout. A total sleep time of less than 3.65 hours and elevated levels of depression were the two most robust predictors of treatment dropout.[39] The role of nonspecific treatment factors on outcomes also was investigated. Findings indicated that among clients with relatively low expectations of change, those who perceived greater affiliation with their therapists had less total wake time at night. Among those with high treatment expectation, therapist affiliation did not relate to treatment outcomes. In addition, those who perceived their therapist as hostile and critically confrontational were less satisfied with treatment and were more likely to drop out.[40] Overall, these findings combine to suggest that both patients' characteristics and therapists' characteristics (including warmth and a nonconfrontational demeanor) interact to affect treatment completion and treatment outcomes. Future research may benefit from examining additional factors in this domain. For example, individuals with an elevated level of fear of sleep may be more likely to actively avoid sleep. To date, there is minimal research on fear and avoidance of sleep, and this may be a component of sleep disruption that impacts the success of sleep treatment.

Comorbidity

There are elevated rates of comorbidity between insomnia (particularly insomnia lasting longer than 6 months) and different types of psychopathology, including major depression, anxiety disorders, and substance use disorders.[41] In fact, 40% of people with chronic insomnia (present for at least 6 months) meet criteria for at least one type of psychiatric comorbidity.[42] Accordingly, the role of comorbidity must be considered and better understood in order to inform approaches to treatment and prevention of insomnia. Some research has demonstrated that CBT for insomnia is effective in reducing insomnia symptoms in the presence of comorbid disorders, including serious mental illness.[43] Currie and colleagues[44] demonstrated that among recovering alcoholics, 7 weeks of CBT for PI (administered by 3 mental health professionals, including a clinical psychologist, social worker, and addictions specialist) reduced self-reported sleep problems compared with a waitlist control group posttreatment through a 6-month follow-up. Treatment, however, did not prevent relapses to using alcohol. Taylor and colleagues[45] investigated the effects of CBT for PI among individuals with mild depression. The 6-week treatment was conducted by doctoral-level graduate students in clinical psychology. Results indicated significant posttreatment improvements in sleep onset latency, frequency and length of awakenings after sleep onset, total sleep time, sleep efficiency, and subjective sleep quality, while a trend toward decreasing depression emerged. At a 3-month follow-up, sleep parameter improvements were maintained and a significant decrease in depression was observed. A separate study investigating CBT for insomnia among individuals with major depressive disorder indicated that supplementing antidepressants with brief CBT for insomnia helped to alleviate both depression and insomnia symptoms.[46] Whereas some results have indicated that CBT for insomnia can be effective in reducing insomnia symptoms among individuals with comorbid disorders, including alcohol dependence, mild depression, major depression, and serious mental illness, other research has demonstrated that treatment targeting comorbid conditions does not always alleviate PI. For example, after successful treatment of posttraumatic stress disorder (PTSD) using PTSD-focused CBT, clients continued to report insomnia. Results indicated self-reported improvements in sleep parameters after adding 5 sessions of CBT for insomnia post-PTSD treatment; however, improvements were often below clinically significant levels.[47] Overall, research on treating comorbid insomnia and psychopathology has begun to demonstrate that the co-occurrence of sleep problems and other types of psychopathology may complicate treatment. Given the initial stages of this research, more investigation is necessary to better understand these likely complex interactions.

There are also elevated rates of comorbidity between insomnia and medical conditions, including chronic pain and cancer. In fact, 50% to 70% of patients with chronic pain report significant sleep problems.[48] Approximately 30% to 50% of people with recent diagnoses of cancer report significant sleep problems, with 23% to 44% of individuals with cancer reporting chronic sleep problems up to 5 years after cancer treatment.[49,50] Not only can pain lead to sleep problems, but some research has indicated that sleep problems can increase pain severity.[51] While this area is relatively understudied,[17] the role of medical comorbidity must be considered to better understand and inform treatments. The majority of research in this area has focused on chronic pain conditions and breast cancer. Currie and colleagues[52] conducted a randomized clinical trial investigating the efficacy of CBT for insomnia secondary to chronic pain. Sixty patients were randomly assigned to a 7-week CBT group for insomnia or waitlist control. Results indicated that CBT for insomnia improved self-reported sleep onset latency, amount of time awake after sleep onset, sleep efficiency, sleep quality, and decreased nocturnal movement. Of note, treatment gains were maintained through a 3-month follow-up.[52] Insomnia is also highly prevalent in patients with breast cancer.[53] An RCT of CBT for insomnia secondary to breast cancer indicated that CBT for insomnia led to improvements in subjective sleep quality while also decreasing psychological distress and increasing global quality of life, with treatment gains being maintained through 12 months.[54] A second study employed a multiple baseline design to examine CBT for insomnia secondary to nonmetastatic breast cancer. Results indicated significant improvements in sleep efficiency and total wake time. In addition, improvements in mood, fatigue, and quality of life were observed.[55] Overall, relatively limited research has investigated the effectiveness of CBT for insomnia secondary to medical conditions. Results from this work suggest that CBT is an efficacious treatment for insomnia secondary to both chronic pain and breast cancer. However, future research is needed to better understand the role of medical conditions on CBT for insomnia.

FUTURE DIRECTIONS

Decades of theoretical inquiry, basic research, and clinical trials have led to the development and refinement of CBT for PI. In fact, research has demonstrated that CBT is an efficacious, effective, and likely cost-effective treatment for insomnia that yields reliable, robust, and long-term benefits among children as well as young, middle-aged, and elderly adults. Based on this backdrop, new questions have emerged informing the future direction of this field. First, future research would benefit from continuing investigation into treatment effects of CBT for PI for different populations, including adolescents and culturally, ethnically, and socioeconomically diverse samples. Further research in this area would better inform the generalizability of CBT for PI. Second, relatively limited information has been collected on the incremental efficacy of individual components of CBT for insomnia. Future research should continue to examine the relative efficacy of individual components of CBT packages (via dismantling designs, for example) to better understand and identify the critical and active components of CBT for insomnia. Similarly, future research would benefit from better understanding insomnia and comorbid psychopathologies. For instance, laboratory-based experimental research has demonstrated that physiological and cognitive arousal relates to elevated self-reported sleep problems. Tang and Harvey[56] experimentally manipulated cognitive (instructed to give a speech after a nap) and physiological (administration of caffeine) arousal and measured the effects on perception of sleep. Results indicated that both elevated cognitive and physiological arousal were associated with greater subjective sleep latency. A separate laboratory-based line of work suggests that sleep deprivation increases anxious and fearful reactivity to bodily arousal (administered via a biological challenge procedure)[57] and that such anxious reactivity is positively associated with self-reported sleep problems.[58] Collectively, these laboratory-based programs of research suggest that anxiety-related processes (eg, elevated arousal, anxiety, and worry) may be bidirectionally related to problems sleeping. Research has also demonstrated that insomnia is elevated among individuals with depression as well as severe psychopathologies including schizophrenia. For example, Hall and colleagues[59] demonstrated that among individuals with PI, elevations in subclinical levels of depression were associated with objective sleep problems as indexed via 2 nights of polysomnography. Relatively less research has investigated PI among individuals with schizophrenia. The research conducted in this area has generally focused on the overlapping changes within the neurotransmitter system, specifically related to the overactivation of the dopaminergic system.[60] Additional research is now needed to better understand the mechanisms involved in the development and maintenance of comorbid insomnia and other psychopathologies.

REFERENCES

1. American Psychiatric Association. Diagnostic and statistical manual of mental disorders. 4th edition—text revision. Washington, DC: American Psychiatric Association; 2000.
2. U.S. Surgeon General. Frontiers of knowledge in sleep & sleep disorders: opportunities for improving health and quality of life. Bethesda (MD): National Institutes of Health; 2004.
3. World Health Organization. The global burden of disease: 2004 update. Geneva (Switzerland): WHO Press; 2008. Annex A.
4. Morin CM, Culbert JP, Schwartz SM. Nonpharmacological interventions for insomnia: a meta-analysis of treatment efficacy. Am J Psychiatry 1994;151: 1172–80.
5. Edinger JD, Means MK. Cognitive-behavioral therapy for primary insomnia. Clin Psychol Rev 2005;25:539–58.
6. Malaffo M, Espie CA. Cognitive and behavioural treatments of primary insomnia. Minerva Psichiatr 2007;48:313–27.
7. Edinger JD, Wohlgemuth WK, Radtke RA, et al. Cognitive behavioral therapy for treatment of chronic primary insomnia: a randomized controlled trial. JAMA 2001; 285:1856–64.
8. Morin CM, Mimeault V, Gagne A. Nonpharmacological treatment of late-life insomnia. J Psychosom Res 1999;46:103–16.
9. Edinger JD, Wohlgemuth WK. The significance and management of persistent primary insomnia. Sleep Med Rev 1999;3:101–18.
10. Wang MY, Wang SY, Tsai PS. Cognitive behavioural therapy for primary insomnia: a systematic review. J Adv Nurs 2005;50:553–64.
11. Smith MT, Neubauer DN. Cognitive behavioral therapy for chronic insomnia. Clin Cornerstone 2003;5:28–40.
12. Harvey AG, Tang NK. Cognitive behavioral therapy for primary insomnia: can we rest yet? Sleep Med Rev 2003;7:237–62.
13. Morin CM. Cognitive-behavioral approaches to the treatment of insomnia. J Clin Psychiatry 2004;65:33–40.
14. Morin CM. Cognitive-behavioral therapy of insomnia. Sleep Med Clin 2006;1: 375–86.
15. Morin CM, Bastien C, Savard J. Current status of cognitive-behavioral therapy for insomnia: evidence for treatment effectiveness and feasibility. In: Perlis ML, Lichstein KL, editors. Treating sleep disorders: principles and practice of behavioral sleep medicine. New York: John Wiley & Sons; 2003. p. 262–85.
16. Cohen J. A power primer. Psychol Bull 1992;112:155–9.

17. Murtagh DR, Greenwood KM. Identifying effective psychological treatments for insomnia: a meta-analysis. J Consult Clin Psychol 1995;63:79–89.
18. Sadeh A. Cognitive-behavioral treatment for childhood sleep disorders. Clin Psychol Rev 2005;25:612–28.
19. Ancoli-Israel S. Insomnia in the elderly: a review for the primary care practitioner. Sleep 2000;23:s23–30.
20. Irwin MR, Cole JC, Nicassio PM. Comparative meta-analysis of behavioral interventions for insomnia and their efficacy in middle aged adults and in old adults 55+ years of age. Health Psychol 2006;25:3–14.
21. Hryshko-Mullen AS, Broeckl LS, Haddock CK, et al. Behavioral treatment of insomnia: the Wilford Hall Insomnia Program. Mil Med 2000;165:200–7.
22. Verbeek I, Schreuder K, Declerck G. Evaluation of short-term nonpharmacological treatment of insomnia in a clinical setting. J Psychosom Res 1999;47:369–83.
23. Espie CA, Inglis SJ, Tessier S, et al. The clinical effectiveness of cognitive behavioral therapy for chronic insomnia: implementation and evaluation of a sleep clinic in general medical practice. Behav Res Ther 2001;39:45–60.
24. Harvey L, Inglis CA, Espie C. Insomniacs' reported use of CBT components and relationship to long-term clinical outcome. Behav Res Ther 2002;40:75–83.
25. Perlman LM, Arnedt JT, Gorman AA, et al. Group cognitive behavioral therapy for insomnia in a VA mental health clinic. Cogn Behav Pract 2008;15:426–34.
26. Backhaus J, Hohagen F, Voderholzer U, et al. Long-term effectiveness of a short-term cognitive behavioral group treatment for primary insomnia. Eur Arch Psychiatry Clin Neurosci 2001;251:35–41.
27. Chambless DL, Ollendick TH. Empirically supported psychological interventions: controversies and evidence. Annu Rev Psychol 2001;52:685–716.
28. National Institutes of Health. National institutes of health state of science conference statement: manifestations and management of chronic insomnia in adults. Sleep 2005;28:1049–57.
29. Morin CM, Kwentus JA. Behavioral and pharmacological treatments for insomnia. Ann Behav Med 1988;10:91–100.
30. Roy-Byrne PP, Hommer DH. Benzodiazepine withdrawal: overview and implications for the treatment of anxiety. Am J Med 1988;84:1041–52.
31. Greenblatt DJ, Hormatz JS, Zinny MA, et al. The effects of gradual withdrawal on the rebound sleep disorder after discontinuation of triazolam. N Engl J Med 1987; 12:722–8.
32. Siversten B, Omvik S, Pallesen S, et al. Cognitive behavioral therapy vs Zopiclone for treatment of chronic primary insomnia in older adults A randomized controlled trial. JAMA 2006;295:2851–8.
33. Morin CM, Colecchi C, Stone J, et al. Behavioral and pharmacological therapies for late-life insomnia. JAMA 1999;281:991–9.
34. Morin CM, Vallieres A, Guay B, et al. Cognitive behavioral therapy, singly and combined with medication, for persistent insomnia a randomized clinical trial. JAMA 2009;301:2005–15.
35. Jansson M, Linton SJ. Cognitive-behavioral group therapy as an early intervention for insomnia: a randomized controlled trial. J Occup Rehabil 2005;15:177–90.
36. Verbeek I, Konings GM, Aldenkamp AP, et al. Cognitive behavioral treatment in clinically referred chronic insomniacs: group versus individual treatment. Behav Sleep Med 2006;4:135–51.
37. Morganthaler T, Kramer M, Alessi C, et al. American Academy of Sleep Medicine. Practice parameters for the psychological and behavioral treatment of insomnia: an update. An American Academy of Sleep Medicine Report. Sleep 2006;29:1415–9.

38. Morgan K, Thompson J, Dixon S, et al. Predicting longer-term outcomes following psychological treatment for hypnotic-dependent chronic insomnia. J Psychosom Res 2003;54:21–9.
39. Ong JC, Kuo TF, Manber R. Who is at risk for dropout from group cognitive-behavioral therapy for insomnia? J Psychosom Res 2008;64:419–25.
40. Constantino MJ, Manber R, Ong J, et al. Patient expectations and therapeutic alliance as predictors of outcome in group cognitive-behavioral therapy for insomnia. Behav Sleep Med 2007;5:210–28.
41. Roth T, Jaeger S, Jin R, et al. Sleep problems, comorbid mental disorders, and role functioning in the National Comorbidity Survey Replication. Biol Psychiatry 2006;60:1364–71.
42. Drake CD, Roehrs T, Roth R. Insomnia causes, consequences, and therapeutics: an overview. Depress Anxiety 2003;18:163–76.
43. Dopke CA, Lehner RK, Wells AM. Cognitive-behavioral group therapy for insomnia in individuals with serious mental illnesses: a preliminary evaluation. Psychiatr Rehabil J 2004;27:235–42.
44. Currie SR, Clark S, Hodgins DC, et al. Randomized controlled trial of brief cognitive-behavioural interventions for insomnia in recovering alcoholics. Addiction 2004;99:1121–32.
45. Taylor DJ, Lichstein KL, Weinstock J, et al. A pilot study of cognitive-behavioral therapy of insomnia in people with mild depression. Behav Ther 2007;38:49–57.
46. Manber R, Edinger JD, Gress JL, et al. Cognitive behavioral therapy for insomnia enhances depression outcome in patients with comorbid major depressive disorder and insomnia. Sleep 2008;31:489–95.
47. DeViva JC, Zayfert C, Pigeon WR, et al. Treatment of residual insomnia after CBT for PTSD: case studies. J Trauma Stress 2005;18:155–9.
48. Atkinson JH, Ancoli-Israel S, Slater MA, et al. Subjective sleep disturbance in chronic back pain. Clin J Pain 1988;4:225–32.
49. Savard J, Morin CM. Insomnia in the context of cancer: a review of a neglected problem. J Clin Oncol 2001;19:895–908.
50. Lindley C, Vasa S, Sawyer WT, et al. Quality of life and preferences for treatment following systemic adjuvant therapy for early-stage breast cancer. J Clin Oncol 1998;16:1380–7.
51. Affleck G, Urrows S, Tennen H, et al. Sequential daily relations of sleep, pain intensity, and attention to pain among women with fibromyalgia. Pain 1996;68:363–8.
52. Currie SR, Wilson KG, Pontefract AJ, et al. Cognitive-behavioral treatment of insomnia secondary to chronic pain. J Consult Clin Psychol 2001;68:407–16.
53. Savard J, Simard S, Blanchet J, et al. Prevalence, clinical characteristics, and risk factors for insomnia in the context of breast cancer. Sleep 2001;24:583–90.
54. Savard J, Simard S, Ivers H, et al. Randomized study on the efficacy of cognitive-behavioral therapy for insomnia secondary to breast cancer, part I: sleep and psychological effects. J Clin Oncol 2005;1:6083–96.
55. Quesnel C, Savard J, Simard S, et al. Efficacy of cognitive-behavioral therapy for insomnia in women treated for nonmetastatic breast cancer. J Consult Clin Psychol 2003;71:189–200.
56. Tang NK, Harvey AG. Effects of cognitive arousal and physiological arousal on sleep perception. Sleep 2004;27:69–78.
57. Babson KA, Feldner MT, Trainor CD, et al. An experimental investigation of the effects of acute sleep deprivation on panic-relevant biological challenge responding. Behav Ther 2009;40:239–50.

58. Babson KA, Feldner MT, Connolly KM, et al. Subjective sleep quality and anxious and fearful responding to bodily arousal among children and adolescents. Cognit Ther Res, in press.

59. Hall M, Buysse DJ, Nowell PD. Symptoms of stress and depression as correlates of sleep in primary insomnia. Psychosom Med 2000;62:227–30.

60. Monti M, Monti D. Sleep disturbance in schizophrenia. Int Rev Psychiatry 2005; 17:247–53.

Behavioral Interventions for Tic Disorders

Shana A. Franklin, BA, Michael R. Walther, MS,
Douglas W. Woods, PhD*

KEYWORDS

- Tic disorders • Tourette syndrome
- Behavior therapy • Habit reversal training

Tic disorders are characterized by the presence of tics: stereotyped, repetitive movements or vocalizations.[1] Motor tics involve specific movements such as eye blinking, head jerking, and muscle tensing, whereas vocal tics are defined by the presence of sounds or vocalizations. Tics are further distinguished based on their complexity: simple tics are rapid and without apparent purpose, whereas complex tics are typically slower, more purposeful in appearance, and may involve a specific sequence of simple tics. Eye blinking and sniffing are examples of simple tics. Making obscene gestures (ie, copopraxia) and repeating others' words (ie, echolalia) are examples of complex tics.

Four distinct categories are used to classify tic disorders: Tourette syndrome (TS), chronic tic disorder (CTD), transient tic disorder, and tic disorder not otherwise specified (NOS).[1] TS is defined by the presence of multiple motor tics and one or more vocal tics occurring over the span of at least 12 months. CTD is defined by either motor or vocal tics (but not both) lasting at least 12 months. Transient tic disorder is diagnosed if tics have been present for at least 4 weeks but not 12 months, and tic disorder NOS is diagnosed when tics are present but do not meet criteria for another tic disorder.

TS was once considered a rare disorder, but recent data suggest the overall prevalence may be as high as 1% in the general population.[2–5] Tic disorders are more common in childhood, and a recent study of grade school children found tics to be present in 18% of the sample, with 3% meeting diagnostic criteria for TS.[6] Onset typically occurs between ages 4 and 6 years, with boys affected approximately 4 times more frequently than girls.[5,7–9] The frequency and severity of tics usually wax and wane,[10] with symptom severity increasing in early adolescence and beginning a general decline as the individual enters adulthood.[5,7] For some, tics remain chronic

Psychology Department, The University of Wisconsin-Milwaukee, 224 Garland Hall, 2441 East Hartford Avenue, Milwaukee, WI 53211, USA
* Corresponding author.
E-mail address: dwoods@uwm.edu

Psychiatr Clin N Am 33 (2010) 641–655
doi:10.1016/j.psc.2010.04.013
0193-953X/10/$ – see front matter © 2010 Elsevier Inc. All rights reserved.

and severe in adulthood, producing significant impairment in academic, social, and occupational functioning.[11,12]

Tic disorders, particularly TS, often co-occur with other psychiatric conditions, the most common of which are obsessive-compulsive disorder (OCD) and attention-deficit/hyperactivity disorder (ADHD).[13] For individuals with TS, the rate of comorbid OCD is approximately 30%, but as many as 80% exhibit OCD or obsessive-compulsive features in the absence of meeting full diagnostic criteria for OCD.[2,14,15] The high rate of obsessive-compulsive symptoms in TS may be attributed in part to the difficulty distinguishing complex tics from compulsions. This distinction may be particularly difficult when a patient describes performing a specific behavior in question to achieve or satisfy a "just right" feeling, which can be a characteristic of OCD and tic disorders. The rate of comorbid ADHD in TS is reported to be close to 50%.[16,17] Depression and anxiety disorders are also more common in TS than in the general population, but it is unclear whether these conditions are independent of TS or occur secondary to the tic disorder.[13] Although tics are a source of significant impairment in certain individuals, many people with tic disorders suffer greater impairment from the comorbid conditions.[5,18]

In addition to the overt symptoms of tics, an important phenomenological aspect of tic disorders involves the premonitory urge, which is described as a feeling of tension or discomfort preceding the tic. As many as 90% of individuals with tics report experiencing this urge for some, if not all, of their tics.[19,20] The premonitory urge is described, and most likely experienced, differently across patients, but often manifests as a physical sensation (eg, muscle tightness, internal or bodily tension, or an itch) or vague mental urge (eg, urge or need to tic, feeling that something is incomplete or needs to be done just right) that is relieved or markedly reduced after performance of the tic.[20–23] Premonitory urges are easily confused with obsessions seen in OCD. However, unlike obsessions in most cases of OCD, the urge is not experienced as physiological signs of anxiety (ie, increased heart rate, perspiration, increased respiration) nor as a thought of specific threat or harm that leads to anxiety. Rather it is a vague sensory discomfort.

One of the earliest descriptions of tic disorders was provided in 1885 by the French physician George Gilles de Tourette, for whom TS is named. Although the pathogenesis was unknown, tic disorders were initially characterized and treated as a neurological disorder.[24] This conceptualization shifted as psychoanalytic theories gained prominence in the early twentieth century, and tics were reconceived as physical expressions in response to the buildup of nervous energy or emotional conflict.[25] As a treatment, psychoanalysis was largely ineffective, but it did lead to a conceptualization of tics as reflective of some underlying psychological disturbance.[13,26] This psychological conceptualization lasted until the 1960s, when antipsychotic medication was introduced as a treatment of tics. The success of medication was seen as evidence for the biological origin of tics, which led to the prevailing conceptualization of tics as a symptom of a neurological disorder.[26] More recently, integrative models have emerged, which assume that underlying biological abnormalities are the root cause of the disorder, but that contextual factors interact with these abnormalities to maintain the disorder and to produce predictable fluctuations in symptom expression.[27,28]

CAUSES

Tics have long been observed to run in families, and research supports the heritability of tic disorders. There is an increased incidence of tic disorders amongst biological relatives, particularly when spectrum disorders like OCD are included.[29–32] When a first-degree relative is afflicted with TS, the risk of having TS, CTD, or OCD is approximately 35%.[33] Twin studies provide further support for the heritability of tic disorders.[32,34] Current evidence suggests a genetic basis for tic disorders, although genomic studies have thus far failed to reliably locate a specific gene. Researchers now postulate that multiple genes are involved in creating the susceptibility to tic disorders.[35,36]

Advances in imaging technology have offered examination into the possible neurobiological and anatomical bases of tic disorders. Researchers have proposed the involvement of several possible areas, particularly those related to the basal ganglia and the corticostriatal-thalamocortical (CSTC) circuit,[35,37] which is highly involved in the selection and inhibition of motoric behavior. The neurotransmitter dopamine has also been implicated in tic disorders, stemming from the observed effect of dopaminergic antagonists on tics.[38] Data supporting a specific structural and neurochemical model for tic disorders have yet to be replicated. In a recent review of the functional neuroimaging findings, Rickards[35(p583)] concluded:

No clear endophenotype has emerged from scanning studies, which could be correlated to factor analyses of symptom clusters or to genetic data. So far, no single finding has been reliably replicated in this area. TS is a dynamic illness involving different systems of the brain, so studies that use specific pharmacological or cognitive stimulation paradigms are more likely to yield success in the future. Although the pathology of TS may be focal, functional brain changes are widespread, involve many different areas and systems, and are extremely complex.

BEHAVIORAL MODEL OF TICS

Although behavioral treatments for tics have existed for nearly 40 years,[39] most have been developed and tested in the absence of a clear and comprehensive behavioral model. In recent years, a behavioral model has begun to emerge, based on clinical observation and experimental studies of contextual influences on tic expression. Although a full review of an entire behavioral model is beyond the scope of this article, a brief summary may be helpful in interpreting the possible usefulness of the treatment alternatives described later.

The behavioral model for tics assumes that the basis for tics and their expression is biological in nature. It is thought that the abnormalities described earlier give rise to neurocognitive deficits including, but not limited to, difficulties in response inhibition,[40–44] which result in an individual who experiences somatosensory signals to move, but who, through normal inhibitory processes, is unable to inhibit the execution of movement stemming from these impulses.

The behavioral model is not offered as an alternative to a biological model, rather the behavioral model seeks to build on the biological model and explain how tics, once present, can be strengthened and shaped to occur with varying levels of frequency across different contexts. According to the behavioral model, there are at least 2 factors that maintain and alter tic expression, including contextual factors occurring outside the person's body (external factors) and contextual factors occurring inside the person's body (internal factors).[28]

Research supports the notion that external factors, such as socially based reactions to tic expression, can alter tic frequency. Tic expression has been found to be strengthened by social attention or escape from demanding situations,[45,46] and tic suppression can also be strengthened through external consequences.[47–50] Furthermore, there is evidence (empirical and clinical) that tics are highly influenced by the situation the individual is in or activity in which he or she is engaged.[27,28,51–54] The effect of these contextual variables (eg, social attention or activities) is highly individ-ualized and affects different individuals in different ways. For example, one child may experience tic decreases while playing sports or singing, whereas playing videogames or sitting in mathematics class may exacerbate tics. For another child, the exact oppo-site pattern may occur. Potential reasons for this situational variability found in tic expression are many, but one explanation that has garnered some empirical support is that with time, certain environmental variables come to predict the availability of reinforcers for tic expression or suppression. As a result, when individuals encounter these various predictive situations throughout the day, their tics fluctuate in frequency and intensity in a pattern that is consistent with their history.[49]

In addition to the external contextual factors influencing tics, there is a growing body of literature showing that internal factors are also important. Most individuals are capable of reporting and do report premonitory urges.[22] These urges are experienced as aversive and are reduced contingent on tics.[47] As a result, tic expression is consis-tently and immediately reinforced via reduction of the urge (ie, negative reinforce-ment). This negative reinforcement process is believed to be a primary factor responsible for the maintenance of tics.[55] In addition to urge reduction, others have suggested that broad emotional states such as anxiety or boredom may significantly increase tic frequency for many persons with TS.[56] How these emotional states affect tic frequency is unclear, but possible explanations include (1) the state allows for heightened awareness of premonitory urges,[57] (2) the state of anxiety mimics the sensation of a premonitory urge (eg, a sense of tension) that then elicits the tic, and (3) anxiety may simply make response inhibition processes more difficult.[58]

A final internal factor that has been posited as being related to tic expression is a particular tendency to process information in ways that have a downstream effect on tic occurrence. O'Connor and colleagues[59] have suggested that persons with TS have a perfectionistic style of action characterized by (1) a belief that it is important to be efficient in one's actions, (2) by a tendency to abandon tasks prematurely, and (3) by a tendency to take on too many tasks at one time.[60] In addition, O'Connor[60] has suggested that persons with TS have a heightened sense of self-awareness, thus making them more adept at detecting internal bodily cues that could trigger tics. There is evidence that persons with TS perceive tic exacerbating situations as particularly frustrating and unsatisfying, perceptions that are believed to contribute to tic exacerbation.[60]

Combined, this emerging behavioral model suggests that a treatment package with multiple contextual targets (internal and external) may be the most useful approach to the nonpharmacological management of the disorder. However, as described later, nonpharmacological treatments do not often address the external and internal contex-tual factors that may be needed to effectively treat persons with tics.

TREATMENT OF TIC DISORDERS

There is no cure for tic disorders, only successful symptom management. Although education, reassurance, and a wait-and-see approach is often the primary treatment modality,[7] drug treatment is the most common active intervention.[61] Haloperidol (Hal-dol), an antipsychotic, was the first medication to be widely used in the treatment of tic disorders.[5,25,35] Haloperidol and other antipsychotics are generally considered to be the most effective medications for the treatment of tic disorder,[5,62–66] although atyp-ical antipsychotics (eg, risperidone) and medications such as clonidine and guanfa-cine have also shown efficacy in reducing tic symptoms.[67–69] In addition to treating tics, guanfacine has the added benefit of treating comorbid ADHD.[69]

The more effective antipsychotic medications are associated with severe side effects including akathisia, bradykinesia, dystonia, and parkinsonism.[64] A large percentage of individuals choose to discontinue such treatment as a result of experiencing side effects.[63,64] The newer medications used for tic disorders have fewer side effects, yet these are still associated with discontinued use.[70] Clonidine and guanfacine have the fewest and least severe side effects and are common first-line medications for mild to moderately severe tics.[24] Atypical and traditional antipsychotics are more commonly used for moderate to severe cases of TS or for cases in which explosive anger outbursts are common.

Deep brain stimulation (DBS) is a surgical treatment reserved for severe cases of TS that have not responded to other behavioral or pharmacological treatments. Because of risks associated with neurosurgery, DBS is used only after all other treatment options have been exhausted.[71] Research on DBS has been promising, with studies showing significant tic reduction, although not necessarily complete symptom remission.[72,73]

Medical interventions are the standard method for managing tics, but may produce undesirable side effects or present unacceptable risks. Considering that many parents are reluctant to medicate their children[74] and DBS is limited to the most extreme cases, there is a need for other treatment options. Psychosocial interventions, primarily behavioral, represent the most viable alternative to medical treatment. However, these interventions have yet to gain prominence in the medical community and the general public is often unaware of their presence.[74]

Several different behavioral therapies have been examined for treatment of tics, each showing varying levels of efficacy. These include: (1) massed practice (MP) (or negative practice), (2) relaxation training, (3) self-monitoring, (4) function-based/contingency management procedures, (5) habit reversal training (HRT), (6) exposure and response prevention (ERP), and (7) cognitive behavioral therapy (CBT). Each of these procedures is described later, along with the evidence supporting their efficacy or lack thereof. Because this literature has been critically evaluated in numerous recent papers,[75,76] the purpose of this work is not to provide a critical empirical review of the literature. Rather, it is to offer a broad description of the evidence base and point clinicians/researchers toward a synthesis of the findings and implications.

MP

MP requires patients to voluntarily reproduce and repeat tics several times a minute over the course of several sessions. This overrepetition of the tic is believed to produce a buildup of inhibition or fatigue, which leads to tic reduction. Despite initial case reports of success using MP, subsequent studies have yielded mixed results[77–79] and were compounded by methodological concerns. In the only randomized controlled study to date involving MP, 17% of subjects treated with the procedure were tic free at the end of treatment compared with 80% of the subjects treated with HRT.[77] Cook and Blacher[75] determined that MP did not have sufficient empirical support to be considered a "well-established" or "probably efficacious" intervention according to the American Psychological Association Task Force for Promotion and Dissemination of Psychological Procedures, which has proposed rigorous criteria for the evaluation of psychological interventions to determine their evidence-based efficacy.[80]

Relaxation Training

Relaxation training has 2 intended purposes in the treatment of tic disorders: to reduce muscle tension and alleviate anxiety. These actions are believed to be beneficial because of the clinical observations that tics worsen during heightened states of anxiety.[54] Various case reports have described moderate decreases in tic frequency with the use of relaxation techniques,[81,82] but in the most well-controlled studies, relaxation has not been proved effective as a monotherapy.[83,84] Nevertheless, because some individuals may experience exacerbation of tic symptoms from environmental stressors or a concurrent anxiety disorder, relaxation is often used as part of a more comprehensive treatment.[50,85]

Self-monitoring

Self-monitoring involves the patient's making an overt action to track tics as they occur. It is often used as an assessment tool or as a strategy to enhance tic awareness. There is limited case-study evidence that self-monitoring alone is successful in treating tics[86–89] and the efficacy of self-monitoring as a monotherapy has never been confirmed in a well-controlled randomized controlled trial. As posited by Woods and colleagues,[88] in patients in whom self-monitoring is effective as a treatment, it is possible that the act of noting tic occurrences (eg, making a checkmark when they happen) functions as a competing response (ie, a behavior that prevents the tic from occurring), which is a core component of habit reversal (see later discussion). Another possibility is that the gains observed during self-monitoring are only temporary, although the durability of gains produced by self-monitoring have not yet been adequately examined. Accordingly, Cook and Blacher[75] concluded that there is no evidentiary support of self-monitoring as a probably efficacious treatment. As with relaxation training, there is currently insufficient evidence to advocate the use of self-monitoring alone, but it is often included as an aspect of several other interventions.

Function-based/Contingency Management Procedures

In developing function-based interventions, clinicians systematically identify the possible contextual variables that function to increase the tics and then implement specific interventions to modify these variables in the service of tic reduction. The purpose of function-based interventions is not to cure the tic disorder. Rather, it is to create a systematic strategy for minimizing tic occurrence. For example, Watson and Sterling[46] found that social attention received when a child was engaging in a tic was the likely reinforcer for the behavior. When the parents were asked to ignore the vocal tic, but provide attention for every 15 seconds the child went without a tic, the tics rapidly diminished to near-zero levels. In another study, a young man's tics were found to differentially occur as a function of his current posture. While he was sitting, his tics were more frequent than while lying down. As part of a larger intervention, it was suggested that the client be given the opportunity to lie down when it was feasible.[90]

Other studies have sought to reinforce the reduction of tics[91] or punish the presence of tics through time-out.[82,92] Such contingency management strategies have often been used in the absence of conducting a full functional assessment of the exacerbating factors. Data on these procedures have come from small uncontrolled studies, the results of which have been positive in the short-term but not tested with long-term maintenance phases. Function-based and contingency management procedures, although consistent with a theoretical understanding of tic disorders, have not been adequately tested as monotherapies for TS.

HRT

HRT is a comprehensive multicomponent intervention first introduced by Azrin and Nunn.[93] The initial version used standard components of behavior therapy, including self-monitoring and relaxation techniques but also added tic-specific techniques of awareness training, competing response training, and social support.

In awareness training, increasing the patient's ability to anticipate tics and detect occurrences in real time are emphasized. The patients are taught to recognize the warning signs or signals that the tic is about to occur. Typically, these include the premonitory urge and early parts of the tic movement. In treatment, the client and therapist practice identifying the tic and the warning signs until the client is able to accurately detect both.

During competing response training, the therapist helps the patient select a behavior that is physically incompatible with the tic and intentionally performed contingent on the urge to tic or the actual tic. Ideally, this competing response is socially covert and sustainable for several minutes, as the patient is instructed to hold the competing response for at least 1 minute or until the urge to tic subsides.[94] The competing response should physically prevent the tic from occurring or at least make tic occurrence more difficult. Examples of suggested competing responses can be found in **Table 1**.

In terms of efficacy, HRT has outperformed most other psychosocial interventions for tics, including MP, relaxation therapy, and self-monitoring.[77,84] In addition, HRT is the best studied of the psychosocial interventions to date. It has been evaluated with the largest number of studies using rigorous methodological standards, including several randomized controlled trials.[75] Results from randomized control trials have reported tic reductions ranging from 32% to 99%,[77,95,96] and follow-up data suggest gains are maintained for up to 10 months.[95,97] Randomized trials have been conducted primarily in adults, and larger-scale trials in children are still needed. Review of these studies led Cook and Blacher[75] to categorize HRT as a well-established treatment of tic disorder.[97]

The successes of HRT led to several subsequent studies examining the contribution made by individual treatment components. Miltenberger and colleagues[98] compared the original HRT with an abbreviated version consisting only of awareness training and competing response training. Results showed both versions were equally successful in reducing tic frequency, suggesting that the core components were awareness training and competing response training. These findings have been confirmed in

Table 1
Suggested competing response

Tic	Competing Response
Eye blinking/eye darting	Smooth, controlled blinking. If needed, focus on one spot in the room
Facial grimacing	Gently purse lips together
Head jerking/head movements	Gently tense neck muscles and fixate eyes. If needed, push chin down into sternum
Mouth opening/mouth movements	Clench jaw and press lips together
Shoulder shrugging	Keep arms at side while pushing elbow toward hip
Hand/finger movements	Push hand against arms of chair, desk, or leg. If needed, make fists and push elbow to side
Nose scrunching	Pull nose or upper lip down. Keep lips pressed together while breathing
Vocal tics	Controlled, diaphragmatic breathing through nose or mouth. Inhalation/exhalation should be opposite of that of the tic (eg, in/out through nose/mouth)

several additional studies.[84,88,99,100] Furthermore, the competing response was most effective when performed contingent on the tic,[101] and the competing response need not be physically incompatible to be effective.[102]

The mechanisms responsible for the success of HRT remain unclear. One possible explanation is that the competing response interrupts the tic and also serves to physically strengthen the opposing muscles.[22] However, this claim has not been supported empirically.[102] Others have proposed that tic reductions occur because the competing response is reinforced through praise administered as part of the social support process.[103] Although the social support component of HRT is believed to be necessary in children, it does not seem necessary for adults to achieve meaningful gains in the treatment of nontic repetitive behavior.[104] This suggests that social reinforcement may not be the primary mechanism of action of HRT. Another hypothesis is that HRT allows the individual to habituate to the premonitory urge, thus decreasing the need to tic. This hypothesis is supported by the preliminary finding that ERP, a treatment based on models of habituation, may yield similar results to HRT.[95,105] Regardless of the precise mechanism of action, HRT remains an efficacious and acceptable treatment of tics.[74]

ERP

Tic disorders are highly comorbid with OCD, and patients with both disorders often report an overlap in tic symptoms and compulsions. As a result, ERP, a leading behavioral treatment of OCD, has also been used to treat tics.[95,106,107] ERP exposes the patient to the premonitory sensations and prevents the individual from performing the tic. This procedure derives from the hypothesis that tic frequency is reduced as the individual habituates to the premonitory urge and learns to tolerate the discomfort without performing the tic.[105] Unlike HRT, patients are not given an alternative to ticcing but rather asked to suppress their tics, ideally for longer and longer periods of time while concentrating on the uncomfortable sensations related to the premonitory urge. Continued exposure is believed to lead to habituation and reduced tic frequency.

There are too few studies examining ERP for the treatment to be considered well established, but the positive results suggest it is a probably efficacious treatment.[75] Additional research is needed to explore ERP as an intervention for tic disorders, as well as the possibility that HRT and ERP share a common therapeutic mechanism: habituation to the premonitory urge. Treatment compliance and acceptability of ERP also require further examination as individuals may be opposed to the intentional and sustained exposure to negative sensations. Alternatively, they may find it physically difficult to suppress a tic without being provided with a behavior (eg, a competing response) to facilitate the process. Examining predictors to treatment response may reveal additional distinctions between the interventions. For example, it is possible that patients with comorbid OCD or primarily mental premonitory urges may respond better to ERP, whereas patients with purely sensory premonitory urges, or no recognizable urge at all, may have more success with HRT.

CBT

CBT combines behavioral strategies such as HRT with a specific cognitive component designed to restructure mental concepts and expectations related to tics. In a case report, Fuata and Griffiths[108] included cognitive therapy as an adjunct to habit reversal for the treatment of an individual with a coughing tic. The cognitive component was deemed important in overcoming the individual's discomfort with the wet sensation in his mouth preceding his tic as well as his irrational belief that his mouth had too much saliva. Another study examining CBT in the treatment of chronic tic and habit disorders found CBT was superior to wait-list in reduction of tic and habit frequency; however, the mixed sample limited the ability to draw conclusions specific to tic disorder.[60] The investigators also reported significant decreases in self-reported anxiety and depression along with increases in reported self-esteem. O'Connor and colleagues[59] conducted a randomized control trial comparing the effects of HRT versus CBT. Results showed that although the CBT group showed significant tic reductions, these were not superior to HRT, suggesting the cognitive component was unnecessary. Current evidence suggests that cognitive components are not likely to be necessary for tic reduction but they may have a therapeutic effect on concurrent depression and anxiety. Further research is needed to explore this issue.

BARRIERS TO BEHAVIORAL INTERVENTIONS FOR TIC DISORDERS

In recent decades, behavioral interventions, HRT in particular, have shown efficacy and acceptability in the treatment of tic disorders. Despite yielding similar reductions in tics, these interventions have not been widely adopted. Reasons for this are speculative, but one possibility for the discrepancy is the apparent lack of knowledge among health care providers and the larger TS community about behavioral interventions for tics.[109] This situation is compounded by the scarcity of health care providers adequately trained in interventions such as HRT.[75] Treatment dissemination, education, and training must remain a top priority for these interventions to be embraced on a larger scale. However, these are not the only obstacles facing the use of behavior therapy for tic disorders.

Another possible explanation for the reluctance to embrace behavior therapy for tics may stem from residual bias against psychological interventions that had been ineffective, but widely used before the rise of pharmacotherapy.[25] In addition, several misconceptions about the nature of tics persist among clinicians and patients alike, and these misconceptions could naturally lead one to argue that behavior therapy would not only fail to be effective, but could produce untoward consequences.

One misconception is that the suppression of tics ultimately leads to an increase in tic symptoms. As many as 77% of health care providers believe in this eventual buildup of tics following suppression, referred to as the rebound effect.[109,110] However, experimental evidence does not support the existence of this phenomenon.[50] A similar misconception, called symptom substitution, is that suppression of one tic results in the worsening of other tics or emergence of new tics.[110] This is not supported by data, because results show that treating one tic either has no effect on other tics or produces a generalized reduction in untreated tics.[50] A third concern is that attention used to suppress or disrupt tics impedes performance on other cognitive activities as a result of depletion of attentional resources.[111,112] Initial evidence suggests that tic suppression does mildly affect performance on attention-demanding tasks.[28] However, this effect may diminish as patients practice suppression or become proficient in implementing the competing response. Further research should address attention and task performance of patients throughout the course of HRT to determine if treatment has a negative effect on these variables.

SUMMARY

Although treatment practices for TS trend toward a singular biologically based treatment strategy, increasing evidence suggests the development and course of TS is likely produced by a complicated interaction of biogenetic influences and contextual factors.[35] As a result, it is plausible that nonpharmacological treatments may also be useful in treating TS. Future research should analyze the additive effects of each individual treatment (ie, medication vs behavior therapy) and establish the most effective sequence of care. Clinical research, particularly in psychiatry, is beginning to use treatment outcome designs that allow for understanding the benefits of individual interventions as well as their additive or sequential effect.[113] This design may be especially useful for severe intractable cases of tics so that individuals may be assured all options are exhausted before being referred for riskier treatments like DBS. In addition, predictors of treatment response should be further explored among the individual interventions (medical and behavioral). This strategy is particularly important so that patients may make the most educated decision regarding risks and benefits of treatment.

The conceptualization of tic disorders has shifted throughout history, from the time of Gilles de Tourette to Freud through the development and use of effective medications. If the history of TS has taught us any lesson it is that no one conceptualization or treatment approach should be held to dogmatically. Various models should be examined objectively and future research should explore the interaction of biology, environment, and behavior. In addition, the barriers hindering the acceptance of behavioral interventions must be addressed. The data suggest that these interventions, particularly HRT, are effective in the treatment of tic disorders but the widespread usage of these treatments is hampered by a lack of awareness in the health care community and the public at large.

REFERENCES

1. American Psychiatric Association. Diagnostic and statistical manual of mental disorders. text revision. 4th edition. Washington, DC: American Psychiatric Association; 2000.
2. Robertson MM. Diagnosing Tourette syndrome: is it a common disorder? J Psychosom Res 2003;55:3–6.
3. Robertson MM, Eapen V, Cavanna AE. The international prevalence, epidemiology, and clinical phenomenology of Tourette syndrome: a cross-cultural perspective. J Psychosom Res 2009;67(6):475–83.
4. Stefanoff P, Wolanczyk T, Gawrys A, et al. Prevalence of tic disorders among schoolchildren in Warsaw, Poland. Eur Child Adolesc Psychiatry 2008;17(3): 171–8.
5. Bloch MH, Leckman JF. Clinical course of Tourette syndrome. J Psychosom Res 2009;67(6):497–501.
6. Kurlan R, McDermott MP, Deeley C, et al. Prevalence of tics in schoolchildren and association with placement in special education. Neurology 2001;57: 1383–8.
7. Leckman JF, Zhang H, Vitale A, et al. Course of tic severity in Tourette syndrome: the first two decades. Pediatrics 1998;102:14–9.
8. Khalifa N, von Knorring AL. Prevalence of tic disorders and Tourette syndrome in a Swedish school population. Dev Med Child Neurol 2003;45:315–9.
9. Kadesjo B, Gillberg C. Tourette's disorder: epidemiology and comorbidity in primary school children. J Am Acad Child Adolesc Psychiatry 2000;39:548–55.
10. Piacentini JC, Pearlman AJ, Peris TS. Characteristics of Tourette syndrome. In: Woods DW, Piacentini JC, Walkup JT, editors. Treating Tourette syndrome and tic disorders: a guide for practitioners. New York: Guilford; 2007. p. 9–21.
11. Pappert EJ, Goetz CG, Louis ED, et al. Objective assessments of longitudinal outcome in Gilles de la Tourette's syndrome. Neurology 2003;61(7):936–40.
12. Elstner K, Selai C, Trimble M, et al. Quality of life (QOL) of patients with Gilles de la Tourette's syndrome. Acta Psychiatr Scand 2001;103(1):52–9.

13. Findley B. Characteristics of tic disorders. In: Woods DW, Miltenberger RG, editors. Tic disorders, trichotillomania, and other repetitive disorders. New York: Springer; 2001. p. 53–72.
14. King R, Leckman J, Scahill L, et al. Obsessive-compulsive disorder, anxiety, and depression. In: Leckman JF, Cohen DJ, editors. Tourette's syndrome-tics, obsessions, compulsions: developmental psychopathology and clinical care. New York: John Wiley; 1999. p. 43–62.
15. Shavitt RG, Hounie GA, Compos MCR, et al. Tourette's syndrome. Psychiatr Clin North Am 2006;29:471–86.
16. Spencer T, Biederman J, Harding M, et al. Disentangling the overlap between Tourette's disorder and ADHD. J Child Psychol Psychiatry 1998;39(7):1037–44.
17. Comings DE, Comings BG. Tourette syndrome: clinical and psychological aspects of 250 cases. Am J Hum Genet 1985;37:435–50.
18. Scahill L, Sukhodolsky DG, Williams SK, et al. Public health significance of tic disorders in children and adolescents. Adv Neurol 2005;96:240–8.
19. Kwak C, Dat Vuong K, Jankovic J. Premonitory sensory phenomenon in Tourette's syndrome. Mov Disord 2003;18(12):1530–3.
20. Bliss J. Sensory experiences of Gilles de la Tourette syndrome. Arch Gen Psychiatry 1980;37(12):1343–7.
21. Prado HS, Rosário MC, Lee J, et al. Sensory phenomena in obsessive-compulsive disorder and tic disorders: a review of the literature. CNS Spectr 2008;13(5):425–32.
22. Leckman JF, Walker DE, Cohen DJ. Premonitory urges in Tourette's syndrome. Am J Psychiatry 1993;150:98–102.
23. Miguel EC, do Rosario-Campos MC, Prado HS, et al. Sensory phenomena in obsessive–compulsive disorder and Tourette's disorder. J Clin Psychiatry 2000;61(2):150–6.
24. Jimenez-Shahed J. Tourette syndrome. Neurol Clin 2009;27:737–55.
25. Kushner HI. A cursing brain? The histories of Tourette syndrome. Cambridge (MA): Harvard University Press; 2000.
26. Chang SW, Piacentini J, Walkup JT. Behavioral treatment of syndrome: past, present, and future. Clin Psychol Sci Pract 2007;14(3):268–73.
27. O'Connor K, Brisebois H, Brault M, et al. Behavioral activity associated with onset in chronic tic and habit disorder. Behav Res Ther 2003;41(2):241–9.
28. Conelea C, Woods D. The influence of contextual factors on tic expression in Tourette's syndrome: a review. J Psychosom Res 2008;65(5):487–96.
29. Eldridge R, Sweet R, Lake R, et al. Gilles de la Tourette's syndrome: clinical, genetic, psychologic, and biochemical aspects in 21 selected families. Neurology 1977;27(2):115–24.
30. Pauls DL, Cohen DJ, Heimbuch R, et al. Familial pattern and transmission of Gilles de la Tourette syndrome and multiple tics. Arch Gen Psychiatry 1981; 38(10):1091–3.
31. Hanna PA, Janjua FN, Contant CF, et al. Bilineal transmission in Tourette syndrome. Neurology 1999;53(4):813–8.
32. Tourette Syndrome Association International Consortium for Genetics. Genome scan for Tourette disorder in affected-sibling-pair and multigenerational families. Am J Hum Genet 2007;80(2):265–72.
33. Pauls DL, Alsobrook JP, Gelernter J, et al. Genetic vulnerability. In: Leckman JF, Cohen DJ, editors. Tourette's syndrome—tics, obsessions, compulsions: developmental psychopathology and clinical care. New York: John Wiley; 1999. p. 194–211.

34. Hyde TM, Aaronson BA, Randolph C, et al. Relationship of birth weight to the phenotypic expression of Gilles de la Tourette's syndrome in monozygotic twins. Neurology 1992;42:652–8.

35. Rickards H. Functional neuroimaging in Tourette syndrome. J Psychosom Res 2009;67(6):575–84.

36. Walkup JT, LaBuda MC, Singer HS, et al. Family study of segregation analysis of Tourette syndrome: evidence for a mixed model of inheritance. Am J Hum Genet 1996;59:684–93.

37. Peterson BS, Thomas P, Kane MJ, et al. Basal ganglia volumes in patients with Gilles de la Tourette syndrome. Arch Gen Psychiatry 2003;60(4):415–24.

38. Anderson GM, Leckman JF, Cohen DJ. Neurochemical and neuropeptide systems. In: Leckman JF, Cohen DJ, editors. Tourette's syndrome—tics, obsessions, compulsions: developmental psychopathology and clinical care. New York: John Wiley; 1999. p. 261–80.

39. Woods DW, Miltenberger RG. Habit reversal: a review of applications and variations. J Behav Ther Exp Psychiatry 1995;26(2):123–31.

40. Castellanos FX, Fine EJ, Kaysen D, et al. Sensorimotor gating in boys with Tourette's syndrome and ADHD: preliminary results. Biol Psychiatry 1996;39:33–41.

41. Casey B, Tottenham N, Fossella J. Clinical, imaging, lesion, and genetic approaches toward a model of cognitive control. Dev Psychobiol 2002;40(3):237–54.

42. Chang S, McCracken J, Piacentini J. Neurocognitive correlates of child obsessive compulsive disorder and Tourette syndrome. J Clin Exp Neuropsychol 2007;29(7):724–33.

43. Channon S, Pratt P, Robertson M. Executive function, memory, and learning in Tourette's syndrome. Neuropsychology 2003;17(2):247–54.

44. Channon S, Sinclair E, Waller D, et al. Social cognition in Tourette's syndrome: intact theory of mind and impaired inhibitory functioning. J Autism Dev Disord 2004;34(6):669–77.

45. Carr J, Taylor C, Wallander R, et al. A functional-analytic approach to the diagnosis of a transient tic disorder. J Behav Ther Exp Psychiatry 1996;27(3):291–7.

46. Watson T, Sterling H. Brief functional analysis and treatment of a vocal tic. J Appl Behav Anal 1998;31(3):471–4.

47. Himle MB, Woods DW, Conelea CA, et al. Investigating the effects of tic suppression on premonitory urge ratings in children and adolescents with Tourette's syndrome. Behav Res Ther 2007;45:2964–76.

48. Woods D, Himle M. Creating tic suppression: comparing the effects of verbal instruction to differential reinforcement. J Appl Behav Anal 2004;37(3):417–20.

49. Woods D, Walther M, Bauer C, et al. The development of stimulus control over tics: a potential explanation for contextually-based variability in the symptoms of Tourette syndrome. Behav Res Ther 2009;47(1):41–7.

50. Woods D, Himle M, Miltenberger R, et al. Durability, negative impact, and neuropsychological predictors of tic suppression in children with chronic tic disorder. J Abnorm Child Psychol 2008;36(2):237–45.

51. Crosland K, Zarcone J, Schroeder S, et al. Use of an antecedent analysis and a force sensitive platform to compare stereotyped movements and motor tics. Am J Ment Retard 2005;110(3):181–92.

52. Malatesta V. Behavioral case formulation: an experimental assessment study of transient tic disorder. J Psychopathol Behav Assess 1990;12(3):219–32.

53. Piacentini J, Himle M, Chang S, et al. Reactivity of tic observation procedures to situation and setting. J Abnorm Child Psychol 2006;34(5):649–58.

54. Silva R, Munoz D, Barickman J, et al. Environmental factors and related fluctuation of symptoms in children and adolescents with Tourette's disorder. J Child Psychol Psychiatry 1995;36(2):305–12.
55. Evers R, van de Wetering B. A treatment model for motor tics based on a specific tension-reduction technique. J Behav Ther Exp Psychiatry 1994; 25(3):255–60.
56. Lin H, Katsovich L, Ghebremichael M, et al. Psychosocial stress predicts future symptom severities in children and adolescents with Tourette syndrome and/or obsessive-compulsive disorder. J Child Psychol Psychiatry 2007;48(2):157–66.
57. Woods DW, Miltenberger RG, Flach AD. Habits, tics and stuttering. Behav Modif 1996;20(2):216–25.
58. Lee H, Yost BP, Telch MJ. Differential performance on the go/no-go task as a function of the autogenous-reactive taxonomy of obsessions: findings from a non-treatment seeking sample. Behav Res Ther 2009;47:294–300.
59. O'Connor K, Gareau D, Borgeat F. Muscle control in chronic tic disorders. Biofeedback Self Regul 1995;20(2):111–22.
60. O'Connor K. A cognitive-behavioral/psychophysiological model of tic disorders. Behav Res Ther 2002;40(10):1113–42.
61. Carpenter LL, Leckman JF, Scahill L, et al. Pharmacological and other somatic approaches to treatment. In: Leckman JF, Cohen DJ, editors. Tourette's syndrome—tics, obsessions, compulsions: developmental psychopathology and clinical care. New York: John Wiley; 1999. p. 370–97.
62. Ross MS, Moldofsky H. A comparison of pimozide and haloperidol in the treatment of Gilles de la Tourette's syndrome. Am J Psychiatry 1978;135:585–7.
63. Shapiro E, Shapiro AK, Fulop G, et al. Controlled study of haloperidol, pimozide, and placebo for the treatment of Gilles de la Tourette's syndrome. Arch Gen Psychiatry 1989;46:722–30.
64. Sallee FR, Nesbitt L, Jackson C, et al. Relative efficacy of haloperidol and pimozide in children and adolescents with Tourette's disorder. Am J Psychiatry 1997; 154:1057–62.
65. Bruggeman R, van der Linden C, Buitelaar JK, et al. Risperidone versus pimozide in Tourette's disorder: a comparative double-blind parallel-group study. J Clin Psychiatry 2001;62:50–6.
66. Gilbert DL, Batterson JR, Sethuraman G, et al. Tic reduction with risperidone versus pimozide in a randomized, double-blind, crossover trial. J Am Acad Child Adolesc Psychiatry 2004;43:206–14.
67. Scahill L, Leckman JF, Schultz RT, et al. A placebo-controlled trial of risperidone in Tourette syndrome. Neurology 2003;60:1130–5.
68. Gaffney GR, Perry PJ, Lund BC, et al. Risperidone versus clonidine in the treatment of children and adolescents with Tourette's syndrome. J Am Acad Child Adolesc Psychiatry 2002;41:330–6.
69. Scahill L, Chappell P, Kim Y, et al. A placebo-controlled study of guanfacine in the treatment of children with tic disorders and attention deficit hyperactivity disorder. Am J Psychiatry 2001;158(7):1067–74.
70. Jagger J, Prusoff BA, Cohen DJ, et al. The epidemiology of Tourette's syndrome: a pilot study. Schizophr Bull 1982;8:276–8.
71. Mink JW, Walkup J, Frey KA. Patient selection and assessment recommendations for deep brain stimulation in Tourette syndrome. Mov Disord 2006; 21(11):1831–8.
72. Welter M, Mallet L, Houeto J, et al. Internal pallidal and thalamic stimulation in patients with Tourette syndrome. Arch Neurol 2008;65(7):952–7.

73. Maciunas RJ, Maddux BN, Riley DE, et al. Prospective randomized double-blind trial of bilateral thalamic deep brain stimulation in adults with Tourette syndrome. J Neurosurg 2007;107(5):1004–14.

74. Woods DW, Conelea CA, Budman C, et al. Priorities as judged by people with TS. In: L Scahill (Chair), Public health. Paper presented at the biannual meeting of the International Scientific Symposium on Tourette Syndrome. New York (NY), June, 2009.

75. Cook CR, Blacher J. Evidence-based psychosocial treatments for tic disorders. Clin Psychol Rev 2007;14:252–67.

76. Carr JE, Chong IM. Habit reversal treatment of tic disorders: a methodological critique of the literature. Behav Modif 2005;29:858–75.

77. Azrin NH, Nunn RG, Frantz SE. Habit reversal vs. negative practice treatment of nervous tics. Behav Ther 1980;11(2):169–78.

78. Nicassio FJ, Liberman RP, Patterson RL, et al. The treatment of tics by negative practice. J Behav Ther Exp Psychiatry 1972;3(4):281–7.

79. Topenhoff M. Massed practice, relaxation and assertion training in the treatment of Gilles de la Tourette's syndrome. J Behav Ther Exp Psychiatry 1973; 4:71–3.

80. Task Force on Promotion and Dissemination of Psychological Procedures. Training in and dissemination of empirically validated psychosocial treatments: report and recommendations. Clin Psychol Rev 1995;48:3–23.

81. Turpin G, Powell G. Effects of massed practice and cue-controlled relaxation on tic frequency in Gilles de la Tourette's syndrome. Behav Res Ther 1984;22(2): 165–78.

82. Canavan A, Powell G. The efficacy of several treatments of Gilles de la Tourette's syndrome as assessed in a single case. Behav Res Ther 1981;19(6): 549–56.

83. Bergin A, Waranch HR, Brown J, et al. Relaxation therapy in Tourette syndrome: a pilot study. Pediatr Neurol 1998;18(2):136–42.

84. Peterson AL, Azrin NH. An evaluation of behavioral treatments for Tourette syndrome. Behav Res Ther 1992;30:167–74.

85. Woods DW. Behavioral interventions for tic disorders. In: Woods DW, Miltenberger RG, editors. Tic disorders, trichotillomania, and other repetitive disorders. New York: Springer; 2001. p. 73–98.

86. Billings A. Self-monitoring in the treatment of tics: a single-subject analysis. J Behav Ther Exp Psychiatry 1978;9(4):339–42.

87. Hutzell R, Platzek D, Logue P. Control of symptoms of Gilles de la Tourette's syndrome by self-monitoring. J Behav Ther Exp Psychiatry 1974;5(1):71–6.

88. Woods DW, Miltenberger RG, Lumley VA. Sequential application of major habit-reversal components to treat motor tics in children. J Appl Behav Anal 1996; 29(4):483–93.

89. Wright K, Miltenberger R. Awareness training in the treatment of head and facial tics. J Behav Ther Exp Psychiatry 1987;18(3):269–74.

90. Roane H, Piazza C, Cercone J, et al. Assessment and treatment of vocal tics associated with Tourette's syndrome. Behav Modif 2002;26(4):482–98.

91. Wagaman J, Miltenberger R, Williams D. Treatment of a vocal tic by differential reinforcement. J Behav Ther Exp Psychiatry 1995;26(1):35–9.

92. Lahey B, McNees M, McNees M. Control of an obscene 'verbal tic' through time-out in an elementary school classroom. J Appl Behav Anal 1973;6(1):101–4.

93. Azrin NH, Nunn RG. Habit-reversal: a method of eliminating nervous habits and tics. Behav Res Ther 1973;11:619–28.

94. Woods DW, Piacentini JC, Chang S, et al. Managing Tourette's syndrome: a behavioral intervention for children and adults. New York (NY): Oxford University Press; 2008.

95. Verdellen CWJ, Keijsers GPJ, Cath DC. Exposure with response prevention versus habit reversal in Tourettes's syndrome: a controlled study. Behav Res Ther 2004;42:501–11.

96. Deckersbach T, Rauch S, Buhlmann U, et al. Habit reversal versus supportive psychotherapy in Tourette's disorder: a randomized controlled trial and predictors of treatment response. Behav Res Ther 2004;44:1079–90.

97. Chambless D, Ollendick T. Empirically supported psychological interventions: controversies and evidence. Annu Rev Psychol 2001;52:685–716.

98. Miltenberger R, Fuqua R, McKinley T. Habit reversal with muscle tics: replication and component analysis. Behav Ther 1985;16(1):39–50.

99. Woods DW, Twohig MP. Using habit reversal to treat chronic vocal tic disorder in children. Behav Interv 2002;17:159–68.

100. Woods DW, Twohig MP, Flessner CA, et al. Treatment of vocal tics in children with Tourette syndrome: investigating the efficacy of habit reversal. J Appl Behav Anal 2003;36:109–12.

101. Miltenberger RG, Fuqua RW. A comparison of contingent vs. non-contingent competing response practice in the treatment of nervous habits. J Behav Ther Exp Psychiatry 1985;16:195–200.

102. Sharenow EL, Fuqua RW, Miltenberger RG. The treatment of muscle tics with dissimilar competing response practice. J Appl Behav Anal 1989;22:35–42.

103. Miltenberger RG, Fuqua RW, Woods DW. Applying behavior analysis to clinical problems: review and analysis of habit reversal. J Appl Behav Anal 1998;31(3): 447–69.

104. Flessner CA, Miltenberger RG, Egemo K. An evaluation of the social support component of simplified habit reversal. Behav Ther 2005;36:35–42.

105. Verdellen C, Hoogduin C, Kato B, et al. Habituation of premonitory sensations during exposure and response prevention treatment in Tourette's syndrome. Behav Modif 2008;32(2):215–27.

106. Wetterneck C, Woods D. An evaluation of the effectiveness of exposure and response prevention on repetitive behaviors associated with Tourette's syndrome. J Appl Behav Anal 2006;39(4):441–4.

107. Woods D, Hook S, Spellman D, et al. Case study: exposure and response prevention for an adolescent with Tourette's syndrome and OCD. J Am Acad Child Adolesc Psychiatry 2000;39(7):904–7.

108. Fuata P, Griffiths R. Cognitive behavioural treatment of a vocal tic. Behav Change 1992;9(1):14–8.

109. Marcks B, Woods D, Teng E, et al. What do those who know, know? Investigating providers' knowledge about Tourette's syndrome and its treatment. Cogn Behav Pract 2004;11(3):298–305.

110. Burd L, Kerbeshian J. Treatment-generated problems associated with behavior modification in Tourette disorder. Dev Med Child Neurol 1987;29:831–3.

111. Silverstein S, Como P, Palumbo D, et al. Multiple sources of attentional dysfunction in adults with Tourette's syndrome: comparison with attention deficit-hyperactivity disorder. Neuropsychology 1995;9(2):157–64.

112. Shimberg E. Living with Tourette syndrome. New York: Fireside Books; 1995.

113. Murphy SA. An experimental design for the development of adaptive treatment strategies. Stat Med 2005;24(10):1455–81.

The Effectiveness of Cognitive Behavioral Therapy for Personality Disorders

Alexis K. Matusiewicz, BA[a,b], Christopher J. Hopwood, PhD[c],
Annie N. Banducci, BA[a,b], C.W. Lejuez, PhD[a,b],*

KEYWORDS

- Cognitive behavioral therapy
- Personality disorders • Psychotherapy

Personality disorders (PDs) are characterized by long-standing patterns of impairment that manifest across multiple domains of functioning, including disturbances in cognition (eg, perceptual abnormalities, disruptions in the experience of self), emotion (eg, excessive reactivity or intensity), interpersonal behavior (eg, social isolation, high-conflict relationships), and difficulties with impulse control (eg, repeated engagement in high-risk or criminal activity).[1,2] The *Diagnostic and Statistical Manual of Mental Disorders-IV-TR* (Fourth Edition, Text Revised) (DSM-IV-TR)[1] officially recognizes 10 PDs, which are grouped on the basis of prominent common features: Cluster A refers to the "odd, eccentric" PDs (schizotypal, schizoid, and paranoid), Cluster B includes the "dramatic, erratic and emotional" disorders (histrionic, narcissistic, borderline, antisocial), and Cluster C refers to the "anxious or fearful" disorders (avoidant, dependent, obsessive-compulsive). Prevalence rates of these disorders, as well as prominent cognitive, behavioral, and interpersonal characteristics, as outlined in the DSM, are included in **Table 1**.

Whereas Axis I clinical disorders (eg, depression, anxiety) generally are considered acute disruptions in otherwise normal functioning, Axis II problems historically have

---

[a] Center for Addictions, Personality and Emotion Research, University of Maryland, 2103 Cole Field House, College Park, MD 20742, USA
[b] Department of Psychology, University of Maryland, 2103 Cole Field House, College Park, MD 20742, USA
[c] Department of Psychology, Michigan State University, 107A Psychology, East Lansing, MI 48824, USA
* Corresponding author. Department of Psychology, University of Maryland, 2103 Cole Field House, College Park, MD 20742.
E-mail address: clejuez@psyc.umd.edu

Psychiatr Clin N Am 33 (2010) 657–685
doi:10.1016/j.psc.2010.04.007
0193-953X/10/$ – see front matter © 2010 Elsevier Inc. All rights reserved.

Table 1
Description and population-based lifetime prevalence of DSM-IV PDs

Disorder	Defining Characteristics	Prevalence
Paranoid	Extreme suspicion and mistrust of others, and tendency to view themselves as superior and unique. Constantly on guard and reactive to real or perceived threats	2.3%–4.4%
Schizoid	Restricted range of affect, interpersonal indifference and isolation	3.1%–4.9%
Schizotypal	Odd, eccentric behavior, distorted thoughts and perceptions, inappropriate affect and discomfort with social relationships	3.3%–3.9%
Narcissistic	Inflated self-importance, inability to empathize with others, and overemphasis on status	0.0%–6.2%
Histrionic	Need to be center of attention, exaggerated/inappropriate emotionality, and seductiveness	0.0%–1.8%
Borderline	Volatile interpersonal relationships, fear of abandonment, self mutilation/suicidality, impulsivity, and emotional instability	1.4%–5.9%
Antisocial	Aggressive interpersonal interactions, impulsivity, lack of remorse, and defiant disregard for safety of self and others	1.0%–3.6%
Obsessive-compulsive	Preoccupation with adherence to rules, orderliness, and control	2.4%–7.9%
Dependent	Persistent and pathological need to be with and gain approval of others	0.5%–0.6%
Avoidant	Low tolerance for negative emotions, few close relationships, and fear of rejection or ridicule in interpersonal interactions	2.4%–2%

been conceptualized as chronic and often intractable patterns of dysfunction.[1,3] However, recent findings suggest that individuals with personality pathology may demonstrate symptomatic improvement over time.[4,5] Furthermore, there is growing evidence that targeted psychotherapy can reduce symptoms and enhance functioning among individuals with PDs.[6–9]

Cognitive behavioral therapy (CBT) is well suited to address the varied and often long-standing problems of patients with PDs for several reasons. From a cognitive behavioral perspective, PDs are maintained by a combination of maladaptive beliefs about self and others, contextual/environmental factors that reinforce problematic behavior and/or undermine effective behavior, and skill deficits that preclude adaptive responding.[10,11] CBT incorporates a wide range of techniques to modify these factors, including cognitive restructuring, behavior modification, exposure, psychoeducation, and skills training. In addition, CBT for PDs emphasizes the importance of a supportive, collaborative, and well-defined therapeutic relationship, which enhances the patient's willingness to make changes and serves as a potent source of contingency.[10–13] In sum, several aspects of CBT's conceptual framework and its technical flexibility make it appropriate to address the pervasive and diffuse impairment commonly observed among patients with PDs.

The empirical focus of CBT has translated into strong interest in evaluating treatment outcomes for CBT, which is compatible with the growing emphasis on evidence-based practice in the fields of psychiatry and clinical psychology.[14,15]

However, despite marked advances in the development, evaluation, and dissemination of empirically supported treatments for Axis I disorders, progress has been slow for most PDs. Treatment evaluation remains in its early stages, and many PDs are only now receiving preliminary empirical attention. In this regard, borderline and avoidant PDs have the most extensive empirical support, including numerous randomized controlled trials (RCTs). In contrast, evidence for CBT for other PDs is limited to a small number of open-label trials and case studies. For this reason, uncontrolled studies (eg, open trials, single-case designs, case reports) are included in this review. Although certainly lacking the rigor of RCTs, uncontrolled studies can provide clinically important information about mechanisms of change and moderators of treatment outcome. In addition to their use for driving theory and hypotheses for testing in future RCTs, uncontrolled studies can be useful for uncovering essential qualities of effective interventions and the effectiveness of CBT as it is delivered "in the field."[16,17]

METHOD

To identify appropriate publications, the authors conducted literature searches using MedLine, PubMed, and PsycInfo using the names of the 10 PDs of interest, variations of the phrase "cognitive behavioral therapy," the names of common CBT components (eg, skills training), and specific cognitive behavioral treatments (eg, Dialectical Behavior Therapy) as keywords. These searches were supplemented with a hand search of relevant journals, review articles, and bibliographies. English-language studies published between 1980 (ie, when the modern multiaxial taxonomy was introduced) and 2009 were included if they had a sample of adult patients with a diagnosis of PD, provided a clear description of a cognitive behavioral intervention, specified diagnostic and outcome measures, and reported outcomes related to Axis II symptoms and symptomatic behavior. Studies were excluded if they were concerned primarily with the effect of comorbid Axis II disorders on Axis I treatment outcomes.

This search yielded 45 publications evaluating the outcome of cognitive behavioral interventions for PDs. **Table 2** summarizes key elements of the study design and significant findings for each publication. To provide consistency with previous reviews, outcomes are divided into 4 categories: symptoms, symptomatic behavior, social functioning, and global functioning.[7] The *symptoms* category consists of measures of symptom severity (including Axis I and Axis II disorders and overall psychiatric symptom ratings), symptom counts, or percentage of patients who met the recovery criterion. *Symptomatic behavior* includes measures of specific cognitive and/or behavioral outcomes, such as extent of dysfunctional cognitions, frequency of nonsuicidal self-injury, or days of abstinence from substances. *Social functioning* includes assessments of overall social functioning or social adjustment, whereas specific interpersonal behaviors (eg, frequency of verbal assault) are coded as symptomatic behavior. Finally, *global functioning* includes measures of overall functioning, (eg, Global Assessment of Functioning Scale).

TREATMENT OUTCOME
Borderline Personality Disorder

Treatments for BPD have been studied more extensively than treatments for any other PD. For example, the authors identified 16 RCTs of cognitive behavioral treatments that specifically target BPD, as well as 10 naturalistic studies and 8 case studies, which provide evidence of the effectiveness of CBT in real-world settings. Of these, dialectical behavior therapy (DBT)[11] has received the most thorough evaluation and

Table 2
Treatment outcomes of CBT for PDs

Citation	Study Type	Subject(s)	Treatment	Duration, Frequency	Findings
Borderline PD					

Linehan et al[18-20]	RCT	Outpatients with BPD and parasuicide
		n = 44
		100% female
			1. TAU
			2. DBT
				12 months of weekly individual DBT and skills group	1. Symptomatic behavior:
					   DBT>TAU
					2. Social functioning:
					   DBT>TAU
					3. Global functioning:
					   DBT>TAU

Turner[21]	RCT	Outpatients with BPD
		n = 24
		76% female
			1. CCT
			2. DBT
				49–84 individual sessions	1. Symptoms: DBT>CCT
					Decreased depression, anger, impulsivity, suicidal ideation
					2. Symptomatic behavior:
					   DBT>CCT
					Decreased suicide, NSSI
					3. Global Functioning:
					   DBT>CCT

Koons et al[22]	RCT	Outpatients with BPD n = 20 100% female	1. TAU 2. DBT	5 months of weekly individual DBT and skills group	1. Symptoms: DBT>TAU 2. Symptomatic behavior: DBT>TAU
Verheul et al[23]	RCT	Outpatients with BPD with and without substance dependence n = 58 100% female	1. TAU 2. DBT	12 months of weekly individual DBT and skills group	1. Symptomatic behavior: DBT>TAU

Study	Design	Sample	Treatments	Duration	Results
Linehan et al[24]	RCT	Outpatients with BPD and parasuicide n = 100 100% female	1. CTBE 2. DBT	12 months of weekly individual DBT and skills group	1. Symptoms: DBT = CTBE 2. Symptomatic behavior: DBT>CTBE
Clarkin et al[25]	RCT	Outpatients with BPD n = 90 83% female	1. ST 2. TFP 3. DBT	52 weekly sessions	1. Symptoms: SC = TFP = DBT 2. Symptomatic behavior: TFP>DBT = SC 3. Social functioning: SC = TFP = DBT 4. Global functioning: SC = TFP = DBT
McMain et al[26]	RCT	Outpatients with BPD with 2+ self-injurious episodes in prior 5 years n = 180 90% female	1. GPM 2. DBT	Weekly sessions for 1 year	1. Symptoms: DBT = GPM 2. Symptomatic behavior: DBT = GPM 3. Social functioning: DBT = GPM
Harley et al[27]	Controlled trial	Outpatients with BPD n = 45 92% female	1. DBT (w/DBT skills) 2. Non-DBT individual + DBT skills	7 months of weekly individual and group sessions	1. Symptoms: Improvement in symptoms regardless of individual treatment 2. Symptomatic behavior: Improvement in symptoms regardless of individual treatment
Brassington and Krowitz[28]	Open trial	Outpatients with BPD n = 10 100% female	DBT	6 months of weekly individual DBT and skills group	1. Symptoms: Decreased BPD, depression, anxiety Improved SCL-90-R
Prendergast and McCausland[29]	Open trial	Outpatients with BPD n = 11 100% female	DBT	6 months of weekly individual and group sessions	1. Symptomatic behavior: Decreased parasuicide and frequency of medically severe suicide attempts

(continued on next page)

Table 2
(continued)

Citation	Study Type	Subject(s)	Treatment	Duration, Frequency	Findings
Comtois et al[30]	Open trial	Outpatients with BPD (community) n = 24 96% female	DBT	1 year	1. Symptomatic Behavior: Reduced self-injurious behaviors, psychiatric inpatient admissions, days, emergency room visits
Ben-Porath et al[31]	Open trial	Patients with DBT and an Axis I diagnosis	DBT	6 months	1. Symptoms: Reduced suicidal thoughts 2. Symptomatic behavior: Reduction in behaviors interfering with quality of life and therapy interfering behaviors
Hopko et al[32]	Case study	Outpatient with BPD, OCPD, and MDD (community) Female	BA + DBT skills in individual therapy	12 weekly sessions	1. Symptoms: Diminished depressive symptoms
Kerr et al[33]	Case study	Outpatient with BPD (community) Female	DBT (no group skills, on-call system, or consultation team)	6 months	1. Symptoms: Decreased suicidality and misery
Bohus et al[34,35]	RCT	Inpatients with BPD n = 50 100% female	1. WL-TAU 2. DBT (inpatient)	3 months inpatient treatment	1. Symptoms: DBT>TAU 2. Symptomatic behavior: DBT>TAU
Barley et al[36]	Controlled trial	Inpatients with BPD	1. Inpatient TAU 2. DBT (inpatient)	Average of 103 inpatient days	1. Symptomatic behavior: Inpatient DBT>TAU
Davidson et al[37]	RCT	Outpatients with BPD n = 106 84% female	1. TAU 2. TAU + CBT	Average of 16 sessions over 52 weeks	1. Symptoms: TAU + CBT>TAU 2. Symptomatic behavior: TAU + CBT>TAU
Cottraux et al[38]	RCT	Outpatients with BPD n = 65	1. SC 2. CBT	12 months of weekly sessions	1. Symptomatic behavior: CBT>SC

Study	Design	Sample	Treatment/Comparison	Duration	Outcomes
Turner[40]	Open trial	Outpatients with BPD n = 4 50% female	CBT + Alprazolam	3 times a week for 3 months, then weekly for 9–18 months	1. Symptoms: reduced BPD symptoms
Evans et al[41] MacLeod et al[42]	RCT	Individuals with Cluster B PDs and a parasuicide attempt in the past 12 months n = 34	1. MACT 2. TAU	6 weekly sessions	Lower suicide attempts, self-rated depressive symptoms, and cost of care in MACT. Improvements in positive future thinking
Weinberg et al[43]	RCT	Borderline personality disorder patients n = 30 100% female	1. TAU 2. TAU + MACT	6 weekly sessions	1. Symptomatic behavior: TAU + MACT>TAU
Nordahl and Nysæter[44]	Single case study series	Outpatients with BPD n = 6 50% female	1. SFP	65–120 weekly sessions	1. Symptoms: 50% of patients no longer met diagnostic criteria for BPD at the end of treatment
Blum et al[45]	RCT	Outpatients with BPD n = 124 83% female	1. TAU 2. TAU + STEPPS	20 weekly group sessions	1. Symptoms: TAU + CBGT>TAU 2. Symptomatic behavior: TAU + STEPPS = TAU
Black et al[46]	Open Trial	Offenders with BPD n = 12 100% female	STEPPS	20 weekly sessions	1. Symptoms: BPD and depression 2. Symptomatic behavior: Decreased engagement in impulsive and self-damaging behaviors, increased positive coping
Gratz and Gunderson[47]	RCT	Outpatients with BPD and nonsuicidal self-injury n = 22 100% female	1. TAU 2. TAU + ERGT	14 weekly sessions	1. Symptoms: TAU + skills group>TAU 2. Symptomatic behavior: TAU + ERGT>TAU

(continued on next page)

Table 2
(continued)

Citation	Study Type	Subject(s)	Treatment	Duration, Frequency	Findings
Avoidant PD					
Alden[48]	RCT	Outpatients with AVPD n = 76 45% female	1. WL 2. CBGT 3. CBGT + social skills 4. CBGT + intimacy skills	10 weekly sessions	1. Symptoms: all CBGTs>WL; addition of skill modules did not improve outcomes beyond CBGT 2. Social functioning: CBGT + intimacy focus>all other CBGTs; all conditions produced improvements
Stravynski et al[49]	RCT	Outpatients with AVPD n = 21	1. CBGT with social skills 2. CBGT with discussion	5 weekly sessions	1. Symptoms: Skills = Discussion 2. Symptomatic behavior: Skills = Discussion
Renneberg et al[50]	Open trial	Outpatients with AVPD n = 17 47% female	CBGT	32 hours over 4 days	1. Symptoms: Modestly improved at posttreatment assessment 2. Symptomatic behavior: Improved at posttreatment assessment
Stravynski et al[39]	Open trial	Outpatients with AVPD n = 28	CBGT	14 weekly sessions	1. Symptoms: Improved at postassessment
Emmelkamp et al[51]	RCT	Outpatients with AVPD n = 62 52% female	1. WL 2. CBT 3. BDT	20 weekly sessions	1. Symptoms: CBT>BDT = WL 2. Symptomatic behavior: CBT>BDT = WL
Strauss et al[52]	Open trial	Outpatients with AVPD n = 24	CBT	Up to 52 weekly sessions	1. Symptoms: Improvements in depressive symptoms and PD symptoms

Study	Design	Sample	Treatment	Length	Outcomes
Hyman and Schneider[53]	Case study	Outpatient with AVPD, GSP Female	CBT	21 weekly sessions	1. Symptoms: Reduced at treatment termination
Hofmann[54]	Case study	Outpatient with AVPD, GSP Male	CBT	27 sessions over 18 months	1. Symptoms: Below clinical cutoff on symptom measures at termination and follow-up 2. Symptomatic behavior: Improved interpersonal and occupational functioning
Obsessive-compulsive PD					
Strauss et al[52]	Open trial	Outpatients with OCPD n = 16	CBT	Up to 52 weekly sessions	1. Symptoms: Improvements in depressive symptoms and PD symptoms
Antisocial PD					
Davidson et al[13]	RCT	Outpatients with ASPD and aggression n = 52 100% male	1. TAU 2. TAU + CBT	15 sessions over 6 months or 30 sessions over 12 months	1. Symptoms: TAU = TAU + CBT; both treatments produced reductions in symptoms 2. Symptomatic behavior: TAU = TAU + CBT; both treatments reduced symptomatic behaviors 3. Social functioning: TAU = TAU + CBT; both treatments produced improvement
Other PDs, comorbid PDs, PDNOS, or mixed PD samples					
Muran et al[55]	RCT	Outpatients with Cluster C or PDNOS n = 128 53% female	1. BRT 2. BDT 3. CBT	30 weekly sessions	1. Symptoms: BRT = BDT = CBT 2. Symptomatic behavior: BRT = BDT = CBT

(continued on next page)

Table 2
(continued)

Citation	Study Type	Subject(s)	Treatment	Duration, Frequency	Findings
Springer et al[56]	RCT	Inpatients with PDs $n = 31$ 68% female	1. ST 2. DBT skills group	10 sessions daily sessions	1. Symptoms: DBT = TAU; both groups exhibited improvements in symptoms during the trial 2. Symptomatic behavior: DBT = TAU; both groups exhibited improvements in symptomatic behaviors during treatment
Lynch et al[57]	RCT	Outpatients with PDs and MDD Study 1: $n = 34$ (46% female) Study 2 $n = 37$ (46% female)	Study 1 1. MED 2. MED + DBT skills Study 2 1. MED 2. MED + DBT	Study 1: 28 weekly group sessions Study 2: 24 weekly group and individual sessions	Study 1 1. Symptoms: MED+ DBT>MED (depression) Study 2 1. Symptoms: MED + DBT>MED (PD)
Williams[58]	Case study	Outpatient with PPD, MDD Male	CBT	11 weekly sessions	1. Symptoms: Remission of depressive symptoms during treatment 2. Symptomatic behavior: Fewer suspicious comments and greater self-disclosure
Lynch and Cheavens[59]	Case study	Outpatient with PPD, OCPD, MDD Male	DBT (mod)	9 months of weekly individual DBT; 6 months of weekly skills group	1. Symptoms: no longer met diagnostic criteria for PPD, OCPD or MDD at follow-up 2. Symptomatic behavior: Diminished interpersonal sensitivity, aggression, improved interpersonal relationships at follow-up

| Busch et al[84] | Single subject | Outpatient with HPD Female | CBT + FAP | 20 weekly sessions | 1. Symptoms: Remission of depressive symptoms 2. Symptomatic behavior: Reduced engagement in aversive interpersonal behaviors in and out of session; greater perceived social support |
| Callaghan et al[60] | Single subject | Outpatient with PDNOS (histrionic, narcissistic features) Male | FAP | 23 weekly sessions | 1. Symptomatic behavior: fewer aversive interpersonal behaviors; greater involvement in prosocial behaviors; improved emotional expression |

Abbreviations: ASPD, antisocial PD; AVPD, avoidant PD; BA, behavioral activation; BDT, brief dynamic therapy; BPD, borderline PD; BRT, brief relational therapy; CBGT, cognitive behavioral group therapy; CBT, cognitive behavioral therapy; CTBE, community treatment by experts; DBT, dialectical behavior therapy; ERGT, emotion regulation group treatment; FAP, functional analytic psychotherapy; GPM, general psychiatric management; GSP, generalized social phobia; HPD, histrionic PD; MACT, Manual-Assisted Cognitive Therapy; MDD, major depressive disorder; MED, medication management; OCPD, obsessive-compulsive PD; PDNOS, PD not otherwise specified; PPD, paranoid PD; SC, supportive counseling; SFP, schema-focused psychotherapy; ST, standard treatment; STEPPS, Systems Training for Emotional Predictability and Problem Solving; TAU, treatment as usual; TFP, transference-focused psychotherapy; WL, waitlist control.

empirical support; however, there have been several studies that evaluate traditional CBT approaches, schema-focused therapy, and skills-based interventions.

Dialectical behavior therapy

DBT is an extensively studied and widely adopted treatment for patients with BPD and parasuicidal behavior (eg, suicide attempts and nonsuicidal self-injury). DBT is informed by a biosocial model of BPD, which suggests that BPD emerges from a biological predisposition to emotional intensity and reactivity coupled with an invalidating childhood environment.[11] Accordingly, DBT emphasizes the importance of acceptance and validation in the therapeutic relationship, and conceptualizes symptomatic behaviors as understandable products of the patient's learning history. In addition, DBT has roots in dialectical philosophy and Eastern spiritual traditions, which place value on the synthesis of opposites (eg, balancing acceptance and change) and creation of a life worth living.[11,17] Standard, outpatient DBT has 4 components, delivered concurrently over the course of a year or more: individual DBT, group skills training, phone consultation for skills coaching, and weekly consultation meetings for the therapists. Individual treatment uses functional analysis, exposure, contingency management, and cognitive restructuring to decrease problematic behaviors and enhance quality of life. Skills training enhances the patient's ability to respond effectively in difficult situations. The DBT-targeted skills include mindfulness, interpersonal effectiveness, emotion regulation, and distress tolerance. Phone consultation is available to patients to support the generalization of skills. Finally, the treatment team participates in weekly supervision to provide support and enhance adherence to the DBT treatment model.[11,17]

The efficacy of the full DBT treatment package (consisting of all 4 treatment elements) has been demonstrated in multiple RCTs, including trials conducted by independent research groups and in diverse patient populations. Because these studies been reviewed in depth elsewhere,[17,61] they are discussed only briefly here. Several trials have compared 12 months of DBT with treatment as usual (TAU). However, the quality of this control condition has varied considerably from minimal (eg, bimonthly clinical management; 19) to intensive (eg, weekly individual and group psychotherapy, and medication management; 20). Despite this variability in the TAU condition, findings suggest that DBT yields significantly greater reductions in the frequency of parasuicidal behavior and anger and higher rates of treatment retention.[18–20,22,23] In addition, findings suggest that, relative to TAU, DBT is associated with fewer emergency room contacts and inpatient days, decreased depression and impulsiveness, and greater social and global adjustment; however, these results have not been replicated across studies.

While these findings are certainly promising, they raise the question of whether treatment effects are specific to DBT, or whether these outcomes can be matched by other active treatment conditions delivered by well-trained clinicians. In one study, Turner[21] randomized outpatients with BPD to either client-centered therapy (CCT; $n = 12$) or modified DBT, which consisted of only individual treatment (with individual skills training) and included a psychodynamic case conceptualization ($n = 12$). At the end of treatment, clients in DBT had significantly fewer suicide attempts, emergency room visits and inpatient days, decreased impulsiveness, depression, and anger, and greater global adjustment, suggesting that the effects of DBT is superior to an active but unstructured control treatment across numerous domains of functioning. Similarly, Linehan and colleagues[24] assigned outpatients with BPD to receive a year of either community treatment by experts (CTBE; $n = 51$) or full-package DBT ($n = 52$), with treatments matched for many nonspecific clinician characteristics (eg, therapist sex, training, supervision, allegiance to treatment). DBT was associated with fewer suicide attempts, fewer emergency contacts and inpatient days, and superior treatment retention, suggesting that DBT's effects cannot be explained by general therapy factors. Overall, there is reliable evidence that DBT is superior to active, nonbehavioral treatments in terms of incidence of suicide attempts, and use of emergency and inpatient psychiatric services; however, there is inconsistent evidence that DBT enhances emotional variables, social adjustment, or global functioning.

Most recently, there have been 2 RCTs that compare the effectiveness of DBT to other empirically supported interventions for BPD. For example, Clarkin and colleagues[25] randomized outpatients with BPD to receive a year of biweekly transference-focused psychotherapy (TFP; $n = 23$), a year of full-package DBT ($n = 17$), or a year of weekly psychodynamic supportive therapy ($n = 21$). In addition, all clients received medication as necessary. Over the course of treatment, patients in all conditions showed significant improvements in depression, anxiety, social adjustment, and global functioning. Both TFP and DBT produced significant reductions in suicidality, whereas supportive treatment did not; on the other hand, TFP and supportive treatment reduced anger, but DBT did not. Furthermore, only TFP was associated with significant reductions in irritability, physical assault, and verbal aggression. Findings indicate that all 3 treatments are effective in reducing symptoms and dysfunction associated with BPD. Consistent with previous findings, DBT did have a positive effect on suicide-related outcomes. However, the most widespread gains were observed among clients in TFP. In another study, McMain and colleagues[26] compared DBT ($n = 90$) with general psychiatric management ($n = 90$), which was based on the American Psychiatric Association recommendations, and consisted of psychodynamic psychotherapy and symptom-targeted medication management. From the baseline assessment to the end of treatment, both groups showed significant improvements in almost every outcome assessed (eg, frequency of suicide attempts and nonsuicidal self-injury, medical severity of these behaviors, emergency room visits and inpatient days, depression, anger, BPD symptom severity, and overall symptom distress). However, contrary to predictions the groups did not differ significantly on any treatment outcome, suggesting that DBT and general psychiatric management are equally effective in addressing symptoms and impairment associated with BPD.

Taken together, findings from RCTs for DBT provide considerable support for its effectiveness as a treatment for BPD across many symptom domains. There is consistent evidence that DBT reduces suicidal and parasuicidal behavior, decreases the medical risk associated with these behaviors, and produces fewer emergency visits and inpatient days. There is also evidence that DBT reduces affective symptoms of BPD (eg, depression, anxiety, anger), and that it enhances global adjustment. It is also noteworthy that the effectiveness of DBT has been demonstrated in a range of real-world clinical settings, including a veterans' affairs hospital,[22] community mental health centers,[30,31] a university training clinic,[33] and among clinicians in private practice.[21,25] Moreover, DBT has been found to be superior to TAU, and generally equivalent to other active, structured, theoretically sound outpatient treatments.

Whereas standard DBT was developed to be a long-term outpatient treatment, there have been efforts to adapt DBT for use inpatients with BPD. In an initial trial, Barley and colleagues[36] compared frequency of nonsuicidal self-injury and overdose before and after a long-term inpatient ward transitioned to DBT. As an additional control, they compared these changes to another general psychotherapy ward. These investigators reported significant reductions in the incidence of nonsuicidal self-injury, and parasuicidal behavior decreased on the DBT unit, whereas no decrease was observed on the comparison unit. Bohus and colleagues[34,35] found similarly promising outcomes following 3-month inpatient DBT-based treatment, designed to jumpstart outpatient DBT. Inpatient DBT consisted of psychoeducation about BPD and mechanisms of treatment, skills training, and contingency management for parasuicidal behavior. In a pilot study, 24 female inpatients were assessed before and after 12 weeks of treatment. Significant improvements were observed in frequency of parasuicidal behavior, depression, anxiety, stress, and overall psychiatric symptoms.[34] Results were replicated in a subsequent RCT, in which women with BPD assigned a waitlist-TAU condition ($n = 31$) or inpatient DBT ($n = 19$). The inpatient group made significant gains in frequency of nonsuicidal self-injury, depression, anxiety, and social and global functioning, whereas the TAU condition did not demonstrate significant improvements in any symptom domain. Overall, 42% of the inpatient DBT group exhibited clinically significant change compared with 0% of the TAU group, and gains were maintained 1 month after treatment. While these findings are promising, there is also evidence that the duration and the extent of its integration into the inpatient program may be critical determinants of its effectiveness. For example, in one study, inpatients with PDs, including BPD, were randomized to receive either 10 sessions of a nontherapuetic discussion group or a DBT-based skills group.[56] Both groups showed similar remission in symptoms, suggesting that the passage of time may account for some of the improvement observed; however, the frequency of acting out actually increased in the DBT group. In sum, findings suggest that inpatient DBT can be effective during longer-term hospitalizations (ie, 3 months), when a DBT approach is reflected in many facets of treatment; however, it appears to be less helpful when a short-term group format is added to inpatient TAU.

Also of note, although DBT was initially developed to target parasuicidal behavior among individuals with BPD, the treatment has also been applied for patients with BPD and substance use disorders[62–66] as well as patients with BPD and bulimia nervosa or binge eating disorder.[67,68] These studies have produced generally favorable results for reducing incidence of specific self-damaging behaviors, with mixed findings as to whether treatment gains generalize to all types of impulsive behavior.

Cognitive behavioral therapy

The Borderline PD Study of Cognitive Therapy (BOSCOT) trial[37] was the first randomized controlled study to evaluate the effectiveness of traditional CBT for BPD. BOSCOT examined clinical outcomes in a sample of 106 patients with BPD, who received either TAU (community-based medication management and emergency services; $n = 52$) or TAU and up to 30 sessions of individual CBT (TAU+CBT; $n = 54$) over 1 year (patients attended an average of 16 sessions). The initial sessions of CBT were used for assessment and development of a cognitive case formulation.[13] Later sessions were devoted to cognitive restructuring (eg, identifying and evaluating negative automatic thoughts and cognitive errors, and modifying dysfunctional schemas and core beliefs) and implementing behavioral change (eg, decreasing self-defeating behaviors and practicing adaptive responding to problems). Gains were observed in both treatment groups over the course of treatment and at follow-up. Participants in TAU+CBT reported fewer suicide attempts during the study period than did participants in TAU. At follow-up, the TAU+CBT group also reported less anxiety, lower symptom distress, and fewer dysfunctional cognitions. However, the conditions did not differ in terms of number of inpatient hospitalizations or emergency room visits, frequency of nonsuicidal self-injury, psychiatric symptoms, interpersonal functioning, and global functioning. Overall, CBT+TAU led to improved treatment outcomes in a handful of critical domains when compared with a low-intensity TAU condition.

A recent study by Cottraux and colleagues[38] found that CBT for BPD was superior to Rogerian supportive counseling (SC) for some outcomes. Outpatients with BPD were randomized to receive 1 year of weekly CBT ($n = 33$) or SC ($n = 32$). Treatment completers were assessed at 6, 12, and 24 months. Participants in CBT and SC did not differ in terms of depression, anxiety, dysfunctional cognitions, suicidal and self-damaging behavior, or quality of life. However, CBT was associated with more rapid improvements in hopelessness and trait-level impulsivity, higher ratings of the therapeutic relationship, and better treatment retention. CBT also was associated with greater improvements in patient- and clinician-rated global symptom severity at the 24-month follow-up, which may suggest continued gains following treatment termination. However, this finding should be interpreted with caution because a high proportion of patients dropped out of treatment or were lost to follow-up, so an intent-to-treat analysis may have produced different results.

Manual-assisted cognitive therapy (MACT) is another CBT package that was developed to address the need for a brief, cost-effective intervention for patients with BPD (and other Cluster B PDs) who engage in nonsuicidal self-injury.[41] MACT is a 6-session manualized treatment that combines traditional components of CBT (eg, thought monitoring, psychoeducation) with elements of DBT (eg, distress tolerance skills, functional analysis of incidents of nonsuicidal self-injury). Treatment material is presented to the patient in the form of a workbook, which contains information about various skills and strategies for reducing episodes of self-damaging behavior. The therapist provides support as the patient completes the worksheets for content area. MACT has been evaluated in several studies. In the preliminary study, patients with a Cluster B PD and a recent episode of nonsuicidal self-injury or suicide attempt were assigned to receive either TAU, which consisted of standard psychiatric care ($n = 16$), or MACT ($n = 18$). Even though patients received, on average, less than 3 of the 6 treatment sessions, patients in MACT demonstrated significant reductions in depression and inpatient days and a significant increase in future-oriented thinking at follow-up.[41,42] In a follow-up to this study, participants with BPD were randomized to receive either TAU ($n = 15$) or MACT+TAU.[43] Treatment uptake was excellent, with all participants completing all 6 MACT sessions. The addition of MACT to TAU was associated with a significant decrease in the frequency and medical severity of nonsuicidal self-injury; however, the treatment groups did not differ in length of time to repeat or suicidal ideation.[43] Of note, these findings contrast with the results of a previous trial of MACT, which used a sample of patients with a recent suicide attempt or episode of nonsuicidal self-injury who did not necessarily have a PD diagnosis. This study failed to find any benefit of MACT beyond the effects of TAU, which may be attributed to the fact that 40% of patients failed to attend a single session (ie, the intervention consisted of the treatment manual alone). In sum, MACT appears to have clinical utility for individuals with BPD when delivered in conjunction with TAU; however, in mixed-diagnosis samples, its effects may be negligible and treatment retention may be problematic.

Schema-focused therapy

Critics of traditional CBT have observed that the demands and assumptions of CBT are at odds with the needs of patients with PDs.[69] Specifically, CBT's structured, instructive, problem-focused approach may be ill suited to patients who present with vague or diffuse problems, cognitive rigidity, poor emotional awareness, or an interpersonal style that undermines collaborative relationships.[70,71]

Schema-focused therapy (SFT) retains a cognitive theoretical framework, and suggests that PDs result from early maladaptive schemas that interfere with the individual's ability to meet his or her core needs. The individual develops patterns of avoidance and compensation to avoid triggering the schema, but these patterns become overgeneralized and rigid. To modify early maladaptive schemas, SFT employs a broad range of techniques, including behavioral, psychodynamic, experiential, and interpersonal strategies. As a result, the treatment is more flexible, elaborative, and emotion-focused than traditional cognitive approaches.[69] SFT treatments also tend to be longer, ranging from 1 to 4 years in duration.[72]

The first systematic investigation of SFT as a treatment for BPD was published as a series of 6 case reports.[44] Outpatients received SFT based on treatment guidelines compiled by McGinn and Young.[69] Patients were assessed periodically over the course of 18 to 36 months of SFT, and again a year after treatment termination. All 6 patients showed progressive improvements in symptoms of depression, social functioning, and global functioning. At follow-up, 5 had maintained treatment gains and 3 no longer met diagnostic criteria for BPD at the end of treatment. As a group, the patients remained mildly impaired at follow-up; however, improvements in symptoms, and social and overall functioning were equivalent to a large effect size.

These findings have been replicated and broadened in 2 RCTs. Giesen-Bloo and colleagues[73] evaluated outcomes of patients who participated in either SFT ($n = 45$) or transference-focused psychotherapy (TFP; $n = 43$), a psychodynamic intervention. Patients received biweekly individual psychotherapy for up to 3 years. Relative to those in TFP, patients in SFT showed greater improvement across BPD symptom domains, including abandonment fears, relationships, identity disturbance, dissociation and paranoia, impulsivity, and parasuicidal behavior. A symptomatic behavior composite, consisting of measures of general symptoms, defense style, and PD-related beliefs, favored SFT over TFP throughout the course of treatment. At treatment termination, the treatment groups did not differ in terms of quality of life; however, patients in SFT made more rapid gains in this domain. Overall, a greater proportion of patients in SFT compared with TFP made clinically significant gains (66% vs 43%) and met the BPD recovery criterion (46% vs 24%), suggesting that long-term, individual SFT is an effective treatment for individuals with BPD, and that it outperforms TFP in terms of symptomatic improvement.[73]

Although SFT findings are promising, a long-term individual treatment may not be feasible in most mental health care settings. To address this concern, Farrell and colleagues[74] adapted SFT to be delivered in a group format over 30 sessions, as an adjunct to individual psychotherapy. The group treatment consisted of psychoeducation about BPD, skills training for emotional awareness and distress tolerance, and schema change work. The latter module focused on weakening maladaptive schemas enough to allow the patients to practice and apply other skills. Similar to individual SFT, in-session activities included cognitive restructuring, experiential activities (eg, empty chair technique) and behavioral skills practice.[74] Women with BPD were randomized to receive either TAU ($n = 16$) or 8 months of group SFT in addition to TAU ($n = 16$). Patients were assessed at baseline, posttreatment, and 6-month follow-up. Findings indicated a significant effect favoring SFT for BPD symptoms, general psychiatric symptom severity, and global functioning. Patients in the SFT group showed improvements in all BPD symptom domains. At posttreatment, 94% of patients in the SFT group no longer met diagnostic criteria for BPD, whereas only 25% of the TAU group reached this criterion. In sum, SFT appears to reduce BPD symptoms and enhance overall functioning, whether it is delivered as a long-term individual psychotherapy or as a shorter-term adjunctive group treatment. Individual SFT compared favorably to long-term psychodynamic psychotherapy, delivered by well-trained and experienced clinicians.

Skills-based interventions

Skills training has emerged as an important component of treatment for patients with BPD. Skills training is based on the assumption that individuals with BPD lack the skills necessary to behave effectively in the situations they encounter. Skills training interventions aim to remediate these deficits by providing direct instruction, modeling, and opportunities for rehearsal and coaching.[17] With skills in hand, patients are better able to avert crises or manage them without resorting to self-damaging behavior, which allows individual therapy to progress. Although DBT skills (described earlier) are widely adopted, 2 additional skills-based groups warrant mention. Like DBT, both interventions aim to reduce self-damaging behavior through the development of emotion regulation and other skills. However, in light of these similarities, there are important practical, conceptual, and empirical differences among these interventions.

Systems Training for Emotional Predictability and Problem Solving (STEPPS) is a manualized skills-based group treatment designed to reduce the self-damaging behaviors associated with BPD. STEPPS is based on the premise that individuals with BPD have limited access to specific strategies to regulate emotions or manage behavior in a way that promotes emotional stability, and that these difficulties are exacerbated by ineffective use of support systems.[75] To address these deficits, STEPPS integrates a systems perspective with a traditional CBT skills training approach. STEPPS consists of 20 weekly group sessions, divided into 4 modules. The first component of treatment has the patient assemble a support system, which may be composed of family members, friends, significant others, and health care providers.[75] Members of the supportive team receive psychoeducation about BPD and are taught how to respond to the patient in a manner that reinforces the new behavioral skills. The second component of treatment involves psychoeducation for the patients, who are taught to identify the thoughts and emotions that contribute to problematic behavior. The next component consists of emotion management skills training, including strategies such as distancing, communicating, and challenging thoughts. The final component consists of behavioral management skills such as goal-setting, sleep hygiene, and avoiding self-damaging behavior. STEPPS assigns homework that includes daily monitoring of emotional intensity and skill use.

STEPPS has been evaluated in 3 RCTs, in which outpatients with BPD were assigned to either TAU or a combination of STEPPS+TAU, and with consistent results across studies.[45,76,77] Compared with TAU, STEPPS+TAU is associated with greater improvements in BPD symptom severity, negative affectivity, trait impulsivity, and global functioning, with gains maintained over a 1-year follow-up. However, STEPPS does not appear to reduce frequency of nonsuicidal self-injury or suicide attempts, nor does it reduce inpatient hospitalizations or emergency room visits. STEPPS also has been piloted in a sample of incarcerated women with BPD ($n = 12$; 56). From pre- to posttreatment, patients showed improvements in BPD symptom severity, negative affectivity, and depression. Suicide attempts and acts of nonsuicidal self-injury occurred too infrequently to identify a potential treatment effect. Taken together, STEPPS appears to reduce symptoms and symptomatic behaviors when used as adjunctive treatment, and there is preliminary evidence that it may be effective as a stand-alone treatment. In addition, findings highlight the feasibility of implementing STEPPS in a range of clinical settings.

Like STEPPS, Emotion Regulation Group Treatment (ERGT) is a brief, manualized skills-based group, developed to reduce nonsuicidal self-injury among women with

BPD.[47] ERGT is based on the premise that individuals with BPD lack basic emotion regulation skills, which leads to self-damaging behavior in an effort to reduce strong negative affect. ERGT draws on an acceptance-based model, which defines emotion regulation as control over behavior while distressed, rather than control over the experience of emotions. This model highlights the functional aspects of emotional experience and the problems associated with attempts to avoid and control emotions.[47,78] Accordingly, ERGT focuses on understanding the functions of behaviors and emotions, reducing avoidant responses to emotion, and promoting emotional acceptance in the service of goal-directed behavior. The treatment consists of 14 weekly sessions. In the initial session, patients identify the functions of nonsuicidal self-injury. Subsequent sessions include psychoeducation about the functions of emotions and the benefits of emotional willingness and skills training to enhance emotional clarity and awareness as well as to promote adaptive emotion regulation skills. The final sessions are used to discuss values and to plan for behavioral change that supports those values. Gratz and Gunderson[47] conducted a small RCT among women with BPD and a recent history of nonsuicidal self-injury. Patients were randomized to receive either TAU ($n = 10$) or 14 weekly sessions of ERGT in addition to TAU ($n = 12$). Following treatment, patients in the ERGT group had significantly reduced their average frequency of nonsuicidal self-injury: 42% of the ERGT+TAU group had reduced their frequency of nonsuicidal self-injury by 75% or more, and 59% had reduced it by 45% or more. Moreover, the ERGT group showed clinically significant reductions in symptoms of BPD, depression, anxiety and stress, emotion dysregulation, and experiential avoidance, whereas patients in TAU failed to show improvements in any of the outcomes of interest. Given the small sample size and absence of follow-up data, findings should be considered preliminary; however, this is one of the first studies to show that a brief, skills-based intervention can produce clinically significant reductions in nonsuicidal self-injury and BPD symptom severity.

Avoidant Personality Disorder

There are a total of 7 studies that evaluate CBT for avoidant PD (AVPD), including 1 RCT and 2 open trials of cognitive behavioral group therapy (CBGT), and 1 RCT, 1 open trial, and 2 case studies of individual CBT. It is noteworthy that given the high rates of comorbidity between AVPD and social phobia (approximately 30% of those with social phobia also meet diagnostic criteria for AVPD[78]), there is a substantial body of research that examines the efficacy of treatment for social phobia among patients with co-occurring AVPD.[79–81] However, this review is limited to treatment outcome studies in which AVPD was targeted specifically (ie, patients were selected on the basis of their AVPD diagnosis, and/or AVPD was considered the primary diagnosis).

Cognitive behavioral group therapy

CBGT interventions for AVPD draw on strategies that have been shown to be effective in treating social phobia and patients with interpersonal problems, including graduated exposure, cognitive restructuring, and social skills training.[48,50] The core of CBGT treatments for AVPD is graduated exposure, in which patients are encouraged to approach situations that are feared or avoided. Group sessions are used to prepare for upcoming exposure exercises and to review previous exposures, while also providing a real-world opportunity for sustained exposure to a social situation.[50] Another element of CBGT interventions is cognitive restructuring, which in this treatment is used primarily facilitate willingness to participate in exposure exercises. Finally, some CBGT approaches include an interpersonal skills training component, based on the assumption that individuals with AVPD lack the social skills necessary to interact effectively or appropriately.[48,49]

Although CBGT interventions for AVPD include multiple treatment elements, findings suggest that multicomponent treatments do not necessarily produce better outcomes. For example, Stravynski and colleagues[39] randomized 22 participants with AVPD and generalized social phobia either to a treatment that included exposure, skills training, and cognitive restructuring ($n = 11$), or to a treatment that included only exposure and skills training ($n = 11$). Treatment consisted of 12 weekly group sessions. Both groups showed significant improvements in symptoms of depression, anxiety, and symptomatic behavior (eg, fewer irrational beliefs, less social isolation); however, the inclusion of cognitive restructuring did not improve outcomes beyond the effects of exposure and skills training. In a subsequent trial, Stravynski and colleagues[49] questioned whether the didactic component of skills training was necessary, or whether informal exposure to skills through group discussions would produce similar improvements in social functioning. Patients with AVPD ($n = 21$) served as their baseline, and participated in 5 sessions of skills training and 5 sessions of group discussions that addressed skills without providing instruction. Exposure homework was assigned in both treatments. In terms of overall social functioning, patients benefited as much from the general discussion group as they did from overt skills training. Findings suggest that patients with AVPD may not require explicit instruction to function effectively in social situations; rather, patients may benefit from the informal modeling of skills, planning, rehearsal, and feedback that occur during group discussions.

Finally, Alden[48] conducted an RCT comparing 3 active CBGT treatments to a waitlist control group ($n = 76$). Standard CBGT included exposure with a limited cognitive component (eg, increasing awareness of fearful thoughts). The second group consisted of standard CBGT in addition to general social skills training (eg, listening skills, assertiveness), and the final group consisted of standard CBGT plus intimacy-focused skills training (eg, how to foster a friendship with an acquaintance). All active treatment conditions produced improvements in symptoms of anxiety and depression, reductions in symptomatic behavior (eg, self-reported shyness, anxious mannerisms), and improvements in social functioning, with gains maintained 3 months after treatment. In general, the addition of skills training did not improve outcomes beyond the effects of the standard CBGT. However, the group that received intimacy-focused skills reported greater involvement in and enjoyment of social activities than patients in the other active treatment conditions. Although patients in all treatment conditions made gains over the course of treatment, it is noteworthy that the majority of patients remained impaired in terms of self-esteem, social reticence, and overall social functioning. Alden[48] suggested that residual symptoms may be due to the brevity of CBGT. Consistent with this suggestion, there is evidence that the efficacy of CBGT may be compromised when treatment is delivered over a short period of time or in a small number of sessions. For instance, Renneberg and colleagues[50] found comparably modest rates of recovery following a very brief but intensive CBGT intervention. The treatment consisted of exposure and skills training delivered over 4- to 8-hour (full-day) group sessions. Although 40% of patients were considered recovered on their basis of one outcome score (fear of negative evaluation), much lower rates of recovery were observed for symptoms of depression (27% recovered), anxiety (25% recovered), social avoidance/distress (22% recovered), and overall social functioning (8% recovered). In sum, there are data to support the efficacy of short-term CBGT in reducing symptoms of AVPD, anxiety, depression, as well as symptomatic behaviors and overall social functioning. Although cognitive restructuring and skills training are both associated with positive gains in treatment, they do not seem to improve outcomes beyond the effect of graduated exposure. However, because many patients continued to experience significant impairment following CBGT, further research is warranted to identify the optimal treatment composition and dose. Longer-term, comprehensive interventions may be necessary to change long-standing cognitive and behavioral patterns.[39,48]

Individual cognitive behavioral therapy

Whereas studies of group treatment for AVPD found the strongest evidence for behavioral treatment components (ie, exposure, skills training, and rehearsal), the 4 published studies on individual CBT for AVPD favor a cognitively oriented approach.[51,52] The cognitive model of AVPD holds that the emotional and behavioral problems associated with the disorder are based on dysfunctional schemata and irrational beliefs.[82] Therefore, CBT emphasizes the identification and modification of negative automatic thoughts and maladaptive schemata using thought monitoring, Socratic dialog, and disputation of irrational beliefs.[10,51,52] In addition to cognitive restructuring, it is notable that the treatment includes a range of behavioral exercises, such as activity monitoring and scheduling, as well as behavioral experiments that are designed to highlight and undermine cognitive distortions. Of note, only one publication, a case study of individual CBT, included social skills training.[52]

Strauss and colleagues[52] conducted an open trial of treatment outcomes among outpatients with AVPD ($n = 24$) and obsessive-compulsive personality disorder (OCPD) ($n = 16$). All patients received up to 52 weekly sessions of individual CBT and were assessed before and after treatment. Among those with AVPD, the majority reported clinically significant improvements across a range of symptoms and problematic behaviors. For example, 67% of patients no longer met diagnostic criteria for AVPD at the end of treatment, and 65% experienced remission of depressive symptoms. These encouraging findings were replicated in an RCT conducted by Emmelkamp and colleagues.[51] Patients were assigned to CBT ($n = 26$), brief dynamic therapy (BDT; $n = 28$), or a waitlist condition ($n = 16$). The 2 active treatments consisted of 20 sessions delivered over 6 months, and patients were assessed at the end of treatment and 6 months after treatment termination. Although both CBT and BDT produced significant improvements in anxiety symptoms, behavioral avoidance, and dysfunctional beliefs at the end of treatment, CBT was significantly superior to BDT on all outcome measures. Moreover, BDT did not differ from the waitlist control condition on any measure at the end of treatment. At follow-up treatment gains were maintained, with 91% of the CBT group and 64% of the BDT group no longer meeting diagnostic criteria for AVPD, a statistically significant difference.

Obsessive-Compulsive Personality Disorder

Individual CBT for OCPD has been evaluated in one open trial. In the study described above, Strauss and colleagues[52] conducted an open trial of traditional individual CBT.[82] The trial, which included 16 patients with OCPD and 24 with AVPD, attended up to 52 weekly sessions of CBT. Results indicated that 53% of patients with OCPD showed clinically significant reductions in depressive symptoms, and 83% exhibited clinically significant reductions in OCPD symptom severity. Of note, the CBT-based approach was equally effective for both disorders.[52]

Antisocial Personality Disorder

Only one treatment outcome study has evaluated CBT for antisocial personality disorder (ASPD). CBT for ASPD is a brief, structured treatment that applies a cognitive formulation to target the dysfunctional beliefs that underlie aggressive, criminal, or self-damaging behaviors. Davidson and colleagues[13] randomized men with ASPD and recent histories of aggression to receive either CBT ($n = 25$) or TAU ($n = 27$). Because of the exploratory nature of this study, patients in the CBT group received either 15 sessions over 6 months or 30 sessions over 12 months. Patients were assessed at baseline and followed up at 12 months. No group differences were observed in terms of depression, anxiety, anger, or negative beliefs about others. Patients in both treatment conditions reported lower frequency of verbal and physical aggression at follow-up, although the groups did not differ from one another. Patients who received 6 months of CBT showed trends for less problematic alcohol use, more positive beliefs about others, and better social functioning, but there was no significant effect for CBT on any of the outcomes assessed.

Comorbid PD, PD Not Otherwise Specified, and Mixed PD Samples

The majority of interventions for PDs are disorder specific and, as a result, treatment outcome research is usually conducted separately for each disorder. However, 3 RCTs have used samples composed of patients with different PDs, co-occurring PDs, or a diagnosis of PD not otherwise specified (PDNOS). For example, Springer and colleagues[56] conducted a small-scale RCT on an inpatient psychiatric unit. Of 31 patients, 6% received a diagnosis of PDNOS. Of the remaining patients, 65% had a primary diagnosis of a Cluster C PD, and 44% had a primary diagnosis of BPD, although co-occurring PDs were common. Patients were randomized to receive either 10 daily sessions of supportive group treatment ($n = 15$) or DBT skills ($n = 16$). The DBT group consisted of emotion regulation skills, interpersonal effectiveness training, and distress tolerance. The control condition was a "lifestyle and wellness" discussion group that was not intended to be therapeutic. Patients were assessed at baseline and at discharge. Both treatment groups improved over the course of treatment, and there were no group differences on measures of hopelessness, depression, suicidal ideation, anger, or coping-skill knowledge. Contrary to expectations, however, patients in the DBT-based group were more likely to "act out" (ie, engaging in self-injurious behavior, threatening to harm oneself or others, attempting to leave the unit, refusing to eat for 1 day or more). Based on these findings, a brief inpatient DBT-based skills intervention may not enhance treatment outcome beyond the effects of a discussion group among a group of patients with mixed personality disorder diagnoses.

Muran and colleagues[55] examined treatment outcomes among outpatients with Cluster C PDs or a diagnosis of PDNOS. The majority of the patients (66%) were diagnosed with PDNOS, 19% met diagnostic criteria for multiple PDs, and 87% had comorbid Axis I psychopathology. Patients were randomly assigned to receive 30 weekly sessions of brief relational therapy (BRT), short-term dynamic therapy (BDT), or traditional CBT (ie, cognitive restructuring, self-monitoring, and behavioral experiments). All 3 treatments produced improvements in symptoms and functioning from pretreatment to posttreatment. In general, the treatments yielded equivalent improvements in global functioning, and depressive and PD symptoms; however, CBT was associated with significantly greater reductions in interpersonal problems, and BRT was associated with significantly better treatment retention. Findings provide evidence that symptoms and dysfunction related to complex personality pathology can be reduced by several treatment approaches, including CBT.

Finally, Lynch and colleagues[57] have applied DBT for outpatients with personality pathology and comorbid MDD. In an initial pilot study, patients were randomized to receive antidepressant medication alone (MED) or antidepressant medication, the DBT skills group, and weekly phone calls for skills coaching (DBT+MED). At the end of treatment, 71% of patients in the DBT group were in remission based on their depression scores, compared with 41% of patients in the medication group. At 6-month follow-up, 75% of the DBT group was in remission compared with 31% of the medication group, a statistically significant difference. In a follow-up study, 65 patients with depression and a PD diagnosis received an 8-week trial of antidepressant medication; of these, 29% were classified as responders and 23% dropped out. The remaining patients were randomized to receive either medication and case management (MED; $n = 14$) or medication and DBT (DBT + MED; $n = 21$). DBT consisted of 24 sessions of standard individual DBT and 28 weekly sessions of group skills training. At the posttreatment and follow-up assessments, the 2 treatment groups did not differ on measures of depressive symptoms; however, the DBT+MED group achieved remission more rapidly than the medication-only group. By the end of treatment, rates of remission from BPD were equivalent in the 2 groups, and patients who received DBT showed greater reductions in BPD symptoms, including interpersonal sensitivity and aggression. In summary, DBT combined with antidepressant medication shows promise as a treatment for comorbid depression and PDs, beyond the effects of medication alone.

Other PDs

At the present time there are neither RCTs nor open trials of CBT for schizotypal, schizoid, paranoid, dependent, narcissistic, or histrionic PDs. However, there are a handful of case and empirical single-subject studies that describe cognitive behavioral interventions for the lesser-studied PDs, which may lay the groundwork for future treatment development.

For example, Williams[58] described cognitive behavioral treatment of a patient with paranoid PD (PPD) and MDD. The 11-session treatment aimed to reduce suspicious thoughts and decrease tension, anxiety, and depressive symptoms. Treatment strategies included behavior and thought monitoring, cognitive restructuring, role playing, and relaxation skills training. By the end of treatment, the patient experienced remission of his depression and diminished anxiety about others' intentions toward him; in addition, both the clinician and the patient noted improvements in symptomatic behavior and social functioning. Lynch and Cheavens[59] reported similarly encouraging outcomes for a patient with PPD, OCPD, and MDD, who was treated with a modified DBT-based treatment. Specifically, whereas DBT for BPD targets emotional dysregulation and impulsive behavior, modified DBT for PDs focuses on reducing features that generally characterize Cluster C PDs such as emotional overcontrol, cognitive rigidity, and risk aversion, The 28-week skills group includes modules on mindfulness, distress tolerance, and radical openness, in addition to a new module that provides skills for forgiveness and expressing loving kindness.[59] The client received 9 months of treatment: the first 3 months of treatment consisted of individual weekly DBT, and the last 6 months consisted of weekly individual DBT and weekly DBT skills training group (using the modified material). Individual treatment goals were to decrease fear and hostility in relationships, to tolerate criticism, and to make decisions in ambiguous situations. Individual sessions involved exposure exercises, and skills included modules on mindfulness, distress tolerance, and radical openness. At the end of treatment the patient was in remission from PPD, OCPD, and MDD, and demonstrated improvements in interpersonal functioning and emotional well-being. Taken together, these studies highlight the potential utility of both CBT and DBT for PPD. These approaches led to distinct case conceptualizations, and different therapeutic strategies were emphasized in each treatment; however, both patients showed symptomatic and functional recovery across multiple symptom domains.

Two single-case designs have been used to describe functional analytic psychotherapy (FAP) for histrionic PD (HPD). FAP is a radical behavioral approach in which the therapist uses principles of reinforcement to modify the patient's behavior.[12] FAP cases are conceptualized in terms of problematic clinically relevant behaviors and desirable clinically relevant behaviors (ie, adaptive alternatives). As target behaviors occur in session, the therapist blocks or reinforces them using natural contingencies (eg, sharing feelings that the patient has evoked in the therapist), with the goal of creating behavioral change that generalizes to daily life.[12,83] Given its interpersonal emphasis, FAP may be well suited to the needs of patients with interpersonal difficulties,[84] including patients with PDs. For example, Busch and colleagues[84] described treatment of a patient with features of histrionic and narcissistic PDs. The patient's difficulties were characterized as involving problems identifying personal needs and values, and identifying and responding to feedback from others. Over the course of 23-sessions, the patient displayed less dramatic behavior in session, was better able to identify and express his emotional experiences, demonstrated greater skill at noticing his impact on others, and became more successful in social interactions. Callaghan and colleagues[60] reported similarly encouraging findings using a FAP-CBT integration to treat a patient with HPD. Traditional CBT techniques were used in the first 11 sessions, and the final 9 sessions used FAP techniques to decrease behaviors driven by attention- and approval-seeking or motivated by fear of disapproval, and to increase genuine responding. During the FAP-focused portion of treatment, the patient experienced significant improvements in depressive symptoms and satisfaction with social relationships.

SUMMARY

Research generally supports the conclusion that CBT is an effective treatment modality for patients with personality disorders. However, further research is warranted to develop specific and unambiguous recommendations for how to treat PD symptoms using CBT principles. Ongoing research is needed to identify specific elements of CBT that contribute to positive patient outcomes, as well common therapeutic factors that appear in CBT and other treatment approaches.

As described in this article, CBT offers several specific treatment techniques that appear to map onto the pathology of PDs well. For example, CBT approaches emphasize the connection between implicit, automatic thoughts and their underlying schemas, which are widely thought to be dysregulated and maladaptive in PDs. CBT approaches focus on practical goals such as skills training to address the common problem of social dysfunction in PDs, homework assignments that promote generalization of skills into regular life, and learning-based procedures designed to inhibit self-defeating or treatment-threatening behaviors common in PDs. Furthermore, because CBT is a practical and technique-based approach, it is generally amenable to selecting packages of treatment methods and augmenting treatments with other approaches to address what are often unique and complex symptom presentations in PDs. However, to test the specific utility of these CBT techniques, elements of CBT treatments that overlap with one another and with other treatments need to be identified and articulated more clearly. RCTs that have been conducted for PDs have generally shown that most well-intentioned treatments designed to treat PDs are similarly effective, and are often usually more effective than TAU.

However, the legacy and strength of behavior therapy is its focus on the functional mapping of specific therapeutic techniques with specific patient problems. Research at this molecular level carries the potential to supplement RCT methods in identifying specific factors and distinguishing them from both common factors as well as the specific factors of other approaches. A first step in the process of distinguishing common from specific factors might involve quantifying the ways in which treatments vary so that these differences can be tested directly, rather than be presumed based on the results of comparisons of overall treatment packages. For example, it has been argued that CBT is more structured than other approaches; if this is so, researchers should be able to quantify the degree of structure for any therapy and test the relation between therapeutic structure and treatment outcomes in specific patient populations. A second step would involve using multiple research methods to test different mechanisms of change implied by different approaches. For example, single-subject and dismantling designs are well suited to test the effectiveness of specific interventions in a way that RCTs cannot accommodate. Again these are complementary methods: single-subject designs often provide a justification for larger and more expensive randomized trials, and dismantling studies are often a logical follow-up to findings from RCTs that suggest the effectiveness of a given treatment package. A third step would involve effectiveness studies in naturalistic settings in which therapists use principles, but not necessarily manuals, from different theoretical approaches. It remains a fairly open question as to how well the results of highly controlled trials generalize to the community, where clinicians tend to be eclectic and typically do not rely closely on manuals. Indeed, common factors may play a particularly important role in naturalistic settings, so such settings represent an important potential arena for testing the effect of adding specific, CBT-based techniques. At the same time, research disseminating treatment manuals is needed to test whether community treatment would be enhanced by increasing consistency with manual-based treatments that have shown empirical promise. Finally, research should anticipate changes to the PD taxonomy proposed for DSM-V, which places greater emphasis on dimensional personality traits (eg, neuroticism, impulsivity) and domains of impairment (eg, cognitive, interpersonal) that transcend diagnostic labels. Thus, future research may focus on the development of interventions that can be applied to maladaptive traits or dysfunctional behavioral patterns regardless of the particular PD. This approach also will facilitate targeted idiographic treatments that can be tailored to the unique needs of individual patients.

Ultimately, this practical and methodologically open-minded approach to studying psychotherapy for PD should lead to more specific recommendations for clinicians and patients who struggle with these common but difficult-to-treat diagnoses. Given the conceptual links between CBT and PD problems described earlier, the authors anticipate that many of these specific factors involve techniques that have long been used in cognitive and behavioral treatments. However, it is also clear that other treatments have specific strengths as well, which may complement CBT approaches. As Branch[85] has argued, there is value in maintaining one's theoretical framework while remaining open to technical eclecticism, such that techniques from a variety of approaches can be integrated as part of a cognitive behavioral intervention. In this way, it is possible to continue to develop interventions that retain a cognitive behavioral framework while allowing flexibility in addressing the empirical and largely undecided question of how best to help patients with PDs.

REFERENCES

1. American Psychiatric Association. Diagnostic and statistical manual of mental disorders. text revised. 4th edition. Washington, DC: American Psychiatric Association; 2000.

2. Skodol AE, Oldham JM, Bender DS, et al. Dimensional representations of DSM-IV personality disorders: relationships to functional impairment. Am J Psychiatry 2005;162(10):1919–25.
3. Oken D. Multiaxial diagnosis and the psychosomatic model of disease. Psychosom Med 2000;62(2):171–5.
4. Zanarini MC, Frankenburg FR, Reich DB, et al. The subsyndromal phenomenology of borderline personality disorder: a 10-year follow-up study. Am J Psychiatry 2007;164(6):929–35.
5. McGlashan TH, Grilo CM, Sanislow CA. Two-year prevalence and stability of individual DSM-IV criteria for schizotypal, borderline, avoidant, and obsessive-compulsive personality disorders: toward a hybrid model of axis II disorders. Am J Psychiatry 2005;162:883–9.
6. Leichsenring F, Leibing E. The effectiveness of psychodynamic therapy and cognitive behavior therapy in the treatment of personality disorders: a meta-analysis. Am J Psychiatry 2003;160:1223–32.
7. Sanislow CA, McGlashan TH. Treatment outcome of personality disorders. Can J Psychiatry 1998;43:237–50.
8. McMain S, Pos AE. Advances in psychotherapy of personality disorders: a research update. Curr Psychiatry Rep 2007;9(1):46–52.
9. Bateman AW, Fonagy P. Effectiveness of psychotherapeutic treatment of personality disorder. Br J Psychiatry 2000;177:138–43.
10. Beck AT, Freeman A, Davis DD. Cognitive therapy of personality disorders. New York: Guilford Press; 2004.
11. Linehan MM. Cognitive-behavioral treatment of borderline personality disorder. New York: Guilford Press; 1993.
12. Kohlenberg RJ, Tsai M. Functional analytic psychotherapy. New York: Plenum; 1991.
13. Davidson KM, Tyrer P, Tata P, et al. Cognitive behaviour therapy for violent men with antisocial personality disorder in the community: an exploratory randomized controlled trial. Psychol Med 2009;39:569–77.
14. Chambless DL, Ollendick TH. Empirically supported psychological interventions: controversies and evidence. Annu Rev Psychol 2001;52:685–716.
15. Westen D, Bradley R. Empirically supported complexity. Curr Dir Psychol Sci 2005;14:266–71.
16. Leichsenring F. Randomized controlled versus naturalistic studies: a new research agenda. Bull Menninger Clin 2004;68(2):137–51.
17. Lynch TR, Trost WT, Salsman N, et al. Dialectical behavior therapy for borderline personality disorder. Annu Rev Clin Psychol 2007;3:181–205.
18. Linehan MM, Armstrong HE, Suarez A, et al. Cognitive-behavioral treatment of chronically parasuicidal borderline patients. Arch Gen Psychiatry 1991;48:1060–4.
19. Shearin EN, Linehan MM. Patient-therapist ratings and relationship to progress in dialectical behavior therapy for borderline personality disorder. Behav Ther 1992;23:730–41.
20. Linehan MM, Tutek DA, Heard HL, et al. Interpersonal outcome of cognitive behavioral treatment for chronically suicidal borderline patients. Am J Psychiatry 1994;151:1771–6.
21. Turner RM. Naturalistic evaluation of dialectical behavior therapy-oriented treatment for borderline personality disorder. Cogn Behav Pract 2000;7:413–9.
22. Koons CR, Robins CJ, Tweed J, et al. Efficacy of dialectical behavior therapy in women veterans with borderline personality disorder. Behav Ther 2001;32:371–90.

23. Verheul R, van den Bosch LMC, Koeter MWJ, et al. Dialectical behaviour therapy for women with borderline personality disorder: twelve month, randomized clinical trial in The Netherlands. Br J Psychiatry 2003;182:135–40.

24. Linehan MM, Comtois KA, Murray AM, et al. Two-year randomized controlled trial and follow-up of dialectical behavior therapy vs therapy by experts for suicidal behaviors and borderline personality disorder. Arch Gen Psychiatry 2006;62:1–10.

25. Clarkin JF, Levy KN, Lenzenweger MF, et al. Evaluating three treatments for borderline personality disorder: a multiwave study. Am J Psychiatry 2007;164: 922–8.

26. McMain SF, Links SF, Gnam WH, et al. A randomized trial of dialectical behavior therapy versus general psychiatric management for borderline personality disorder. Am J Psychiatry 2009;166(12):1365–75.

27. Harley RM, Baity MR, Blais MA, et al. Use of dialectical behavior therapy skills training for borderline personality disorder in a naturalistic setting. Psychother Res 2007;17(3):362–70.

28. Brassington J, Krawitz R. Australasian dialectical behaviour therapy pilot outcome study: effectiveness, utility and feasibility. Australas Psychiatry 2006; 14(3):313–21.

29. Prendergast N, McCausland J. Dialectic behaviour therapy: a 12-month collaborative program in a local community setting. Behav Change 2007;24(1):25–35.

30. Comtois KA, Elwood L, Holdcraft LC, et al. Effectiveness of dialectical behavior therapy in a community mental health center. Cogn Behav Pract 2007;14:406–14.

31. Ben-Porath D, Peterson GA, Smee J. Treatment of individuals with borderline personality disorder using dialectical behavior therapy in a community mental health setting: clinical application and a preliminary investigation. Cogn Behav Pract 2004;11:424–34.

32. Hopko DR, Sanchez L, Hopko SD, et al. Behavioral activation and the prevention of suicidal behaviors in patients with borderline personality disorder. J Pers Disord 2003;17(5):460–78.

33. Kerr PL, Muehlenkamp JJ, Larsen MA. Implementation of DBT-informed therapy at a rural university training clinic: a case study. Cogn Behav Pract 2009;16: 92–100.

34. Bohus M, Haaf B, Simms T, et al. Effectiveness of inpatient dialectical behavioral therapy for borderline personality disorder: a controlled trial. Behav Res Ther 2004;42(5):487–99.

35. Bohus M, Haaf B, Stiglmayr C, et al. Evaluation of inpatient dialectical-behavioral therapy for borderline personality disorder—a prospective study. Behav Res Ther 2000;38:875–87.

36. Barley WD, Buie SE, Peterson EW, et al. Development of an inpatient cognitive-behavioral treatment program for borderline personality disorder. J Personal Disord 1993;7:232–40.

37. Davidson K, Norrie J, Tyrer P, et al. The effectiveness of cognitive behavior therapy for borderline personality disorder: results from the borderline personality disorder study of cognitive therapy (BOSCOT) trial. J Personal Disord 2006;20(5): 450–65.

38. Cottraux J, Note I, Boutitie F, et al. Cognitive therapy versus Rogerian supportive therapy in borderline personality disorder: two-year follow-up of a controlled pilot study. Psychother Psychosom 2009;78(5):307–16.

39. Stravynski A, Marks I, Yule W. Social skills problems in neurotic outpatients: social skills training with and without cognitive modification. Arch Gen Psychiatry 1982; 39(12):1378–85.

40. Turner RM. Case study evaluations of a bio-cognitive-behavioral approach for the treatment of borderline personality disorder. Behav Ther 1989;20:477–89.
41. Evans K, Tyrer P, Catalan J, et al. Manual-assisted cognitive behavior therapy (MACT): a randomized controlled trial of a brief intervention with bibliotherapy in the treatment of recurrent deliberate self-harm. Psychol Med 1999;29:19–25.
42. MacLeod AK, Tata P, Evans K, et al. Recovery of positive future thinking within a high-risk suicide group: results from a pilot randomized controlled trial. Br J Clin Psychol 1998;37:371–9.
43. Weinberg I, Gunderson JG, Hennen J, et al. Manual assisted cognitive treatment for deliberate self-harm in borderline personality disorder. J Personal Disord 2006;20(5):482–92.
44. Nordahl H, Nysæter T. Schema therapy for patients with borderline personality disorder: a single case series. J Behav Ther Exp Psychiatry 2005;36(3):254–64.
45. Blum N, St. John D, Pfohl B, et al. Systems Training for Emotional Predictability and Problem Solving (STEPPS) for outpatients with borderline personality disorder: a randomized controlled trial and 1-year follow-up. Am J Psychiatry 2008;165(4):468–78.
46. Black D, Blum N, Eichinger L, et al. STEPPS: Systems Training for Emotional Predictability and Problem Solving in women offenders with borderline personality disorder in prison—a pilot study. CNS Spectr 2008;13(10):881–6.
47. Gratz K, Gunderson J. Preliminary data on acceptance-based emotion regulation group intervention for deliberate self-harm among women with borderline personality disorder. Behav Ther 2006;37(1):25–35.
48. Alden L. Short-term structured treatment for avoidant personality disorder. J Consult Clin Psychol 1989;57(6):756–64.
49. Stravynski A, Belise M, Marcouiller M, et al. The treatment of avoidant personality disorder by social skills training in the clinic or in real-life settings. St J Nerv Ment Dis 1994;39(8):377–83.
50. Renneberg B, Goldstein A, Phillips D, et al. Intensive behavioral group treatment of avoidant personality disorder. Behav Ther 1990;21(3):363–77.
51. Emmelkamp P, Benner A, Kuipers A, et al. Comparison of brief dynamic and cognitive-behavioural therapies in avoidant personality disorder. Br J Psychiatry 2006;189(1):60–4.
52. Strauss J, Hayes A, Johnson S, et al. Early alliance, alliance ruptures, and symptom change in a nonrandomized trial of cognitive therapy for avoidant and obsessive-compulsive personality disorders. J Consult Clin Psychol 2006; 74(2):337–45.
53. Hyman S, Schneider B. The short-term treatment of a long-term interpersonal avoidance. Clin Case Stud 2004;3(4):313–32.
54. Hofmann SG. Avoidant personality disorder: the case of Paul. J Cogn Psychother 2007;21(4):346–52.
55. Muran J, Safran J, Samstag L, et al. Evaluating an alliance-focused treatment for personality disorders. Psychother Theor Res Pract Train 2005;42(4):532–45.
56. Springer T, Lohr N, Buchtel HA, et al. A preliminary report of short-term cognitive-behavioral group therapy for inpatients with personality disorders. J Psychother Pract Res 1996;5:57–71.
57. Lynch T, Cheavens J, Cukrowicz K, et al. Treatment of older adults with co-morbid personality disorder and depression: a dialectical behavior therapy approach. Int J Geriatr Psychiatry 2007;22(2):131–43.
58. Williams J. Cognitive intervention for a paranoid personality disorder. Psychother Theor Res Pract Train 1988;25(4):570–5.

59. Lynch T, Cheavens J. Dialectical behavior therapy for comorbid personality disorders. J Clin Psychol 2008;64(2):154–67.

60. Callaghan G, Summers C, Weidman M. The treatment of histrionic and narcissistic personality disorder behaviors: a single-subject demonstration of clinical improvement using functional analytic psychotherapy. J Contemp Psychother 2003;33(4):321–39.

61. Robins CJ, Chapman AL. Dialectical behavior therapy: current status, recent developments, and future directions. J Personal Disord 2004;18:73–89.

62. Linehan MM, Schmidt H, Dimeff LA, et al. Dialectical behavior therapy for patients with borderline personality disorder and drug dependence. Am J Addict 1999;8: 279–92.

63. Linehan MM, Dimeff LA, Reynolds SK, et al. Dialectical behavior therapy versus comprehensive validation therapy plus 12-step for the treatment of opioid dependent women meeting criteria for borderline personality disorder. Drug Alcohol Depend 2002;67:13–26.

64. Dimeff L, Rizvi SL, Brown M, et al. Dialectical behavior therapy for substance abuse: A pilot application to methamphetamine-dependent women with borderline personality disorder. Cogn Behav Pract 2000;7:457–69.

65. van den Bosch LMC, Verheul R, Schippers GM, et al. Dialectical behavior therapy of borderline patients with and without substance use problems: implementation and long-term effects. Addict Behav 2002;27:911–23.

66. van den Bosch LMC, Koeter MWJ, Stijnen T, et al. Sustained efficacy of dialectical behavior therapy for borderline personality disorder. Behav Res Ther 2005;43: 1231–41.

67. Palmer RL, Birchall H, Damani S, et al. A dialectical behavior therapy program for people with an eating disorder and borderline personality disorder: description and outcome. Int J Eat Disord 2003;33(3):281–6.

68. Chen EY, Matthews L, Allen C, et al. Dialectical behavior therapy for clients with binge-eating disorder or bulimia nervosa and borderline personality disorder. Int J Eat Disord 2008;41(6):505–12.

69. McGinn LK, Young JE. Schema-focused therapy. In: Salkovskis PM, editor. Frontiers of cognitive therapy. New York: The Guilford Press; 1996. p. 182–207.

70. Young JE. Cognitive therapy for personality disorders: a schema-focused approach. Sarasota (FL): Professional Resource Press; 1999.

71. Young JE, Lindemann M. An integrative schema-focused model for personality disorders. In: Leahy RL, Dowd ET, editors. Clinical advances in cognitive psychotherapy: theory and application. New York: Springer Publishing Company; 2002. p. 93–109.

72. Young J, Klosko J, Weishaar M. Schema therapy: a practitioner's guide [e-book]. New York: Guilford Press; 2003.

73. Giesen-Bloo J, van Dyck R, Spinhoven P, et al. Outpatient psychotherapy for borderline personality disorder: randomized trial of schema-focused therapy vs transference-focused psychotherapy. Arch Gen Psychiatry 2006;63(6): 649–58.

74. Farrell J, Shaw I, Webber M. A schema-focused approach to group psychotherapy for outpatients with borderline personality disorder: a randomized controlled trial. J Behav Ther Exp Psychiatry 2009;40(2):317–28.

75. Blum N, Pfohl B, St. John D, et al. STEPPS: a cognitive-behavioral systems-based group treatment for outpatients with borderline personality disorder—a preliminary report. Compr Psychiatry 2002;43(4):301–10.

76. Freije H, Dietz B, Appelo M. Borderline persoonlijkheidsstoornis met de VERS: de vaardigheidstraining emotionele regulatiestoornis. Directieve Therapies 2002;4: 367–78 [in Dutch].
77. Van Wel B, Kockmann I, Blum N, et al. STEPPS group treatment for borderline personality disorder in the Netherlands. Ann Clin Psychiatry 2006;18(1):63–7.
78. Hayes SC, Wilson KG, Gifford EV, et al. Experiential avoidance and behavioral disorders: a functional dimensional approach to diagnosis and treatment. J Consult Clin Psychol 1996;64(6):1152–68.
79. Grant BF, Hasin DS, Stinson FS, et al. Co-occurrence of 12-month mood and anxiety disorders and personality disorders in the US: results from the national epidemiologic survey on alcohol and related conditions. J Psychiatr Res 2004; 39(1):1–9.
80. Brown EJ, Heimberg RG, Juster HR. Social phobia subtype and avoidant personality disorder: effect of severity of social phobia, impairment and outcome of cognitive behavioral treatment. Behav Ther 1995;26(3):467.
81. Hoffman SG, Newman MG, Becker E, et al. Social phobia with and without avoidant personality disorder: preliminary behavior therapy outcome findings. J Anxiety Disord 1995;9(5):427.
82. Beck A, Freeman A. Cognitive therapy of personality disorders. New York: Guilford Press; 1990.
83. Skodol AE, Bender DS. The future of personality disorders in DSM-V. Am J Psychiatry 2009;166(4):388–92.
84. Busch A, Kanter J, Callaghan G, et al. A micro-process analysis of functional analytic psychotherapy's mechanism of change. Behav Ther 2009;40(3):280–90.
85. Branch MN. Behavior analysis: a conceptual and empirical base for behavior therapy. Behav Ther 1987;10:79–84.

Augmentation of Cognitive Behavioral Therapy with Pharmacotherapy

K.A. Ganasen, MBChB*, J.C. Ipser, MA, D.J. Stein, MD, PhD

KEYWORDS

- D-Cycloserine (DCS)
- Augmentation of cognitive behavioral therapy (CBT)
- Fear extinction • Anxiety disorders
- Combining medication with psychotherapy

There has long been in interest in combining pharmacotherapy and psychotherapy.[1] Once cognitive behavioral therapy (CBT) became established as effective for a range of psychiatric disorders, an immediate next question was whether it could be used to augment pharmacotherapy in the many patients who failed to respond, or responded only partially to medication.[2] In the anxiety disorders, however, there have also been concerns that certain medications, such as the benzodiazepines, may negatively affect the effects of CBT.[3] Most recently, basic research on the mechanisms underlying fear extinction has led to interest in the question of whether particular medications that enhance fear extinction may be useful in augmenting CBT.[4]

In this article, the literature on clinical trials that have combined pharmacotherapy and CBT is briefly reviewed, focusing particularly on the anxiety disorders.[5] The literature on CBT and D-cycloseri ne (DCS) is then systematically reviewed.[6] Several related issues, including the relevance of addressing cognitive distortions about the use of medication during psychotherapy and the gradual emergence of a neurobiology of CBT, are also discussed.

PubMed and psycINFO databases were searched up to December 2009 to retrieve published, randomized, placebo-controlled trials of DCS augmentation of psychotherapy for anxiety disorders. The search query included the following terms: "D-cycloserine," "psychotherapy," "cognitive behavioral therapy," "combined treatment."

Department of Psychiatry, University of Cape Town, Anzio Road, Observatory, Cape Town 7925, South Africa
* Corresponding author.
E-mail address: keithganasen@gmail.com

Psychiatr Clin N Am 33 (2010) 687–699
doi:10.1016/j.psc.2010.04.008
0193-953X/10/$ – see front matter © 2010 Elsevier Inc. All rights reserved.

COMBINING CBT AND MEDICATION

The introduction of CBT as an effective treatment of a range of psychiatric disorders raised the question of whether CBT and pharmacotherapy could be successfully combined.[7] In clinical practice, CBT and pharmacotherapy are each effective for only a subset of patients, and it is possible that CBT and pharmacotherapy achieve their effects via different mechanisms.[8] Thus, an early hypothesis was that combined treatment would be more effective than either modality.[2] Here, the authors briefly review studies of combined pharmacotherapy and CBT for anxiety disorders, and note some of the literature on combined treatment of depression, although combined treatments have also been studied in a broad range of other disorder.[9–12] Results from the combination studies discussed are summarized in **Table 1**.

Studies of combined treatment in obsessive-compulsive disorder (OCD) include work on CBT with fluvoxamine and clomipramine.[13–17] These studies showed a numeric advantage for combined treatment over unimodal treatment that did not reach statistical significance. However, the study conducted by Hohagen and colleagues[15] showed that obsessive and secondary depressive symptoms were significantly improved in the group receiving combined fluvoxamine with CBT compared with the group receiving placebo with CBT. Thus, it is possible that additional research may identify subgroups of patients who are more responsive to combined treatment than to unimodal treatment.

Studies of combined treatment in panic disorder include work on CBT with imipramine, buspirone, and alprazolam.[3,18,19] Some data on panic disorder suggest that adding benzodiazepines to CBT may weaken the effects of CBT. For example, in the study of CBT combined with alprazolam, the gains made during alprazolam and placebo treatment were lost after cessation of treatment, whereas the gains made with exposure therapy and placebo were maintained. Furthermore, although the combination of exposure therapy and alprazolam led to increased gains during treatment, these gains were impaired during follow-up. It has been suggested that benzodiazepines interfere with CBT by blocking the fear response during exposure, and so negatively affecting therapeutic cognitive changes.[7]

Studies of combined treatment in posttraumatic stress disorder (PTSD) include work on exposure therapy in combination with sertraline.[20] This study included participants who already had a poor response to sertraline alone. When combined with CBT, however, participants showed a substantial improvement in PTSD symptoms. Southwick and Yehuda[21] have discussed the complexities of combining pharmacotherapy and psychotherapy in PTSD, arguing that medication is most helpful when it is integrated into therapy rather than being viewed as a separate issue. Medication, for example, can reduce involuntary re-experiencing symptoms such as flashbacks and nightmares, which surface during insight-oriented therapy. This may potentially be beneficial to patients and allow them to better work through their trauma without becoming defensive and avoidant.

Studies of combined treatment of social anxiety disorder include work on CBT with sertraline, fluoxetine, and phenelzine.[22–24] The study by Blomhoff and colleagues[22] with sertraline was important in that it was conducted in a real-world setting. Although there were no significant differences between the groups treated with sertraline alone or in combination with exposure therapy, the results seem to suggest that combined treatment may enhance treatment efficacy in this setting. A recent study with phenelzine by Blanco and colleagues[24] showed that the combination of phenelzine and CBT was superior to either treatment alone.

Prevalent anxiety disorders in children and adolescents include separation anxiety, generalized anxiety, and social anxiety disorder. Walkup and colleagues[25] found that sertraline and CBT treatment alone were significantly more effective than placebo, and the combination of sertraline and CBT was significantly more effective than either therapy alone. These findings suggest that developmental considerations may affect the question of whether to use combined treatment and it is possible that a combined approach is particularly useful earlier in life.

Withdrawal of benzodiazepines after prolonged use can be difficult as anxiety symptoms may return and hinder successful discontinuation of treatment. Addition of CBT during the withdrawal phase may alleviate such symptoms and improve the outcome.[26] A study conducted by Otto and colleagues[26] in participants with panic disorder showed that subjects who were tapered from benzodiazepines in combination with group CBT had significantly higher rates of success compared with patients who were tapered without CBT.

Studies of combined treatment of major depression include work on CBT with nefazodone and sertraline.[27–29] Both nefazodone studies found that the combination of medication and therapy was significantly more effective than either treatment alone. The study conducted by Nemeroff and colleagues[28] also showed that in participants with a history of childhood trauma, psychotherapy alone was more effective that medication alone. Combining medication and psychotherapy in this group had a significantly better outcome than psychotherapy alone. This finding points to the possibility that different groups of patients may have differentially improved response to pharmacotherapy, CBT, or the combination. As in the case of anxiety disorders, combined treatment may also be particularly useful in children and adolescents.[30]

Despite some positive findings for combined treatment approaches in some groups of patients, many of the data do not support such an approach. However, combined treatment is often used in clinical practice. This is partly because of a need for better treatments than those offered by either pharmacotherapy or psychotherapy alone; each of these modalities is effective for only a subset of patients. There is also the consideration that even though trials of simultaneous pharmacotherapy and psychotherapy may not be more effective than either agent alone, it is possible that the sequenced use of pharmacotherapy and psychotherapy can optimize therapy by converting a partial response to a full response and by preventing recurrence of symptoms.[31] Similarly, switching from one treatment to another after a good response to the first has also shown some benefit in some disorders.[32]

An important consideration that emerges when reviewing the combined study of CBT and pharmacotherapy is whether CBT is able to address cognitive distortions about medications. Such distortions may reflect characteristic symptoms (eg, patients with OCD may view certain medications as "contaminated"), or they may reflect early maladaptive schemas (eg, patients with a mistrust/abuse schema may fear that medication is being prescribed to hurt them) and so negatively affect adherence or even efficacy. There has been surprisingly little systematic work in this area, despite the possibility that addressing maladaptive thoughts about medication may be valuable.[33]

There has been ongoing interest in the psychobiological mechanisms underlying the combined use of CBT and medication. There is growing evidence that anxiety disorders are mediated by abnormalities within fear response neurocircuitry.[34] This circuitry includes prefrontal areas, as well as more limbic regions.[35,36] A recent meta-analysis of brain imaging studies, for example, revealed increased activity in the amygdala and insula in patients with PTSD, social anxiety disorder and specific phobia, relative to healthy subjects.[37] An immediate hypothesis, therefore, is that psychotherapy acts to improve frontal control over limbic circuitry, whereas pharmacotherapy acts directly on brainstem neurotransmitter systems to reduce limbic activity.

Table 1
Studies combining psychotherapy and medication

	Psychotherapy	Medication	Combination Treatment
Panic Disorder Studies			
Imipramine[18]	Similar efficacy to medication	Similar efficacy to psychotherapy	Slightly more effective than both treatments alone
Buspirone[19]	Significantly better efficacy than placebo	Significantly better efficacy than placebo	Better outcome on general anxiety and agoraphobia symptoms
Alprazolam[3]	Similar efficacy to placebo	Similar efficacy to placebo	Enhanced gains during treatment but not sustained
OCD Studies			
Fluvoxamine[13]	Improved efficacy but similar to placebo	Improved efficacy but similar to placebo	Not significantly improved efficacy with combination
Clomipramine[14]	Better efficacy than placebo but similar to medication	Better efficacy than placebo but similar to psychotherapy	Superior efficacy in combination compared with medication alone
Fluvoxamine[15]	Significantly better efficacy than placebo but similar to treatment	Significantly better efficacy than placebo but similar to psychotherapy	Combination therapy improved obsessive symptoms better than the monotherapies
Fluvoxamine[16]	More effective than placebo but similar to treatment	More effective than placebo but similar to psychotherapy	Similar effect to that of treatment and psychotherapy alone

Social Anxiety Disorder Studies			
Sertraline[22]	Not significantly better than placebo	Significantly more effective than placebo	Combination may enhance efficacy in primary care
Fluoxetine[23]	More effective than placebo but similar to medication	More effective than placebo but similar to psychotherapy	No further advantage with combined treatment
Phenelzine[24]	More effective than placebo	More effective than placebo	Superior efficacy in combination compared with either treatment alone
Posttraumatic Stress Disorder Studies			
Sertraline[20]	Participants improved on psychotherapy	Not much improvement in this treatment-refractory sample	Significant improvement with combination treatment
Anxiety Disorder Studies in Children			
Sertraline[25]	Significantly more effective than placebo	Significantly more effective than placebo	Combination was significantly more effective compared with monotherapy
Depression Studies			
Nefazodone[27]	As effective as medication	As effective as psychotherapy	Significantly more effective than both treatments alone
Nefazodone[28]	As effective as medication	As effective as psychotherapy	Significantly more effective than both treatments alone
Sertraline[29]	Significant improvement in depression	Significant improvement in depression	No advantage in combining treatments

Gorman and colleagues,[8] for example, in their series of reviews on the neuro-anatomy of panic disorder suggested that CBT works via frontal control of limbic structures that mediate anxiety, whereas medications useful in panic disorder work directly on the brainstem to result in anxiolysis. Similarly, Mayberg[38] has argued that in depression, CBT and medications act on different neurocircuits. Certainly, advances in functional imaging have provided growing evidence to support the hypothesis that CBT is able to normalize abnormal neurocircuitry in anxiety disorders and depression.[39] Direct comparisons of the effects of CBT and medication on functional imaging in anxiety disorders have provided useful data on the overlapping and differential effects of each modality in OCD,[40] social anxiety disorder,[41,42] and specific phobia.[43] Although this field is at an early stage, preliminary findings that particular functional imaging abnormalities may predict responsiveness to pharmacotherapy or psychotherapy,[44] seem worth pursuing in future research.

THE NEUROBIOLOGY OF DCS AND PSYCHOTHERAPY

A particularly important set of studies on the neurobiology of psychotherapy emerged not from imaging research but from animal studies on the neurobiology of fear extinction in rodent models. It was found that fear extinction involved the lateral and basolateral amygdaloid nuclei.[45] A second finding was that agents that acted on NMDA receptors in these circuits could enhance fear extinction.[46] NMDA antagonists, for example, were shown to prevent the acquisition and extinction of conditioned responses.[47–49]

As a partial agonist of the NMDA receptor glycine binding site, DCS has a modulatory role and enhances the NMDA receptor function by stimulation of this site, which leads to the overall increase in glutamatergic activity of the receptor.[6,50] DCS also seems to desensitize the NMDA receptor with chronic use, which leads to enhanced fear extinction.[51–53] This work raised the question of whether DCS would be effective in enhancing fear extinction during CBT. The clinical trials that have examined this issue are reviewed in the next section.

RANDOMIZED CONTROLLED STUDIES INVESTIGATING AUGMENTATION OF CBT WITH DCS
OCD

Wilhelm and colleagues[54] used DCS to augment CBT in the treatment of OCD. This was a randomized, double-blind, placebo-controlled augmentation trial of 23 participants with OCD. The participants received 10 behavior therapy sessions twice a week. One hour before each of the sessions, the participants received 100 mg of either DCS or a placebo pill. The study included a mid-treatment assessment after session 5, a posttreatment session after session 10, and a 1-month follow-up assessment after the study. OCD was diagnosed using the Structured Clinical Interview for DSM-IV,[55] with the primary outcome measure being the clinician administered Yale-Brown Obsessive Compulsive Scale (Y-BOCS).[56] In addition, the Beck Depression Inventory-II was used to assess depressive symptoms.[57]

The groups had similar pretreatment Y-BOCS and Beck Depression Inventory-II scores. The DCS group had a significant improvement in OCD symptoms compared with the placebo group at mid-treatment. There were no significant differences between the groups after treatment and at the 1-month follow-up. The DCS group showed significantly improved depressive symptoms after treatment, but no significant change at mid-treatment or the 1-month follow-up. The finding that DCS had an effect on OCD symptoms after 5 CBT sessions suggests that it may be a useful augmentation strategy for OCD.

Another study conducted by Storch and colleagues[58] used 250 mg of DCS to augment exposure and response prevention therapy in OCD. This was a randomized, double-blind, placebo-controlled trial on 24 participants with OCD. Participants received 12 weekly sessions of exposure and response prevention therapy. They received 250 mg of DCS or placebo 4 hours before each therapy session. OCD was diagnosed using the DSM-IV with the primary outcome measure being the clinician administered Y-BOCS. There was no difference between the 2 groups as measured on the primary outcome measure.

Kushner and colleagues[59] conducted a double-blind, placebo-controlled, augmentation study on 25 participants with OCD. Participants received 10 twice weekly exposure-based behavior therapy sessions and received 125 mg of either DCS or placebo 2 hours before the therapy sessions. OCD was diagnosed using the DSM-IV with the Yale-Brown Obsessive Compulsive Scale as the primary outcome measure. Assessments were done at baseline, after the fourth session, at the last session, and at a 3 month follow-up visit.

OCD symptom severity was similar across the experimental and placebo groups at baseline. After 4 sessions, the obsession-related fear ratings declined more rapidly, as determined on the Y-BOCS, in the DCS group, with a significant difference compared with the placebo group. By the last session, the Y-BOCS score was still better, but not significantly different from the placebo group. The Y-BOCS score was not significantly better than the placebo group at the 3-month follow-up visit. These findings seem to indicate that the DCS effects were concentrated in the earlier psychotherapy sessions.

In these OCD studies, differences between the DCS and placebo groups were found when DCS was administered 1 to 2 hours before the therapy sessions, but not when administered 4 hours before. This is consistent with the findings from previous animal research that DCS is more effective when given immediately before or even after extinction exercises.[52] Additional work is needed to determine whether this difference in dosing is the only factor that accounted for the inconsistent findings across these studies.

Panic Disorder

Otto and colleagues[60] conducted a randomized, double-blind, placebo-controlled augmentation study on 31 participants using DCS with brief exposure-based CBT. The participants were given either 50 mg of DCS or a placebo pill 1 hour before the CBT sessions. Participants received 5 sessions of CBT with treatment offered from session 3 to session 5. Participants were diagnosed with panic disorder with or without agoraphobia using the Structured Clinical Interview for DSM-IV (SCID-IV).[61] The primary outcome measure was the Panic Disorder Severity Scale (PDSS).[62] The Clinician Global-Impression-Severity Scale was modified for patients with panic disorder.[63] The PDSS scores were significantly lower in the DCS group after treatment and at a 1-month follow-up assessment.

Social Anxiety Disorder

Hoffman and colleagues[64] conducted a randomized, double-blind, placebo-controlled augmentation study of DCS with exposure therapy in 27 participants with social anxiety disorder with significant public speaking anxiety. Participants received 5 weekly sessions of individual or group therapy. From session 2 to session 5, participants received either 50 mg of DCS or a placebo pill 1 hour before the therapy session. Participants were diagnosed using the Anxiety Disorders Interview Schedule[65] and the Structured Clinical Interview for DSM-IV.[66] The primary outcome measures included scores on the Social Phobia and Anxiety Inventory (SPAI)[67] and the Liebowitz Social Anxiety Scale (LSAS).[68]

Participants in the DCS group showed significantly greater reductions in general social anxiety symptoms as measured by the Stait-Trait Anxiety Inventory (STAI) and LSAS scores compared with the group that received the placebo. This general improvement in social anxiety symptoms occurred even though therapy was focused on the common performance situation of public speaking. The findings of this study provide support for the augmentation of exposure-based exercises with DCS in social anxiety disorder.

Guastella and colleagues[69] recently conducted a randomized, double-blind, placebo-controlled augmentation trial on 56 participants with social anxiety disorder. All participants received 5 group exposure therapy sessions, 1 week apart. From session 2 to session 5, participants were given either 50 mg of DCS or a placebo pill 1 hour before exposure-based therapy. Participants were diagnosed with social anxiety disorder using the Anxiety Disorder Interview Schedule for Adults.[70] Participants also reported a fear of public speaking on a self-report measure. The self-report measures to assess social anxiety disorder symptoms included the SPAI, the LSAS, the Brief Fear of Negative Evaluation Scale (BFNE),[71] and the Life Interference Scale (LIS).[72] These self-report measures were administered before treatment, after session 5, and at 1 month after treatment. In addition, the LSAS and the Speech Performance Questionnaire (SPQ)[73] were administered weekly.

Although exposure therapy reduced symptoms in both groups, the participants treated with DCS showed a greater reduction in social anxiety disorder symptoms on all self-report measures except the SPAI, from before to after treatment. This improvement was maintained at the 1-month follow-up visit. Significant improvements were observed on the weekly measures in the DCS group but not the placebo group by the third week of combined DCS and exposure therapy. Thus, DCS improved the response time to therapy compared with placebo.

Specific Phobia

Ressler and colleagues[4] conducted a randomized, double-blind, placebo-controlled study using DCS with behavioral exposure therapy in 27 participants with acrophobia. Acrophobia is a subtype of a specific phobia and is characterized by an excessive or unreasonable fear of heights. Participants were assigned to 3 groups. One group received Virtual Reality Therapy (VRE) plus 50 mg of DCS, another group received VRE plus 500 mg of DCS, and a third group received VRE plus a placebo pill. Participants underwent 2 therapy sessions and were diagnosed using the Structured Clinical Interview for DSM-III-R.[74] The measures used included the Acrophobia Questionnaire with Avoidance (AAVQ),[75] the Attitudes Toward Heights Inventory (ATHI),[76] and the STAI.[77] There were no differences in scores before treatment.

After treatment, both DCS-treated groups showed significantly better scores on most outcome measures than the placebo control. There were no significant differences in scores between the groups treated with 50 mg and 500 mg. This study showed that DCS facilitated exposure therapy in the treatment of acrophobia after 2 therapy sessions and 2 doses of DCS. At a 3-month follow-up assessment, the DCS group continued to show significant improvements on general acrophobia measures.

DCS AND OTHER DISORDERS
Substance Use Disorders

Exposure therapy has been used to treat individuals with substance use disorders.[78] Such therapies aim to reduce drug-seeking behavior and relapse by desensitizing patients to certain cues from the environment and from drug paraphernalia. To date, these treatments have been at most, moderately successful, depending on the substance of abuse.[78] Given the ability of DCS to facilitate extinction learning via the NMDA receptor, this agent may prove useful in augmenting CBT for substance use disorders. Although human studies have not yet been undertaken, recent animal studies have provided some rationale for such work to proceed. DCS showed efficacy in facilitating the extinction of alcohol-seeking behavior in rats.[79] Similarly, in rats and squirrel monkeys trained to self-administer cocaine,[80] DCS combined with extinction training led to reduced reacquisition of cocaine self-administration.

SUMMARY

It may seem intuitively correct to combine psychotherapy and pharmacotherapy, and in depression there is some evidence for the value of combined treatment.[81] In studies of anxiety disorders, however, the data on combined use of CBT and standard medications are mixed.[7,82,83] Nevertheless, several consistent findings emerge. First, there is preliminary evidence that simultaneous prescription of certain agents, such as benzodiazepines, may interfere with the positive effects of exposure. Second, there is preliminary evidence that sequenced use of pharmacotherapy and CBT may be a useful approach to the treatment-refractory anxiety disorder patient. Third, there is some evidence that combining therapy with medication is useful in improving adherence to pharmacotherapy.[84,85] Fourth, in particular populations, such as children and adolescents with anxiety disorders, combined therapy may be useful. Fifth, some research has indicated the possibility of establishing particular determinants, for example, the exposure to childhood trauma, and certain neuroimaging findings that predict differential responses to pharmacotherapy or CBT, or medication.

Work on DCS combined with CBT has been particularly exciting given its solid foundation in the neuroscience of fear extinction. The studies reviewed here provide evidence that DCS is effective in augmenting CBTs that incorporate exposure and desensitization techniques in several anxiety disorders. DCS seems to be effective at low doses (50 mg) and has no more side effects than placebo, and DCS may be most effective when administered between 1 and 2 hours before CBT. Nevertheless, additional studies are needed to ascertain predictors of response, to determine the longer-term outcome of DCS augmentation, and to assess the effectiveness of DCS and CBT in real-world settings. However, the fact that such work is based on translational work on fear extinction already represents a significant advance in therapeutics.

REFERENCES

1. Riba MB, Balon R. Competency in combining pharmacotherapy and psychotherapy: integrated and split treatment. 1st edition. Washington, DC: American Psychiatric Publishing; 2005.
2. Friedman R, Sedler M, Myers P, et al. Behavioral medicine, complementary medicine and integrated care. Economic implications. Prim Care 1997;24(4):949–62.
3. Marks IM, Swinson RP, Basoglu M, et al. Alprazolam and exposure alone and combined in panic disorder with agoraphobia. A controlled study in London and Toronto. Br J Psychiatry 1993;162:776–87.
4. Ressler KJ, Rothbaum BO, Tannenbaum L, et al. Cognitive enhancers as adjuncts to psychotherapy: use of D-cycloserine in phobic individuals to facilitate extinction of fear. Arch Gen Psychiatry 2004;61(11):1136–44.
5. Hollifield M, Mackey A, Davidson J. Integrating therapies for anxiety disorders. Psychiatr Ann 2006;35(5):329–38.

6. Norberg MM, Krystal JH, Tolin DF. A meta-analysis of D-cycloserine and the facilitation of fear extinction and exposure therapy. Biol Psychiatry 2008;63(12):1118–26.

7. Black DW. Efficacy of combined pharmacotherapy and psychotherapy versus monotherapy in the treatment of anxiety disorders. CNS Spectr 2006; 11(10 Suppl 12):29–33.

8. Gorman JM, Kent JM, Sullivan GM, et al. Neuroanatomical hypothesis of panic disorder, revised. Am J Psychiatry 2000;157(4):493–505.

9. Basco MR, Ladd G, Myers DS, et al. Combining medication treatment and cognitive-behavior therapy for bipolar disorder. J Cogn Psychother 2007;21(1):7–15.

10. Bowers W, Andersen A. Cognitive-behavior therapy with eating disorders: the role of medications in treatment. J Cogn Psychother 2007;21(1):16–27.

11. Kingdon D, Rathod S, Hansen L, et al. Combining cognitive therapy and pharmacotherapy for schizophrenia. J Cogn Psychother 2007;21(1):28–36.

12. Morin CM, Vallieres A, Guay B, et al. Cognitive behavioral therapy, singly and combined with medication, for persistent insomnia: a randomized controlled trial. JAMA 2009;301(19):2005–15.

13. Cottraux J, Mollard E, Bouvard M, et al. A controlled study of fluvoxamine and exposure in obsessive-compulsive disorder. Int Clin Psychopharmacol 1990;5(1):17–30.

14. Foa EB, Liebowitz MR, Kozak MJ, et al. Randomized, placebo-controlled trial of exposure and ritual prevention, clomipramine, and their combination in the treatment of obsessive-compulsive disorder. Am J Psychiatry 2005;162(1):151–61.

15. Hohagen F, Winkelmann G, Rasche-Ruchle H, et al. Combination of behaviour therapy with fluvoxamine in comparison with behaviour therapy and placebo. Results of a multicentre study. Br J Psychiatry Suppl 1998;35:71–8.

16. van Balkom AJ, de Haan E, van Oppen P, et al. Cognitive and behavioral therapies alone versus in combination with fluvoxamine in the treatment of obsessive compulsive disorder. J Nerv Ment Dis 1998;186(8):492–9.

17. Marks IM, Stern RS, Mawson D, et al. Clomipramine and exposure for obsessive-compulsive rituals: i. Br J Psychiatry 1980;136:1–25.

18. Barlow DH, Gorman JM, Shear MK, et al. Cognitive-behavioral therapy, imipramine, or their combination for panic disorder: a randomized controlled trial. JAMA 2000;283(19):2529–36.

19. Cottraux J, Note ID, Cungi C, et al. A controlled study of cognitive behaviour therapy with buspirone or placebo in panic disorder with agoraphobia. Br J Psychiatry 1995;167(5):635–41.

20. Otto MW, Hinton D, Korbly NB, et al. Treatment of pharmacotherapy-refractory posttraumatic stress disorder among Cambodian refugees: a pilot study of combination treatment with cognitive-behavior therapy vs sertraline alone. Behav Res Ther 2003;41(11):1271–6.

21. Southwick SM, Yehuda R. The interaction between pharmacotherapy and psychotherapy in the treatment of posttraumatic stress disorder. Am J Psychother 1993;47(3):404–10.

22. Blomhoff S, Haug TT, Hellstrom K, et al. Randomised controlled general practice trial of sertraline, exposure therapy and combined treatment in generalised social phobia. Br J Psychiatry 2001;179:23–30.

23. Davidson JR, Foa EB, Huppert JD, et al. Fluoxetine, comprehensive cognitive behavioral therapy, and placebo in generalized social phobia. Arch Gen Psychiatry 2004;61(10):1005–13.

24. Blanco C, Heimberg RG, Schneier FR, et al. A placebo-controlled trial of phenelzine, cognitive behavioral group therapy, and their combination for social anxiety disorder. Arch Gen Psychiatry 2010;67(3):286–95.

25. Walkup JT, Albano AM, Piacentini J, et al. Cognitive behavioral therapy, sertraline, or a combination in childhood anxiety. N Engl J Med 2008;359(26):2753–66.
26. Otto MW, Pollack MH, Sachs GS, et al. Discontinuation of benzodiazepine treatment: efficacy of cognitive-behavioral therapy for patients with panic disorder. Am J Psychiatry 1993;150(10):1485–90.
27. Keller MB, McCullough JP, Klein DN, et al. A comparison of nefazodone, the cognitive behavioral-analysis system of psychotherapy, and their combination for the treatment of chronic depression. N Engl J Med 2000;342(20): 1462–70.
28. Nemeroff CB, Heim CM, Thase ME, et al. Differential responses to psychotherapy versus pharmacotherapy in patients with chronic forms of major depression and childhood trauma. Proc Natl Acad Sci U S A 2003;100(24):14293–6.
29. Melvin GA, Tonge BJ, King NJ, et al. A comparison of cognitive-behavioral therapy, sertraline, and their combination for adolescent depression. J Am Acad Child Adolesc Psychiatry 2006;45(10):1151–61.
30. March J, Silva S, Vitiello B. The Treatment for Adolescents with Depression Study (TADS): methods and message at 12 weeks. J Am Acad Child Adolesc Psychiatry 2006;45(12):1393–403.
31. Fava GA, Ruini C, Rafanelli C. Sequential treatment of mood and anxiety disorders. J Clin Psychiatry 2005;66(11):1392–400.
32. Segal Z, Vincent P, Levitt A. Efficacy of combined, sequential and crossover psychotherapy and pharmacotherapy in improving outcomes in depression. J Psychiatry Neurosci 2002;27(4):281–90.
33. Julius RJ, Novitsky MA Jr, Dubin WR. Medication adherence: a review of the literature and implications for clinical practice. J Psychiatr Pract 2009;15(1): 34–44.
34. Shin LM, Liberzon I. The neurocircuitry of fear, stress, and anxiety disorders. Neuropsychopharmacology 2010;35(1):169–91.
35. Anderson KC, Insel TR. The promise of extinction research for the prevention and treatment of anxiety disorders. Biol Psychiatry 2006;60(4):319–21.
36. Grillon C. Startle reactivity and anxiety disorders: aversive conditioning, context, and neurobiology. Biol Psychiatry 2002;52(10):958–75.
37. Etkin A, Wager TD. Functional neuroimaging of anxiety: a meta-analysis of emotional processing in PTSD, social anxiety disorder, and specific phobia. Am J Psychiatry 2007;164(10):1476–88.
38. Mayberg H. Depression, II: localization of pathophysiology. Am J Psychiatry 2002;159:1979.
39. Frewen PA, Dozois DJ, Lanius RA. Neuroimaging studies of psychological interventions for mood and anxiety disorders: empirical and methodological review. Clin Psychol Rev 2008;28(2):228–46.
40. Brody AL, Saxena S, Schwartz JM, et al. FDG-PET predictors of response to behavioral therapy and pharmacotherapy in obsessive compulsive disorder. Psychiatry Res 1998;84(1):1–6.
41. Furmark T, Tillfors M, Marteinsdottir I, et al. Common changes in cerebral blood flow in patients with social phobia treated with citalopram or cognitive-behavioral therapy. Arch Gen Psychiatry 2002;59(5):425–33.
42. Furmark T, Appel L, Michelgard A, et al. Cerebral blood flow changes after treatment of social phobia with the neurokinin-1 antagonist GR205171, citalopram, or placebo. Biol Psychiatry 2005;58(2):132–42.
43. Stein DJ, Matsunaga H. Specific phobia. A disorder of fear conditioning and extinction. CNS Spectr 2006;11(4):248–51.

44. Saxena S, Brody AL, Ho ML, et al. Differential brain metabolic predictors of response to paroxetine in obsessive-compulsive disorder versus major depression. Am J Psychiatry 2003;160(3):522–32.
45. Davis M, Falls WA, Campeau S, et al. Fear-potentiated startle: a neural and pharmacological analysis. Behav Brain Res 1993;58(1–2):175–98.
46. Davis M, Myers KM. The role of glutamate and gamma-aminobutyric acid in fear extinction: clinical implications for exposure therapy. Biol Psychiatry 2002;52(10): 998–1007.
47. Lee H, Kim JJ. Amygdalar NMDA receptors are critical for new fear learning in previously fear-conditioned rats. J Neurosci 1998;18(20):8444–54.
48. Lee JL, Milton AL, Everitt BJ. Reconsolidation and extinction of conditioned fear: inhibition and potentiation. J Neurosci 2006;26(39):10051–6.
49. Szapiro G, Vianna MR, McGaugh JL, et al. The role of NMDA glutamate receptors, PKA, MAPK, and CAMKII in the hippocampus in extinction of conditioned fear. Hippocampus 2003;13(1):53–8.
50. Gomperts SN, Rao A, Craig AM, et al. Postsynaptically silent synapses in single neuron cultures. Neuron 1998;21(6):1443–51.
51. Walker DL, Ressler KJ, Lu KT, et al. Facilitation of conditioned fear extinction by systemic administration or intra-amygdala infusions of D-cycloserine as assessed with fear-potentiated startle in rats. J Neurosci 2002;22(6):2343–51.
52. Ledgerwood L, Richardson R, Cranney J. Effects of D-cycloserine on extinction of conditioned freezing. Behav Neurosci 2003;117(2):341–9.
53. Ledgerwood L, Richardson R, Cranney J. D-Cycloserine facilitates extinction of learned fear: effects on reacquisition and generalized extinction. Biol Psychiatry 2005;57(8):841–7.
54. Wilhelm S, Buhlmann U, Tolin DF, et al. Augmentation of behavior therapy with D-cycloserine for obsessive-compulsive disorder. Am J Psychiatry 2008;165(3): 335–41.
55. American Psychiatric Association. Diagnostic and statistical manual of mental disorders. text revision DSM-IV-TR. 4th edition. Washington, DC: American Psychiatric Association; 2000.
56. Goodman WK, Price LH, Rasmussen SA, et al. The Yale-Brown Obsessive Compulsive Scale. I. Development, use, and reliability. Arch Gen Psychiatry 1989;46(11):1006–11.
57. Beck AT, Steer RA, Ball R, et al. Comparison of Beck Depression Inventories -IA and -II in psychiatric outpatients. J Pers Assess 1996;67(3):588–97.
58. Storch EA, Merlo LJ, Bengtson M, et al. D-Cycloserine does not enhance exposure-response prevention therapy in obsessive-compulsive disorder. Int Clin Psychopharmacol 2007;22(4):230–7.
59. Kushner MG, Kim SW, Donahue C, et al. D-Cycloserine augmented exposure therapy for obsessive-compulsive disorder. Biol Psychiatry 2007;62(8):835–8.
60. Otto MW, Tolin DF, Simon NM, et al. Efficacy of D-cycloserine for enhancing response to cognitive-behavior therapy for panic disorder. Biol Psychiatry 2010;67(4):365–70.
61. First MB. Structured clinical interview for DSM-IV axis I disorders-patient edition (SCID I/P, version 2.0). New York: Biometrics Research Department; 1995.
62. Shear MK. Multicenter collaborative panic disorder severity scale. Am J Psychiatry 1997;154:1571–5.
63. Pollack MH. Combined paroxetine and clonazepam treatment strategies compared to paroxetine monotherapy for panic disorder. J Psychopharmacol 2003;17:276–82.

64. Hofmann SG, Meuret AE, Smits JA, et al. Augmentation of exposure therapy with D-cycloserine for social anxiety disorder. Arch Gen Psychiatry 2006;63(3): 298–304.
65. DiNardo PA. Anxiety disorders interview schedule for DSM-IV: lifetime version (ADIS-IV-L). New York: Graywind Publicatons; 1994.
66. First MB. Structured clinical interview for DSM-IV (Axis I Disorders). Arlington (VA): American Psychiatric Publishing; 1997.
67. Beidel DC, Borden JW, Turner SM, et al. The Social Phobia and Anxiety Inventory: concurrent validity with a clinic sample. Behav Res Ther 1989;27(5):573–6.
68. Liebowitz MR. Social phobia. Mod Probl Pharmacopsychiatry 1987;22:141–73.
69. Guastella AJ, Richardson R, Lovibond PF, et al. A randomized controlled trial of D-cycloserine enhancement of exposure therapy for social anxiety disorder. Biol Psychiatry 2008;63(6):544–9.
70. Brown T. Anxiety disorders interview schedule adult version (ADIS-IV). San Antonio (TX): Psychological Corporation/Graywind Publications; 1994.
71. Leary MR. A brief version of the fear of negative evaluation scale. Pers Soc Psychol Bull 1983;9:371–6.
72. Rapee RM. Treatment of social phobia through pure self help and therapist-augmented self help. Br J Psychiatry 2007;191:246–52.
73. Rapee RM. Discrepancy between self- and observer ratings of performance in social phobics. J Abnorm Psychol 1992;101:728–31.
74. American Psychiatric Association. Diagnostic and statistical manual of mental disorders. Washington, DC: American Psychiatric Association; 1987.
75. Cohen D. Comparison of self-report and overt-behavioral procedures for assessing acrophobia. Behav Ther 1977;8:17–23.
76. Rothbaum BO. Effectiveness of computer-generated (virtual reality) graded exposure in the treatment of acrophobia. Am J Psychiatry 1995;152:626–8.
77. Spielberger C. Manual for the state-trait anxiety inventory (self-evaluation questionnaire). Palo Alto (CA): Consulting Psychologists Press; 1970.
78. Dutra L, Stathopoulou G, Basden SL, et al. A meta-analytic review of psychosocial interventions for substance use disorders. Am J Psychiatry 2008; 165(2):179–87.
79. Vengeliene V, Kiefer F, Spanagel R. D-Cycloserine facilitates extinction of conditioned alcohol-seeking behaviour in rats. Alcohol Alcohol 2008;43(6):626–9.
80. Nic Dhonnchadha BA, Szalay JJ, Achat-Mendes C, et al. D-Cycloserine deters reacquisition of cocaine self-administration by augmenting extinction learning. Neuropsychopharmacology 2010;35(2):357–67.
81. Cuijpers P, Dekker J, Hollon SD, et al. Adding psychotherapy to pharmacotherapy in the treatment of depressive disorders in adults: a meta-analysis. J Clin Psychiatry 2009;70(9):1219–29.
82. Mitte K. Meta-analysis of cognitive-behavioral treatments for generalized anxiety disorder: a comparison with pharmacotherapy. Psychol Bull 2005;131(5):785–95.
83. Furukawa TA, Watanabe N, Churchill R. Combined psychotherapy plus antidepressants for panic disorder with or without agoraphobia. Cochrane Database Syst Rev 2007;1:CD004364.
84. Lingam R, Scott J. Treatment non-adherence in affective disorders. Acta Psychiatr Scand 2002;105(3):164–72.
85. Paykel ES. Psychotherapy, medication combinations, and compliance. J Clin Psychiatry 1995;56(Suppl 1):24–30.

The Empirical Status of the "New Wave" of Cognitive Behavioral Therapy

Stefan G. Hofmann, PhD*, Alice T. Sawyer, MA, Angela Fang, BA

KEYWORDS

- New wave • Third wave • Mindfulness
- Cognitive behavioral therapy
- Acceptance and commitment therapy • Efficacy

In recent years, the terms "new wave," "third wave," "next generation," and "third generation" of behavior and cognitive behavioral therapy (CBT) have appeared with increasing frequency in the literature (eg,[1–3]). Proponents of the "new wave" argue that this "third generation" of behavior therapies adopts a more contextualistic approach than traditional behavior therapy and CBT. Steven Hayes, one of the leading advocates of this perspective, argued that the advent of the "new wave" represents a dramatic change within behavior therapy. For example, he wrote: "This is a time of upheaval in behavioral and cognitive therapy, particularly due to the rapid increase of acceptance and mindfulness-based interventions."[1] Unlike traditional CBT, Hayes argues, the "third wave" behavioral therapies focus on changing the function of psychological events that people experience, rather than on changing or modifying the perception of the events. This change in functionality is achieved through a variety of approaches including acceptance, cognitive defusion, and mindfulness.[1] Hayes considers several interventions to fall under the category of "new wave" treatments, including acceptance and commitment therapy (ACT),[1] dialectical behavior therapy (DBT),[4] mindfulness-based cognitive therapy (MBCT),[5] and metacognitive therapy (MCT).[6]

As discussed elsewhere,[7] we beg to differ from Hayes' perspective. We have argued that, despite sharing common therapeutic strategies, not all of these interventions can be considered "new wave" as defined by Hayes. Indeed, the researchers responsible for developing DBT and MCT posit that their treatments are not part of

Disclosure: S.G.H. is a paid consultant by Merck/Schering-Plough and is supported by NIMH grant 1R01MH078308 and 1R01MH081116 for studies unrelated to the present investigation.
Department of Psychology, Boston University, 648 Beacon Street, Sixth Floor, Boston, MA 02215-2002, USA
* Corresponding author.
E-mail address: shofmann@bu.edu

Psychiatr Clin N Am 33 (2010) 701–710
doi:10.1016/j.psc.2010.04.006
0193-953X/10/$ – see front matter © 2010 Elsevier Inc. All rights reserved.

the "third wave" movement, but rather are firmly grounded in the traditional CBT approach. Adrian Wells (personal communication, August 23, 2007) considers his intervention, MCT, to be a direct extension of CBT because it specifically targets metacognitive content and cognitive processes. Likewise, Marsha Linehan (personal communication, August 28, 2007) considers DBT to be an extension of CBT that integrates acceptance strategies.

Given the stance of these researchers, this discussion of the "new wave" of CBT focuses on ACT and mindfulness-based treatments. Mindfulness-based interventions are included because of the similarities between the acceptance component of ACT and the nonjudgmental awareness component of mindfulness practices. Limiting the discussion to these two forms of treatment is arbitrary and potentially misleading. We do not view CBT as a single treatment, but rather as a family of interventions based on the notion that modifying maladaptive cognitions can lead to a decrease in emotional distress and problematic behaviors. Therefore, because "new wave" treatments are fundamentally related to CBT and share several therapeutic principles, we do not see the need to adopt a separate classification for these interventions, and in fact are in favor of abandoning the term "new wave" entirely (see Refs.[7–9] for a detailed discussion on this topic).

CBT: A FAMILY OF APPROACHES

Since the introduction of Beck's original CBT formulation for depression, many CBT protocols have been developed to address a variety of emotional disorders. Although each of these protocols uses distinct therapeutic techniques, all CBT protocols share several important similarities.[10,11] Therefore, as noted above, CBT should be thought of as a family of interventions rather than as one single treatment.

A major similarity across protocols is the assumption that maladaptive cognitions are causally linked to emotional distress, and therefore, by modifying cognitions emotional distress and maladaptive behaviors will decrease. Research has shown that modifying CBT techniques and tailoring protocols to address specific types of psychopathology improves treatment efficacy for a variety of disorders including post-traumatic stress disorder,[12] social anxiety disorder,[13] generalized anxiety disorder,[14] obsessive-compulsive disorder,[15] panic disorder,[16] and health anxiety,[17] to name only a few.

Beck's content-specificity hypothesis states that each emotional disorder can be characterized by cognitive content specific to that disorder[18]; this is likely one of the main reasons why tailoring CBT techniques to different types of psychopathology has proven so effective. In the case of anxiety disorders, maladaptive cognitions are typically focused on the future possibility of danger or threat, and each disorder is characterized by specific cognitions about the uncontrollability of symptoms or situations. For example, the CBT model of panic disorder[19] assumes that patients with the disorder misinterpret the physical symptoms associated with anxiety as harmful. By contrast, social anxiety is characterized by self-focused cognitions and scrutiny coupled with a fear of embarrassment and humiliation,[20] whereas generalized anxiety disorder and obsessive-compulsive disorder are characterized by excessive obsessions[21] or worry about future undesirable events or the consequences of worry itself.[6]

Modifying maladaptive cognitions is of paramount importance in treating emotional disorders; however, in recent years the validity of the cognitive behavioral model has been questioned. For example, a recent component analysis showed no significant difference between interventions that employed formal cognitive restructuring techniques and those that employed behavioral techniques alone (ie, without directly challenging maladaptive cognitions).[22] The investigators concluded from these find-ings that changes in cognitions do not mediate changes in symptom severity. This conclusion, however, fails to acknowledge that a component analysis is insufficient to make such a determination.[8] As described by one of us (S.G.H.),[23] cognitive change can occur through means other than explicitly challenging maladaptive cognitions; cognitions can mediate treatment change even when cognitions are not explicitly addressed in treatment. Conducting cognitive mediation analyses is the more appro-priate method to study the mechanism of treatment change. Numerous studies to date have provided support for this model in a variety of psychiatric disorders including panic disorder,[24] social anxiety disorder,[25,26] obsessive-compulsive disorder,[27] depression,[28,29] and pain.[30] Although these studies strongly suggest that changes in cognitions mediate treatment change, future studies that employ strict statistical tests are needed to conclusively demonstrate mediation.

MINDFULNESS-BASED TREATMENTS
Overview

Mindfulness-based treatments emphasize achieving a mental state characterized by present-moment focus and nonjudgmental awareness.[31–34] A major aim of such inter-ventions is to improve emotional well-being by increasing awareness of how auto-matic behavioral and cognitive reactions to thoughts, sensations, and emotions can cause emotional distress. Patients are encouraged to gently acknowledge and accept their thoughts, sensations, feelings, and surroundings with an open and curious mind-set. Mindfulness has been defined as "the awareness that emerges through paying attention on purpose, in the present moment, and nonjudgmentally to the unfolding of experience moment by moment."[32(p145)] By focusing on the present, rather than ruminating on the past or worrying about the future, patients can more effectively deal with life stressors that frequently lead to feelings of anxiety and depression.[32]

Mindfulness-based interventions are believed to counter experiential avoidance strategies that maintain and exacerbate emotional disorders, in part by teaching patients to respond reflectively rather than reflexively to stressful situations and nega-tive emotions.[31] Mindful meditation also decreases physical symptoms of distress by balancing sympathetic and parasympathetic responses through meditation exercises such as slow and deep breathing.[32] In the case of mindfulness-based stress reduction (MBSR),[35] alleviation of physical distress is achieved through techniques such as sitting meditation, Hatha Yoga, and body scan.[32]

Efficacy

In recent years, several reviews have examined the efficacy of mindfulness-based interventions,[36–39] especially for physical and psychosomatic problems in chronic diseases such as chronic pain and fibromyalgia,[37] and as a stress reduction method for cancer patients.[38] Two additional reviews examined the effect of mindfulness-based interventions on the reduction of symptoms of anxiety and depression, and arrived at disparate conclusions.[36,39]

To clarify whether mindfulness-based interventions are effective in alleviating symp-toms of anxiety and depression, we conducted a quantitative meta-analysis of studies examining mindfulness-based interventions in psychiatric and medical populations.[40] A total of 39 studies ($n = 1140$) were included in the meta-analysis, and effect size esti-mates suggested that mindfulness-based interventions were moderately effective at reducing symptoms of anxiety (Hedges' $g = 0.63$, 95% confidence interval [CI]: 0.53–0.73) and depression (Hedges' $g = 0.59$, 95% CI: 0.51–0.66) in clinical samples.

These effect sizes are significantly greater than the effect sizes of psychological placebo conditions in anxiety disorder trials (Hedges' g = 0.45, 95% CI: 0.35–0.46) as determined in a previous meta-analytical review.[41] Mindfulness-based interventions proved most effective for reducing anxiety symptoms among patients with anxiety disorders (Hedges' g = 0.97) and for reducing depressive symptoms among patients with mood disorders (Hedges' g = 0.5). To determine whether baseline symptom severity influenced the results, pretreatment mean scores on measures of anxiety and depression were compared with clinical threshold cutoffs. The results showed that studies including patients with elevated levels of anxiety at pretreatment showed a comparable effect size (Hedges' g = 0.67, 95% CI: 0.47–0.87) to those studies including patients without elevated levels at pretreatment (Hedges' g = 0.53, 95% CI: 0.42–0.64). These results suggest that mindfulness-based interventions are effective at reducing symptoms of anxiety and depression across a wide range of severity levels and patient populations.

Comparison with Traditional CBT

MBCT is a direct extension of traditional CBT. MBCT was initially developed to prevent relapse among patients who had recovered from depression.[5] The premise behind using MBCT as a relapse prevention strategy is that by focusing more on the present moment, patients with a history of depression are less likely to fall into the ruminative patterns of negative and hopeless thinking that characterized previous episodes of major depressive disorder. It is assumed that the main reason for relapse is that patients associate negative mood states with self-deprecating and hopeless cognitions. Therefore, patients react to dysphoria by reverting back to maladaptive thinking patterns, which in turn maintain and intensify their dysphoric mood state and subsequently increase the risk of future major depressive episodes.[42] By employing both mindfulness and cognitive techniques, MBCT encourages patients to increase their awareness of and break free from this self-perpetuating cycle. In addition to continued use as a relapse prevention strategy, mindfulness-based interventions have also been applied as an acute treatment for a variety of psychiatric disorders including generalized anxiety disorder,[43,44] panic disorder,[45–47] social anxiety disorder,[48,49] and depression[50–53] (for review, see Refs.[36,40,54,55]).

Another therapy that extends from the CBT framework while integrating mindfulness-based techniques is DBT, a form of therapy that is typically used to treat borderline personality disorder.[56] The basis of DBT is the dialectical worldview, which refers to a perspective that reconciles both acceptance and change as an integral aspect of improving one's ability to regulate his or her own affect. Patients learn to change their behaviors to emotional stimuli by accepting their suffering, with the ultimate goal of adapting the dialectical worldview. To achieve this specific goal, DBT offers numerous mindfulness exercises that are traditionally taught in a weekly skills group.[4] These exercises encourage the development of "what" skills, which allow the patient to observe, describe, and participate, and "how" skills, which allow the patient to do this nonjudgmentally, one-mindfully, and effectively.[4] In addition to mindfulness exercises, DBT offers therapeutic procedures that directly target cognitions, behaviors, or emotions,[36] thereby unifying mindfulness-based strategies to help the patient achieve acceptance, and traditional CBT procedures to help the patient improve dysfunctional behavior.

Although mindfulness-based treatments and CBT interventions are closely related, subtle and important differences exist. In MBCT, for example, the focus is less about changing the content of thoughts, but rather about teaching patients to adopt a broader "decentered" perspective of their thoughts as "mental events" that do not necessarily reflect the self or reality.[34] The concept of "decentering" is closely related to "distancing" in traditional CBT. As Beck has previously described, distancing refers to the process of gaining objectivity toward thoughts.[57] Specifically, distancing involves learning to distinguish between thoughts and reality, and that simply thinking something does not necessarily mean that it is true. It is also generally believed to be a necessary step before the patient can successfully consider alternative explanations for having a particular thought. Gaining a decentered perspective of one's thoughts, rather than necessarily changing the content of one's thoughts, seems to be at the core of mindfulness-based treatments.

ACCEPTANCE AND COMMITMENT THERAPY
Approach

ACT derives its theoretical basis from relational frame theory (RFT),[58] which is a framework for understanding the relationship between cognition and language. RFT extends from a philosophical view called functional contextualism,[59,60] which uses a behavioral analytical model to integrate cognition and language. Therefore, ACT is not an extension of the CBT model, but is rather a reformulation of Skinnerian radical behaviorism,[61] as it rejects the tripartite model and its basic premise of the causative interplay between cognitions, behaviors, and emotions.

Although ACT and CBT differ fundamentally in terms of their theoretical underpinnings, they share many similarities with regard to technique. For example, the set of techniques used in ACT (known as acceptance, cognitive defusion, being present, self as context, values, and committed action) are intended to target experiential avoidance, which is the reluctance to experience negative emotions, physical sensations, and thoughts.[61] These techniques are believed to work by increasing one's psychological flexibility, which refers to the ability to adopt an awareness of the present moment while concurrently adapting this awareness in light of meeting valued goals.[1]

One major aspect of the ACT approach is the notion of acceptance. By encouraging patients to embrace negative thoughts and feelings, such as anxiety, pain, and guilt, rather than attempting to change and eliminate them, patients begin to learn that acceptance can be an important alternative to experiential avoidance. To gain acceptance, individuals become skilled at practicing cognitive defusion which, as mentioned earlier, is a strategy used to target experiential avoidance by relinquishing one's control over one's thoughts and feelings. Cognitive defusion also enables patients to develop a more nonjudgmental and mindful perspective of themselves as well as their external environments. Such strategies ultimately serve to facilitate one's commitment to the pursuit of important life goals.

Efficacy

Two major meta-analyses have examined the efficacy of ACT.[3,62] The first meta-analysis[3] included 29 randomized controlled trials (RCTs) in various third-wave treatments: 13 in ACT, 13 in DBT, 1 in Cognitive Behavioral Analysis System of Psychotherapy, and 2 in Integrative Behavioral Couple Therapy. The results revealed a moderate effect size for the ACT trials ($d = 0.68$), with a fail-safe analysis indicating that 65 unpublished ACT studies would be required for results to reach an insignificant level. These findings, however, are tempered by additional results showing that the methodological rigor of the third-wave RCTs was significantly less stringent than the CBT studies, based on several sample, design, and therapist characteristics, such as representativeness of the sample, reliability of the diagnosis, therapist adherence and competence, and handling of attrition. This finding remained true even after controlling for publication year and journal. Furthermore, the 13 ACT studies included in this review differed greatly with regard to the type of comparison group used—whether it was a control group (ie, treatment as usual) or an active treatment (eg, cognitive therapy). The studies also varied widely in the disorders that were treated, ranging from math anxiety and depression to epilepsy, diabetes, and psychosis. In addition, none of these therapies fulfilled the criteria for empirically supported treatments as defined by the American Psychological Association Division 12 Task Force. The methodology of the meta-analysis was recently criticized[63] and rebutted.[64]

Another meta-analysis[62] examined 18 RCTs ($n = 917$) of ACT for a range of mental and physical problems including anxiety, depression, psychosis, and smoking cessation. This analysis included 3 studies not included in the previous review.[58] Results indicated that ACT outperformed control conditions (Hedges' $g = 0.42$), but was not significantly more effective than established treatments (Hedges' $g = 0.18$, $P > .1$). Based on their analysis, Powers and colleagues[62] cautioned the widespread application of ACT in routine clinical care before it is compared with empirically supported treatments for specific disorders.

Comparison with Traditional CBT

ACT and traditional CBT overlap to a large extent in shared techniques and strategies, particularly with respect to the use of behavioral interventions.[7] For example, both ACT and CBT use behavioral strategies, such as exposure exercises, problem-solving skills, role playing, modeling, and homework, while setting clear and observable goals. In addition, both therapies encourage greater awareness of thoughts, feelings, and sensations without attempting to control or hold onto them. Finally, both approaches target specific concerns and fears, as well as broader improvements in overall quality of life. Consistent with this view, Hayes and colleagues observed that "ACT looks very much like traditional behavior therapy, and almost any behaviorally coherent behavior change method can be fitted into an ACT protocol, including exposure, skills acquisition, shaping methods, goal setting, and the like."[1(p9)] However, major theoretical differences exist between ACT and CBT regarding the role of cognitions. Specifically, ACT views cognitions as a form of behavior, which is "a term for all forms of psychological activity, both public and private, including cognition."[1(p2)] A theoretical discrepancy thus arises between ACT and CBT, whereby the focus in ACT is to identify and alter the function of the cognition, rather than both the content and function as in CBT. As a result of this difference, ACT does not attempt to identify and refute maladaptive cognitions with the goal of changing the emotional response associated with them. Instead, patients are taught in ACT to accept undesirable emotions in the same way that they accept any negative thoughts, whether these thoughts are adaptive or maladaptive. Therefore, ACT and CBT depart in their views of the appropriate types of emotion regulation strategies to foster. As we described elsewhere,[7] some of these discrepancies can be conceptualized as differences in the emotion regulation strategies the two treatments primarily focus on and promote. More specifically, some models of emotions distinguish between antecedent-focused and response-focused emotion regulation strategies, based on the differential processing of internal and external emotional cues.[65–68] Whereas antecedent-focused strategies attempt to regulate emotions prior to the processing of emotional cues, response-focused strategies attempt to do so after emotional responses have already been activated and processed. This distinction emphasizes the main difference between CBT and ACT in their respective approaches to developing beneficial emotion regulation strategies, as CBT tends to promote strong antecedent-focused emotion regulation skills and ACT primarily targets maladaptive response-focused strategies.

SUMMARY AND FUTURE RESEARCH DIRECTIONS

CBT is a family of interventions that attempts to modify maladaptive cognitions in order to improve a patient's emotion regulation, goal setting, and ability to make more adaptive appraisals of situations and events. These goals are achieved through the use of techniques that help the patient foster behavioral, experiential, and cognitive skills.

The basic premise of CBT is that cognitions play an important role in the maintenance of an emotional disorder, primarily through its causal influence on one's emotions and behaviors. In this way, the target of change in CBT is often (but not exclusively) the content of such cognitions. In contrast, mindfulness-based treatments and ACT focus on the function of thoughts and promote emotion regulation strategies that counter experiential avoidance.

Despite some differences on the theoretical level concerning the definition and function of cognitions, treatment-specific techniques between mindfulness-based treatments, ACT, and CBT are not incompatible. However, before embracing these more novel strategies for routine clinical care, they will need to be subjected to empirical tests. Although it may be difficult to test entire treatment protocols against each other, it is certainly possible to isolate specific techniques under controlled laboratory environments and examine differences from a more technical perspective. As empirical data do not yet favor one treatment over another, further testing is needed. By testing the efficacy of a CBT treatment package that includes mindfulness-based and ACT-based techniques, evidence may become more available to help elucidate the necessary components to effect change. One particular avenue of research that warrants further exploration is whether different emotion regulation strategies have an additive beneficial effect and whether outcomes may be maximized by tailoring emotion regulation strategies on an individual or diagnostic basis. To answer the important questions about the mechanism of treatment changes, mediational analyses are essential because they cannot be replaced by efficacy studies or component analyses. Future research on mediation analyses should not be limited to treatment process research but should also include investigations to isolate and experimentally study adaptive and maladaptive emotion regulation strategies in a laboratory.

REFERENCES

1. Hayes SC, Luoma JB, Bond FW, et al. Acceptance and commitment therapy: model, processes, and outcomes. Behav Res Ther 2006;44:1–26.
2. Hayes SC. Acceptance and commitment therapy, relational frame therapy, and the third wave of behavioural and cognitive therapies. Behav Ther 2004;35: 639–65.
3. Öst LG. Efficacy of the third wave of behavioral therapies: a systematic review and meta-analysis. Behav Res Ther 2008;46:296–321.
4. Linehan MM. Skills training manual for treating borderline personality disorder. New York: Guilford Press; 1993.
5. Segal ZV, Williams JMG, Teasdale JD. Mindfulness-based cognitive therapy for depression: a new approach to preventing relapse. New York: Guilford Press; 2002.
6. Wells A. A cognitive model of generalized anxiety disorder. Behav Modif 2000;38: 319–45.

7. Hofmann SG, Asmundson GJ. Acceptance and mindfulness-based therapy: new wave or old hat? Clin Psychol Rev 2008;28:1–16.
8. Hofmann SG. Common misconceptions about cognitive mediation of treatment change: a commentary to Longmore and Worrell (2007). Clin Psychol Rev 2008;28:67–70.
9. Hofmann SG. ACT: new wave or Morita therapy? Clin Psychol 2008;15:280–5.
10. Hofmann SG, Asmundson GJ. The science of cognitive behavioral therapy. Behav Ther, in press.
11. Ellis A. Rational-emotive therapy and cognitive behavior therapy: similarities and differences. Cognit Ther Res 1980;4:325–40.
12. Ehlers A, Clark DM, Hackmann A, et al. Cognitive therapy for post-traumatic stress disorder: development and evaluation. Behav Res Ther 2005;43:413–31.
13. Clark DM, Ehlers A, McManus F, et al. Cognitive therapy versus fluoxetine in generalized social phobia: a randomized placebo-controlled trial. J Consult Clin Psychol 2003;71:1058–67.
14. Wells A, King P. Metacognitive therapy for generalized anxiety disorder. J Behav Ther Exp Psychiatry 2006;37:206–12.
15. Freeston MH, Ladouceur R, Gagnon F, et al. Cognitive-behavioral treatment of obsessive thoughts: a controlled study. J Consult Clin Psychol 1997;65:405–13.
16. Clark DM, Salkovskis PM, Hackman A, et al. Brief cognitive therapy for panic disorder: a randomized controlled trial. J Consult Clin Psychol 1999;67:583–9.
17. Salkovskis PM, Warwick HM, Deale AC. Cognitive-behavioral treatment for severe and persistent health anxiety (hypochondriasis). Brief Treat Crisis Interv 2003;3:353–67.
18. Beck AT. Cognitive therapy and the emotional disorders. New York: International Universities Press; 1976.
19. Clark DM. A cognitive approach to panic. Behav Res Ther 1986;24:461–70.
20. Clark DM, Wells A. A cognitive model of social phobia. In: Heimberg RG, Liebowitz MR, Hope DA, et al, editors. Social phobia: diagnosis, assessment and treatment. New York: Guilford Press; 1995. p. 69–93.
21. Salkovskis PM. Obsessional-compulsive problems: a cognitive-behavioral analysis. Behav Res Ther 1985;23:571–83.
22. Longmore RJ, Worrell M. Do we need to challenge thoughts in cognitive behavioral therapy? Clin Psychol Rev 2007;27:173–87.
23. Hofmann SG. Cognitive processes during fear acquisition and extinction in animals and humans: implications for exposure therapy of anxiety disorders. Clin Psychol Rev 2008;28:200–11.
24. Hofmann SG, Meuret AE, Rosenfield D, et al. Preliminary evidence for cognitive mediation during cognitive behavioral therapy for panic disorder. J Consult Clin Psychol 2007;75:374–9.
25. Hofmann SG, Moscovitch DA, Kim HJ, et al. Changes in self-perception during treatment of social phobia. J Consult Clin Psychol 2004;72:588–96.
26. Smits JAJ, Rosenfield D, Telch MJ, et al. Cognitive mechanisms of social anxiety reduction: an examination of specificity and temporality. J Consult Clin Psychol 2006;74:1203–12.
27. Moore EL, Abramowitz JS. The cognitive mediation of thought-control strategies. Behav Res Ther 2007;45:1949–55.
28. Kaysen D, Scher CD, Mastnak J, et al. Cognitive mediation of childhood maltreatment and adult depression in recent crime victims. Behav Ther 2005;36:235–44.
29. Tang TZ, DeRubeis RJ, Beberman R, et al. Cognitive changes, critical sessions, and sudden gains in cognitive-behavioral therapy for depression. J Consult Clin Psychol 2005;73:168–72.

30. Price DD. Psychological and neural mechanisms of the affective dimension of pain. Science 2000;288:1769–72.
31. Bishop M, Lau S, Shapiro L, et al. Mindfulness: a proposed operational definition. Clin Psychol 2004;11:230–41.
32. Kabat-Zinn J. Mindfulness-based interventions in context: past, present, and future. Clin Psychol 2003;10:144–56.
33. Melbourne Academic Mindfulness Interest Group. Mindfulness-based psycho-therapies: a review of conceptual foundations, empirical evidence and practical considerations. Aust N Z J Psychiatry 2006;40:285–94.
34. Teasdale JD, Segal ZV, Williams JMG, et al. Prevention of relapse/recurrence in major depression by mindfulness-based cognitive therapy. J Consult Clin Psychol 2000;68:615–23.
35. Kabat-Zinn J. An outpatient program in behavioral medicine for chronic pain patients based on the practice of mindfulness meditation: theoretical consider-ations and preliminary results. Gen Hosp Psychiatry 1982;4:33–47.
36. Baer R. Mindfulness training as a clinical intervention: a conceptual and empirical review. Clin Psychol 2003;10:125–43.
37. Grossman P, Niemann L, Schmid S, et al. Mindfulness-based stress reduction and health benefits: a meta-analysis. J Psychosom Res 2004;57:35–43.
38. Ledesma D, Kumano H. Mindfulness-based stress reduction and cancer: a meta-analysis. Psychooncology 2009;18:571–9.
39. Toneatto T, Nguyen L. Does mindfulness meditation improve anxiety and mood symptoms? a review of the controlled research. Can J Psychiatry 2007;52:260–6.
40. Hofmann SG, Sawyer AT, Witt A, et al. The effect of mindfulness-based therapy on anxiety and depression: a meta-analytic review. J Consult Clin Psychol 2010;78:169–83.
41. Hofmann SG, Smits JAJ. Cognitive-behavioral therapy for adult anxiety disorders: a meta-analysis of randomized placebo-controlled trials. J Clin Psychiatry 2008;69:621–32.
42. Teasdale JD. Cognitive vulnerability to persistent depression. Cogn Emot 1988;2:247–74.
43. Craigie MA, Rees CS, Marsh A. Mindfulness-based cognitive therapy for gener-alized anxiety disorder: a preliminary evaluation. Behav Cogn Psychother 2008;36:553–68.
44. Evans S, Ferrando S, Findler M, et al. Mindfulness-based cognitive therapy for generalized anxiety disorder. J Anxiety Disord 2008;22:716–21.
45. Kabat-Zinn J, Massion AO, Kristeller J, et al. Effectiveness of a meditation-based stress reduction program in the treatment of anxiety disorders. Am J Psychiatry 1992;149:936–43.
46. Kim YW, Lee SH, Choi TK, et al. Effectiveness of mindfulness-based cognitive therapy as an adjuvant to pharmacotherapy in patients with panic disorder or generalized anxiety disorder. Depress Anxiety 2009;26:601–6.
47. Lee SH, Ahn SC, Lee YJ, et al. Effectiveness of a meditation-based stress management program as an adjunct to pharmacotherapy in patients with anxiety disorder. J Psychosom Res 2007;62:189–95.
48. Bögels SM, Sijbers GFVM, Voncken M. Mindfulness and task concentration training for social phobia: a pilot study. J Cogn Psychother 2006;20:33–44.
49. Koszycki D, Benger M, Shlik J, et al. Randomized trial of a meditation-based stress reduction program and cognitive behavior therapy in generalized social anxiety disorder. Behav Res Ther 2007;45:2518–26.

50. Ramel W, Goldin PR, Carmona PE, et al. The effects of mindfulness meditation on cognitive processes and affect in patients with past depression. Cognit Ther Res 2004;28:433–55.
51. Barnhofer T, Crane C, Hargus E, et al. Mindfulness-based cognitive therapy as a treatment for chronic depression: a preliminary study. Behav Res Ther 2009; 47:366–73.
52. Kingston T, Dooley B, Bates A, et al. Mindfulness-based cognitive therapy for residual depressive symptoms. Psychol Psychother 2007;80:193–203.
53. Williams JMG, Alatiq Y, Crane C, et al. Mindfulness-based cognitive therapy (MBCT) in bipolar disorder: preliminary evaluation of immediate effects on between-episode functioning. J Affect Disord 2008;107:275–9.
54. Bishop SR. What do we really know about mindfulness-based stress reduction? Psychosom Med 2002;64:71–83.
55. Salmon P, Lush E, Jablonski M, et al. Yoga and mindfulness: clinical aspects of an ancient mind/body practice. Cogn Behav Pract 2009;16:59–72.
56. Linehan MM, Amstrong H-E, Suarez A, et al. Cognitive-behavioral treatment of chronically suicidal borderline patients. Arch Gen Psychiatry 1991;48:1060–4.
57. Beck AT. Cognitive therapy: nature and relation to behavior therapy. Behav Ther 1970;1(2):184–200.
58. Hayes SC, Barnes-Holmes D, Roche B. Relational frame theory: a post-Skinnerian account of human language and cognition. New York: Kluwer Academic; 2001.
59. Gifford EV, Hayes SC. Functional contextualism: a pragmatic philosophy for behavioral science. In: O'Donohue W, Kitchener R, editors. Handbook of behaviorism. San Diego (CA): Academic Press; 1993. p. 287–328.
60. Pepper SC. World hypotheses: a study in evidence. Berkeley (CA): University of California Press; 1942.
61. Hayes SC, Masuda A, Bissett R, et al. DBT, FAP and ACT: how empirically oriented are the new behavior therapy technologies? Behav Ther 2004;35:35–54.
62. Powers MB, Zum Vorde Sive Vording MB, Emmelkamp PM. Acceptance and commitment therapy: a meta-analytic review. Psychother Psychosom 2009;78: 73–80.
63. Gaudiano BA. Öst's (2008) methodological comparison of clinical trials of acceptance and commitment therapy versus cognitive therapy: matching apples with oranges? Behav Res Ther 2009;47:1066–70.
64. Öst LG. Inventing the wheel once more or learning form the history of psychotherapy research methodology: reply to Gaudiano's comments on Öst's (2008) review. Behav Res Ther 2009;47:1071–3.
65. Gross JJ. Antecedent- and response-focused emotion regulation: divergent consequences for experience, expression, and physiology. J Pers Soc Psychol 1998;74:224–37.
66. Gross JJ. Emotion regulation: affective, cognitive, and social consequences. Psychophysiology 2002;39:281–91.
67. Gross JJ, John OP. Individual differences in two emotion regulation processes: implications for affect, relationships, and well-being. J Pers Soc Psychol 2003; 85:348–62.
68. Gross JJ, Levenson RW. Hiding feelings: the acute effects of inhibiting negative and positive emotion. J Abnorm Psychol 1997;106:95–103.

The Future and Promise of Cognitive Behavioral Therapy: A Commentary

Richard E. Zinbarg, PhD[a,b,]*, Nehjla M. Mashal, MA[a], Danielle A. Black, PhD[b], Christoph Flückiger, PhD[c]

KEYWORDS

- Cognitive behavioral therapy • Information processing
- Biological integration • Mechanism research

In this article, the authors present their view of the future and promise of cognitive behavioral therapy (CBT). As the Academy for Psychological Clinical Science and the independent accrediting entity it created, the Psychological Clinical Science Accreditation system, have recently launched a movement aimed at reforming all of clinical psychology, the article begins with a discussion of this movement's view of the future of clinical psychology and the implications of that vision for CBT. In short, if this movement is successful, it will result in a greater emphasis on empirical science in the practice of clinical psychology. As CBT is the approach to therapy that currently has the greatest number of controlled scientific studies supporting it, if clinical practice indeed becomes more deeply rooted in science, this should be an impetus for CBT to grow. The very same scientific evidence that supports the efficacy of CBT, however, also shows that CBT is far from fully efficacious. Thus, several recent trends are discussed that the authors believe hold great promise to enhance the effectiveness of CBT. In particular, there have been recent signs of greater integration of CBT with biological approaches, cognitive science, systemic approaches, motivational interviewing, and strengths-based approaches. As depicted in **Fig. 1**, the authors believe that each of these tends toward greater integration must continue and grow for CBT to realize its full potential. Greater attention to mechanism research is also warranted.

[a] Department of Psychology, Northwestern University, 102 Swift Hall, 2029 Sheridan Road, Evanston, IL 60208-2710, USA
[b] The Family Institute at Northwestern University, 618 Library Place, Evanston, IL 60201, USA
[c] Department of Clinical Psychology and Psychotherapy, University of Bern, Gesellschaftsstr 49, Bern 3012, Switzerland
* Corresponding author. Department of Psychology, Northwestern University, 102 Swift Hall, 2029 Sheridan Road, Evanston, IL 60208-2710.
E-mail address: rzinbarg@northwestern.edu

Psychiatr Clin N Am 33 (2010) 711–727
doi:10.1016/j.psc.2010.04.003
0193-953X/10/$ – see front matter © 2010 Elsevier Inc. All rights reserved.

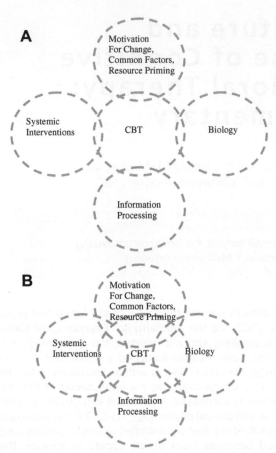

Fig. 1. (A) The current state of CBT and its integration with other approaches. (B) The more integrated future of CBT.

THE FUTURE OF CLINICAL PSYCHOLOGY: IMPLICATIONS FOR CBT

Baker and colleagues[1] have argued that clinical psychology currently operates in a pre-scientific mode much as was true of medicine before the publication of the Flexner[2] Report in 1910. Baker and colleagues[1] base their conclusion largely on 2 facts. First, surveys indicate that many clinical psychologists value clinical experience and expert opinion more than scientific evidence in making clinical decisions.[3] Second, although there has been a great deal of progress over the past 3 to 4 decades in the development of empirically supported treatments (ESTs) for various psychological problems that are also disseminable and cost-effective, many patients receiving psychological services do not receive ESTs.[1] Finally, a growing number of clinical psychologists are being trained in free-standing professional schools, many of which do not offer high-quality, science-based training.[4]

Although the current status of clinical psychology is troubled, a movement is underway to try to achieve similar reforms to those triggered by the Flexner Report[2] that helped move medicine from a pre-scientific state to its more scientific current state. The Academy for Psychological Clinical Science has recently launched a new system for accrediting doctoral programs in clinical psychology, the Psychological Clinical Science Accreditation System (PCSAS). It is hoped that graduation from a PCSAS accredited doctoral program will enable the public, insurers, and public policy decision makers to be able to distinguish psychologists who base their clinical practice on science to the fullest extent possible from those who do not.

Such "branding" by itself might not become the impetus for major reforms. However, the effects of such branding should be magnified by growing market pressures for cost-effectiveness and accountability, as mental health care costs have escalated dramatically and are being increasingly diverted to insurers and the government.[1] As a result of these forces, it is hoped that many of the free-standing schools of professional psychology will be forced to either fold or merge with university-based programs, as happened in medicine subsequent to the publication of the Flexner Report.[2]

Whereas this view of the future of clinical psychology should obviously not be welcomed at many free-standing schools of professional psychology, it should be received more positively at training programs that have a strong CBT orientation or component, given that most lists of ESTs are dominated by CBT interventions (eg, Refs.[1,5]). At the same time, we (the authors of this article) believe that even if PCSAS does trigger reforms leading to the demise of free-stranding schools of professional psychology, reforms will also be needed within university-based CBT oriented doctoral training programs. That is, it is our impression that many faculty members within university-based doctoral training programs do not place as much value on training practitioners who apply scientific knowledge as on training clinical scientists who generate such knowledge. It is certainly the case that in the 2 doctoral programs of the faculty on which the first author has served, the one way that an applicant to the program could be assured to be denied admission would be to state on his or her application that his or her aspiration was to be a full-time clinician (and it is not our intention to point fingers at others—the first author himself has been no less likely to reject an applicant on these grounds than any other faculty member with whom he has served). Yet, it seems to us that if the next generation of practitioners is to be trained in a science-based approach, the current generation of clinical scientists is going to have to develop a greater willingness to be involved in that training.

What is unclear to us is exactly what role the current generation of clinical scientists will play in the training of the next generation of science-based practitioners. One possibility is that clinical scientist PhD programs will need to start accepting more students with aspirations of becoming full-time clinicians. A second possibility seems more likely to be based on another current trend in mental health service delivery. As reviewed by Baker and colleagues,[1] there is evidence indicating that therapy is increasingly being delivered by providers other than psychologists, including by Masters-level individuals. Thus, if this trend continues it may be that clinical scientists will need to partner with faculty and administrators of Masters programs, at least in the design of those programs, to ensure that they have an adequate basis in science. In either case, what we are suggesting is that the divide between science and practice that has long been lamented in clinical psychology may not solely require change on the part of practitioners but rather will also require greater willingness on the part of clinical scientists to become more involved in the training of practitioners than many of us have done in the past. CBT clinical scientists have done an excellent job in establishing a firm foundation for CBT to become a dominant approach in a mental health care market that will be increasingly shaped by accountability and cost-effectiveness considerations. To realize this potential, we believe that CBT clinical scientists must also take a leadership role in the training of full-time practitioners.

We conclude this section by also pointing out that no EST is 100% effective and there is not a recognized EST for every presenting problem. Thus, in addition to training in ESTs, routine training in single-case design methodology will also be essential for science-based practitioners of the future. As CBT clinical scientists have made important contributions to single-case design methodology,[6] this is another reason why CBT clinical scientists are well positioned to assume a leadership role in the training of science-based practitioners.

INTEGRATION WITH BIOLOGY

There is a small but growing body of work that integrates CBT with biological approaches and outcome measures. Indeed, given that it is rooted in learning and cognitive theory,[7] there is great potential for CBT to be enhanced by our increasingly sophisticated understanding of the basic neurochemistry of learning and memory. Integrative treatment approaches are already underway; recent efforts have examined whether D-cycloserine (DCS) enhances exposure therapy for anxiety and phobias.[8,9]

DCS is a partial N-methyl-D-aspartate (NMDA) agonist, which enhances activity in NMDA receptors that support learning and memory.[10,11] Several studies conducted by different research groups have now shown that DCS augments the effects of exposure therapy and CBT for phobia of heights,[8] social phobia,[12,13] and obsessive compulsive disorder (OCD).[14–16]

Not every study that has tested the effect of DCS on exposure therapy has reported significant enhancement effects.[16,17] A recent meta-analysis[11] suggests that DCS is most effective with lower and less frequent doses that are administered immediately before or after exposure. These conditions increase the likelihood that the drug effect would peak either contiguous with or immediately after the learning.[11] Although more work needs to be done to further elucidate and maximize the effects of DCS on exposure therapy, it is clear that it does have some beneficial effects on exposure. Given this, we expect DCS to be used routinely in clinical practice in conjunction with exposure therapy in the not too distant future.

The full promise of DCS may stretch far beyond the realm of exposure therapy, however, to include other portions of CBT protocols. That is, DCS may well boost the effects of other learning that takes place in CBT such as during cognitive restructuring or various forms of skill training. Thus, research testing of whether DCS enhances other CBT interventions in addition to exposure therapy should commence shortly if such studies have not been initiated already. If such work demonstrates DCS's efficacy in these areas, we would expect DCS to be used as a means of enhancing a wide array of CBT interventions in clinical practice in the future.

The small but growing body of literature combining neuroimaging methods and CBT indicates that successful CBT is associated with changes in neuronal activity as well as symptom reduction in individuals with MDD,[18] panic disorder,[19] social anxiety disorder,[20] spider phobia,[21–23] posttraumatic stress disorder (PTSD),[24] and OCD.[25–27] Investigators have also examined how neural responses compare with healthy controls before and after CBT treatment. Participants' neural activity post CBT treatment (for spider phobia) did not differ from that of the nonpsychiatric control group.[23] Still others have successfully examined how neural activity in specific regions predicts response to CBT in patients with PTSD[28] and in depressed patients.[29–31]

At present, neuroimaging work on the correlates, predictors, and mechanisms of successful CBT treatment is in its infancy. Neuroimaging might serve as a useful outcome measure in CBT protocols in the future, although the costs of neuroimaging will have to decrease significantly before such methods become commonplace. With the increased use of high-precision techniques and as methodological rigor increases (see Ref.[32] for a comprehensive review of the methodological shortcomings of the extant literature and recommendations), future neuroimaging work has great potential to illuminate our understanding both of the neural underpinnings of the disorders we treat and the mechanisms that underlie CBT and its mediators. For example, although we know that exposure therapy and CBT are efficacious, we do not yet understand the mechanism(s) by which these techniques are successful. Thus, it is unclear whether exposure involves an unlearning of original, aversive associations or the acquisition of new, inhibitory associations that compete with the original ones. We believe that neuroimaging will play an important role in answering this and related questions regarding the mechanisms mediating the effects of CBT interventions.

INTEGRATION WITH INFORMATION PROCESSING

One of the cornerstones of cognitive and CBT models of psychological problems has been the assumption that information processing mechanisms including biases in attention, interpretation, and memory are involved in problem development and/or maintenance (eg, Refs.[33–38]). Whereas traditional cognitive therapy techniques involve engaging patients in the willful alteration of their interpretations of information, the past decade has witnessed exciting progress in the direct modification of attentional biases, memory biases, and interpretation biases in a more automatic fashion (eg, Refs.[39–49]). Indeed, Amir and colleagues[37] found that training patients with generalized anxiety disorder to decrease their attention to threat led to a decrease in their anxiety symptoms as indicated by both self-report and interviewer measures. Similarly, Schmidt and colleagues[46] reported that training patients with social anxiety disorder to disengage their attention from pictures of disgusted faces led to a reduction in social anxiety and trait anxiety, with 72% of patients in the treatment condition no longer meeting diagnostic criteria for social anxiety disorder after training (compared with only 11% of the patients in a control condition). Amir and colleagues[38] showed that such reductions can be relatively long lasting. These investigators trained patients diagnosed with generalized social anxiety disorder to direct attention away from pictures of disgusted faces, and the resulting symptom reductions were maintained during a 4-month follow-up assessment interval.

We believe cognitive bias modification (CBM) paradigms have tremendous promise for 2 applications. First, as CBM paradigms typically are implemented by computer programs, they can be disseminated quite widely, including to areas with no mental health workers trained in CBT and to those individuals who cannot afford therapy. Second, given that not all high-risk individuals will actually go on to develop psychological problems and knowledge that one has been identified as a high-risk individual might constitute a stressor that triggers the onset of a psychological problem, an ideal preventive intervention would be one that can be delivered without alerting the individual to the fact that they have been designated as being at high risk. CBM paradigms might be very useful in this regard, given that they can be delivered with many individuals not even realizing that they are receiving an intervention.[38]

Thus, we envision a future in which CBM paradigms are used as clinical tools on a large-scale basis. To realize this potential, however, additional research is required either to understand how to implement CBMs in a manner that leads to lasting benefits or to establish the parameters of booster schedules that will maintain their effects.

A recent study has demonstrated that memory consolidation occurs during sleep and can be systematically influenced via simple auditory stimulation.[49] Before napping, participants were taught to associate random locations on a computer screen with 50 images that were also presented with a related sound. Half of these sounds were presented while participants slept (specifically, during slow-wave sleep).

Memory testing showed greater accuracy for those objects cued by their associated sounds during sleep than for the stimuli that were not cued during sleep.

These results have exciting translational potential for CBT. An analogous sleep protocol applied to exposure or cognitive restructuring sessions may serve to enhance consolidation of those therapeutic memories and augment CBT in a similar manner to DCS. If so, patients with difficulty adhering to a CBT protocol (ie, completing thought records, behavioral experiments, and/or exposures in-between sessions) or those who would otherwise be nonresponders might still improve with the addition of this intervention. Sleep rehearsal might also increase the efficiency and cost-effectiveness with which CBT is delivered, reducing the amount of work the client must complete outside of therapy and/or the number of sessions to achieve symptom reduction. Successful application of sleep rehearsal to exposure therapy may also be a useful tool to investigate the mechanism underlying exposure therapy. If sleep rehearsal is mediated by memory consolidation (as opposed to memory pruning), then the augmenting effects of sleep rehearsal on exposure therapy would provide further evidence that exposure works via the acquisition of new inhibitory learning.

INTEGRATION WITH MINDFULNESS APPROACHES

Jon Kabat-Zinn[50] introduced the first mindfulness-based intervention to the psychological field in the late 1970s. By the late 1990s, over 240 hospitals in the United States and Europe offered mindfulness-based stress reduction programs.[51] Mindfulness-based interventions reduce the risk of relapse for depression,[52] decrease binge eating for people suffering from binge-eating disorders,[53] and reduce anxiety symptoms for people suffering from panic disorder, generalized anxiety disorder, and social phobia.[54,55] In addition, mindfulness interventions have reduced suicidal behaviors in individuals with borderline personality disorder.[56] Mindfulness is also an important cornerstone of several individual CBT packages, including dialectical behavior therapy for borderline personality disorder (DBT[57,58]), mindfulness-based cognitive therapy for depression (MBCT[59]), and acceptance and commitment therapy for a variety of conditions (ACT[60]).

The assumptions underlying cognitive restructuring and mindfulness-based interventions may seem incompatible at first glance. For example, traditional cognitive restructuring assumes change occurs by modifying dysfunctional thoughts, whereas mindfulness interventions do not attempt to change thoughts but to observe thoughts. On the other hand, the incompatibility of restructuring and mindfulness may be more apparent then real. That is, it seems to us that cognitive restructuring can be used in the service of acceptance—in our view, for example, this is what good cognitive therapy for panic disorder is all about (reducing the tendency to misinterpret physical sensations such that the individual can be more accepting of them). We also assume that approaches that incorporate mindfulness make a distinction between accepting thoughts and "buying into them" to use the vernacular of ACT. If so, it seems to us that traditional cognitive restructuring skills might be helpful for a patient who is having trouble refraining from buying into a negative judgment to help them get to the point of saying to themselves something like "oh look, I just had the thought 'I am bad'—I no longer have to distract myself from that thought as I don't believe it anymore." Put differently, we assume that when we talk of acceptance of some negative self-judgment that we are talking about acceptance of its occurrence as opposed to its truth value and that cognitive restructuring is only relevant to the latter. Thus, we see mindfulness and cognitive restructuring as being complementary; mindfulness can be useful for working on the acceptance of the occurrence of a negative thought and cognitive restructuring can be useful for disputing the truth value of the negative thought.

We not only believe that mindfulness and more traditional CBT approaches can be integrated but that such integration holds tremendous promise for future interventions. First, we need a better understanding of what works for whom. Are some patients more likely to benefit from a traditional CBT approach compared with others who may benefit from a mindfulness-based approach? Second, we need an understanding of how traditional CBT may be augmented or combined with mindfulness-based approaches. As noted above, one possibility is that mindfulness appears to be useful for working on the acceptance of a negative thought whereas cognitive restructuring appears to be useful for disputing the truth value of the negative thought (which in turn might help prepare the patient to accept rather than distract from the thought when it recurs in the future). Future research investigating how the two approaches might be optimally combined would be very useful.

INTEGRATION WITH SYSTEMIC APPROACHES

The majority of CBT approaches focus on the individual rather than the family system. Integrating systemic interventions with CBT approaches may improve CBT treatment outcome. Most of the major mental disorders are significantly correlated with marital distress, including PTSD,[61–63] generalized anxiety disorder (GAD),[62–65] panic disorder with agoraphobia (PDA),[66] social phobia,[62,63] bipolar disorder,[63] major depressive disorder,[67,68] and alcohol dependence and drug use disorders.[69,70] Problematic communication styles between family members (eg, expressed emotion, negative reciprocity, and so forth) significantly predict worse treatment outcome for several disorders including depression,[71,72] panic disorder,[54] generalized anxiety disorder (GAD),[73] PTSD,[74] OCD,[75] and alcohol and drug use disorders.[69] Systemic CBT approaches perform as well as individually based treatment for depression,[76–78] PDA,[63] and PTSD.[79] However, systemic CBT approaches are more efficacious at improving marital distress or decreasing expressed emotion compared with individual approaches for depression.[76–78,80] Thus, systemic interventions may include the benefit of improving 2 co-occurring problems—the mental disorder and marital distress. Further, systemic CBT approaches for alcohol and drug use disorders produce better long-term results compared with individual CBT.[81]

The future of CBT systemic interventions for mental disorders needs to address several issues. First, although several CBT systemic interventions target several disorders; there exist several disorders that may clearly benefit from a systemic approach. GAD and bipolar disorders strongly correlate with marital distress[65]; Although Miklowitz and colleagues[82] found family-focused therapy is effective for bipolar disorder; a clinical trial investigating a CBT systemic approach has not been completed for either GAD or bipolar disorders. Second, the majority of systemic CBT interventions target behaviors, and we know relatively little regarding cognitive targets at the systemic level (eg, targeting attributions of partners or family members). Third, relationship functioning may moderate the effectiveness of systemic interventions, and we must gain an understanding of what type of intervention (eg, spouse assisted therapy vs targeting martial functioning) works for what population. Finally, even in the most well-developed CBT systemic interventions for disorders (eg, alcohol and drug use disorders), we know relatively little regarding the mechanisms of change.

INTEGRATION WITH MOTIVATIONAL INTERVIEWING

Whereas CBT tends to be effective for many people who comply with treatment, noncompliance has long been a problem in CBT. Zinbarg[83] wrote that patient motivation to comply with therapy was CBT's abused step-child. That is, Zinbarg noted that one of the primary CBT interventions for preventing and dealing with failure to comply up to the time of the writing of his 2000 article was threatening the noncompliant patient with termination. Zinbarg further opined that this approach "never succeeded at anything other than removing noncompliant cases from one's caseload"[83(p397)] and called for greater integration into CBT of motivational interviewing techniques developed by Miller and Rollnick[84] for working with client resistance.[85]

We are very pleased to note that, since the article by Zinbarg,[83] several investigators have been developing specific applications of motivational interviewing for working with populations such as those with various anxiety disorders, depression, or eating disorders for whom we know that CBT tends to be effective when complied with (eg, Refs.[86-98]). This is a trend that we believe needs to continue and strengthen in the future, as both common sense and empirical evidence tell us that if a patient does not practice CBT techniques, he or she is unlikely to benefit from them.[99,100] Indeed, we believe that all CBT therapists in the future need to be trained in basic motivational interviewing principles and techniques to be maximally effective.

INTEGRATION WITH STRENGTHS-BASED APPROACHES

In our view, a topic that is closely related to the need for integration with motivational interviewing is the fact that CBT, especially as it is practiced in North America, is often very focused on patients' problems and their maintaining factors with little to no focus on patient strengths.[101,102] Whereas treatment models focusing on highlighting strengths (capitalization models) have often been contrasted with treatment models that focus on remediating weaknesses (compensation models[103]), capitalization and compensation can be conceptualized in an interactive way. According to Grawe,[104-106] focusing on strengths ("resource activation") can initiate and maintain positive feedback circuits that foster the therapeutic alliance, increase the patient's receptiveness, and support mastery and clarification experiences, all of which result in the implementation of novel coping strategies to remediate the patient's weaknesses.[104-106]

Through resource-activating interventions, therapists actively reinforce patients' positive expectations for change as well as their individual abilities, and use them as a catalyst for therapeutic change[104-106] (for examples of resource-activating interventions see Ref.[107]). It is believed that interventions that focus on strengths and self-worth are particularly important at the beginning of therapy when it is important to induce hope and foster positive expectations for change.[108-112]

In the context of CBT therapies, the benefits of early resource-activating microinterventions or resource priming[113,114] has been demonstrated in patients with social anxiety,[115] human immunodeficiency virus,[116] and in mixed samples of outpatients.[117] Subsequent extensions have demonstrated positive results integrating resource priming within an integrative CBT, solution-focused Training Center[118] and in an inpatient chat group.[119] Related interventions that focus on patients' strengths have been shown to be associated with positive outcomes with a heterogeneous sample of community patients[101] and when integrated within a CBT trial for patients with social phobia.[120] It is our belief that the problem-focus that is so typical of CBT in North America can be very profitably integrated with resource priming and similar interventions that capitalize on patients' and therapists' strengths.[121,122] Indeed, we believe such integration is necessary for CBT to realize its full potential.

NEED FOR MECHANISM RESEARCH

Although many CBT interventions are associated with considerable evidence supporting their efficacy and are therefore considered ESTs,[4] we have little to no good evidence regarding the mechanisms of action mediating the effects of their active ingredients. Moreover, even those CBT interventions that are considered ESTs do not produce clinically significant change in many patients and therefore still leave room for further improvement and development. As an example from our own area of research, Borkovec and Whisman[123] obtained an average clinically significant change figure of 50% from their meta-analysis of CBT trials for GAD. Similar results have been reported for CBT for panic disorder[124,125] and for CBT for depression.[126] It is our belief that furthering our understanding of the mechanisms underlying effective CBT will be very helpful in our efforts to further improve CBT.

In calling for more mechanism research, we want to be careful to note that in our minds our focus on mechanisms should include not only those that are specific to CBT interventions but rather should also include common factors. Indeed, there is empirical evidence that the therapist's empathy and the quality of the therapeutic alliance accounts for significant portions of the variance in outcome in CBT.[127–129] As the first author often tells his supervisees, you can know everything there is to know about CBT but if your patient thinks you are a jerk, he or she is not going to listen to you. Similarly, we are strong adherents of the view that expectation for improvement is a factor to be capitalized on and maximized rather than a nuisance variable to be controlled for when conducting psychotherapy.[130]

Although we believe there is a place for common factors within CBT and CBT research, for CBT to continue to develop, evolve, and mature we also need more research into mechanisms that are likely to be unique to CBT. Such research is difficult to do, and requires sophisticated and intensive methods. Approaches that we believe have great promise in this regard and that we hope to see used more often in future CBT research are sudden gains/critical sessions[131,132] and functional magnetic resonance imaging. In addition, analyses of therapist effects deserve greater attention in future CBT research than they have been accorded in the past.[133]

SUMMARY

Given that most lists of ESTs are dominated by CBT interventions (eg, Refs.[1,5]), we believe that CBT is well positioned to become a dominant approach in a mental health care market that will be increasingly shaped by accountability and cost-effectiveness considerations. The very same scientific evidence that supports the efficacy of CBT, however, also shows that CBT is far from fully efficacious. Although we do not believe it is realistic to expect that CBT, or any other health care intervention, will become 100% effective, several recent trends hold great promise to move us closer to that ideal. As we review in this article, there have been recent signs of greater integration of CBT with biological approaches, cognitive science, systemic approaches, motivational interviewing, and strengths-based approaches. We hope that these trends, along with an increased emphasis on mechanism research, will be nurtured and pursued further as we believe them to be necessary for CBT to realize its full potential.

REFERENCES

1. Baker TB, McFall RM, Shoham V. Current status and future prospects of clinical psychology. Psychol Sci 2009;9:67–103.
2. Flexner A. Medical education in the United States and Canada (No. 4). New York: Carnegie Foundation; 1910.
3. Groopman J. How doctors think. Boston: Houghton Mifflin; 2007.
4. McFall RM. Doctoral training in clinical psychology. Annu Rev Clin Psychol 2006; 2:21–49.

5. Chambless DL, Ollendick TH. Empirically supported psychological interventions: controversies and evidence. Annu Rev Psychol 2001;52:685–716.

6. Barlow DH, Nock MK, Hersen M. Single case experimental designs: strategies for studying behavior change. Boston: Pearson; 2009.

7. Craske M. Theory. Cognitive-behavioral therapy. Washington, DC: US: American Psychological Association; 2010. p. 19–52. Retrieved from PsycINFO database.

8. Ressler K, Rothbaum B, Tannenbaum L, et al. Cognitive enhancers as adjuncts to psychotherapy: use of D-cycloserine in phobic individuals to facilitate extinction of fear. Arch Gen Psychiatry 2004;61(11):1136–44.

9. Otto M, Basden S, Leyro T, et al. Clinical perspectives on the combination of D-cycloserine and cognitive-behavioral therapy for the treatment of anxiety disorders. CNS Spectr 2007;12(1):51–6 59-61. Retrieved from PsycINFO database.

10. Davis M, Ressler K, Rothbaum B, et al. Effects of D-cycloserine on extinction: translation from preclinical to clinical work. Biol Psychiatry 2006;60(4):369–75.

11. Norberg M, Krystal J, Tolin D. A meta-analysis of D-cycloserine and the facilitation of fear extinction and exposure therapy. Biol Psychiatry 2008;63(12): 1118–26.

12. Hofmann S, Meuret A, Smits J, et al. Augmentation of exposure therapy with D-cycloserine for social anxiety disorder. Arch Gen Psychiatry 2006;63(3): 298–304.

13. Guastella A, Richardson R, Lovibond P, et al. A randomized controlled trial of D-cycloserine enhancement of exposure therapy for social anxiety disorder. Biol Psychiatry 2008;63(6):544–9.

14. Kushner M, Kim S, Donahue C, et al. D-Cycloserine augmented exposure therapy for obsessive-compulsive disorder. Biol Psychiatry 2007;62(8): 835–8.

15. Wilhelm S, Buhlmann U, Tolin D, et al. Augmentation of behavior therapy with D-cycloserine for obsessive-compulsive disorder. Am J Psychiatry 2008; 165(3):335–41.

16. Storch E, Merlo L, Bengtson M, et al. D-Cycloserine does not enhance exposure-response prevention therapy in obsessive-compulsive disorder. Int Clin Psychopharmacol 2007;22(4):230–7.

17. Guastella A, Dadds M, Lovibond P, et al. A randomized controlled trial of the effect of D-cycloserine on exposure therapy for spider fear. J Psychiatr Res 2007;41(6):466–71.

18. Goldapple K, Segal Z, Garson C, et al. Modulation of cortical-limbic pathways in major depression. Arch Gen Psychiatry 2004;61(1):34–41.

19. Praško J, Horácek J, Zálesky R, et al. The change of regional brain metabolism (^{18}FDG PET) in panic disorder during the treatment with cognitive behavioral therapy or antidepressants. Neuroendocrinol Lett 2004;25(5):340–8.

20. Furmark T, Tillfors M, Marteinsdottir I, et al. Common changes in cerebral blood flow in patients with social phobia treated with citalopram or cognitive-behavioral therapy. Arch Gen Psychiatry 2002;59(5):425–33.

21. Paquette V, Levesque J, Mensour B, et al. Change the mind and you change the brain: effects of cognitive-behavioral therapy on the neural correlates of spider phobia. Neuroimage 2003;18(2):401–9.

22. Schienle A, Schäfer A, Hermann A, et al. Symptom provocation and reduction in patients suffering from spider phobia: an fMRI study on exposure therapy. Eur Arch Psychiatry Clin Neurosci 2007;257(8):486–93.

23. Straube T, Glauer M, Dilger S, et al. Effects of cognitive-behavioral therapy on brain activation in specific phobia. Neuroimage 2006;29(1):125–35.

24. Felmingham K, Kemp A, Williams L, et al. Changes in anterior cingulate and amygdala after cognitive behavior therapy of posttraumatic stress disorder. Psychol Sci 2007;18(2):127–9.

25. Baxter L, Schwartz J, Bergman K, et al. Caudate glucose metabolic rate changes with both drug and behavior therapy for obsessive-compulsive disorder. Arch Gen Psychiatry 1992;49(9):681–9.

26. Nakatani E, Nakgawa A, Ohara Y, et al. Effects of behavior therapy on regional cerebral blood flow in obsessive-compulsive disorder. Psychiatr Res Neuroimaging 2003;124(2):113–20.

27. Schwartz J, Stoessel P, Baxter L, et al. Systematic changes in cerebral glucose metabolic rate after successful behavior modification treatment of obsessive-compulsive disorder. Arch Gen Psychiatry 1996;53(2):109–13.

28. Bryant R, Felmingham K, Kemp A, et al. Amygdala and ventral anterior cingulate activation predicts treatment response to cognitive behaviour therapy for posttraumatic stress disorder. Psychol Med 2008;38(4):555–61.

29. Costafreda S, Khanna A, Mourao-Miranda J, et al. Neural correlates of sad faces predict clinical remission to cognitive behavioural therapy in depression. Neuroreport Rapid Comm Neurosci Res 2009;20(7):637–41.

30. Fu C, Williams S, Cleare A, et al. Neural responses to sad facial expressions in major depression following cognitive behavioral therapy. Biol Psychiatry 2008; 64(6):505–12.

31. Siegle G, Carter C, Thase M. Use of fMRI to predict recovery from unipolar depression with cognitive behavior therapy. Am J Psychiatry 2006;163(4): 735–8.

32. Frewen P, Dozois D, Lanius R. Neuroimaging studies of psychological interventions for mood and anxiety disorders: empirical and methodological review. Clin Psychol Rev 2008;28(2):228–46.

33. Beck AT. Depression: clinical, experimental, and theoretical aspects. New York: Harper and Row; 1967.

34. Beck AT. Cognitive therapy of depression: new perspectives. In: Clayton PJ, Barrett JE, editors. Treatment of depression: old controversies and new approaches. New York: Raven Press; 1983. p. 265–90.

35. Teasdale JD, Barnard PJ. Affect, cognition and change: re-modelling depressive thought. Hillsdale (NJ): Lawrence Erlbaum Associates; 1993.

36. Williams JM, Watts FN, MacLeod C, et al. Cognitive psychology and emotional disorders. 2nd edition. New York: Wiley; 1997.

37. Amir N, Beard C, Burns M, et al. Attention modification program in individuals with generalized anxiety disorder. J Abnorm Psychol 2009;118:28–33.

38. Amir N, Beard C, Taylor CT, et al. Attention training in individuals with generalized social phobia: a randomized controlled trial. J Consult Clin Psychol 2009; 77:961–73.

39. Grey S, Mathews A. Effects of training on interpretation of emotional ambiguity. Q J Exp Psychol 2000;53(A):1143–62.

40. Hirsch CR, Hayes S, Mathews A. Looking on the bright side: accessing benign meanings reduces worry. J Abnorm Psychol 2009;118:44–54.

41. Holmes EA, Lang TJ, Shah DM. Developing interpretation bias modification as a "cognitive vaccine" for depressed mood: imagining positive events makes you feel better than thinking about them verbally. J Abnorm Psychol 2009; 118:76–88.

42. Joormann J, Hertel PT, LeMoult J, et al. Training forgetting of negative material in depression. J Abnorm Psychol 2009;118:34–43.
43. MacLeod C, Rutherford E, Campbell L, et al. Selective attention and emotional vulnerability: assessing the causal basis of their association through the experimental manipulation of attentional bias. J Abnorm Psychol 2002;111: 107–23.
44. Mathews A, Mackintosh B. Induced emotional interpretation bias and anxiety. J Abnorm Psychol 2000;109:602–15.
45. Schartau PE, Dalgleish T, Dunn BD. Seeing the bigger picture: Training in perspective broadening reduces self-reported affect and psychophysiological response to distressing films and autobiographical memories. J Abnorm Psychol 2009;118:15–27.
46. Schmidt NB, Richey JA, Buckner JD, et al. Attention training for generalized social anxiety disorder. J Abnorm Psychol 2009;118:5–14.
47. See J, MacLeod C, Bridle R. The reduction of anxiety vulnerability through the modification of attentional bias: a real-world study using a home-based cognitive bias modification procedure. J Abnorm Psychol 2009;118:65–75.
48. Watkins ER, Baeyens CB, Read R. Concreteness training reduces dysphoria: proof-of-principle for repeated cognitive bias modification in depression. J Abnorm Psychol 2009;118:55–64.
49. Rudoy J, Voss J, Westerberg C, et al. Strengthening individual memories by reactivating them during sleep. Science 2009;326:1079.
50. Kabat-Zinn J. An outpatient program in behavioral medicine for chronic pain patients based on the practice of mindfulness meditation: theoretical considerations and preliminary results. Revision 1984;7(1):71–2.
51. Salmon PG, Santorelli SF, Kabat-Zinn J. Intervention elements promoting adherence to mindfulness-based stress reduction programs in the clinical behavioral medicine setting. In: Shumaker SA, Schoron EB, Ockene JK, et al, editors. Handbook of health behavior change. 2nd edition. New York: Springer; 1998. p. 239–68.
52. Teasdale JD, Segal ZV, Williams JM, et al. Prevention of relapse / re-occurrence in major depression by mindfulness-based cognitive therapy. J Consult Clin Psychol 2000;68:615–23.
53. Kristeller JL, Hallett B. Effects of a meditation-based intervention in the treatment of binge eating. J Health Psychol 1999;4(3):357–63.
54. Kabat-Zinn J, Massion AO, Kristeller J, et al. Effectiveness of a meditation-based stress reduction program in the treatment of anxiety disorders. Am J Psychiatry 1992;149:936–43.
55. Koszycki D, Benger M, Shlik J, et al. Randomized trial of a meditation-based stress reduction program and cognitive behavior therapy in generalized social anxiety disorder. Behav Res Ther 2007;45:2518–26.
56. Linehan MM, Armstrong HE, Suarez A, et al. Cognitive-behavioural treatment of chronically parasuicidal borderline patients. Arch Gen Psychiatry 1991;48: 1060–4.
57. Linehan MM. Cognitive behavioral treatment of borderline personality disorder. New York: Guilford Press; 1993.
58. Linehan MM. Skills training manual for treating borderline personality disorder. New York: Guilford Press; 1993.
59. Teasdale JD, Segal ZV, Williams JM. How does cognitive therapy prevent depressive relapse and why should attentional control (mindfulness) training help? Behav Res Ther 1995;33:25–39.

60. Hayes SC, Stroshal KD, Wilson KG. Acceptance and commitment therapy: an experimental approach to behavior change. New York: Guilford Press; 1999.

61. Forbes D, Creamer M, Allen N, et al. MMPI-2 as a predictor of change in PTSD symptom clusters: a further analysis of the Forbes et al (2002) data set. J Pers Assess 2003;81:183–6.

62. Whisman M. Marital dissatisfaction and psychiatric disorders: results from the national comorbidity survey. J Abnorm Psychol 1999;108(4):701–6.

63. Whisman M. Marital distress and DSM-IV psychiatric disorders in a population-based national survey. J Abnorm Psychol 2007;116(3):638–43.

64. McLeod JD. Anxiety disorders and marital quality. J Abnorm Psychol 1994;103: 767–76.

65. Whisman M, Sheldon C, Goering P. Psychiatric disorders and dissatisfaction with social relationships: does type of relationship matter? J Abnorm Psychol 2000;109(4):803–8.

66. Bryne M, Carr A, Clark M. The efficacy of couple-based interventions for panic disorder with agoraphobia. J Fam Ther 2004;26:105–25.

67. Beach SR, Katz J, Kim S, et al. Prospective effects of marital satisfaction on depressive symptoms in established marriages: a dyadic model. J Soc Pers Relat 2003;20:355–71.

68. Christian JL, O'Leary KD. Depressive symptomatology in maritally discordant spouses: discrimination and prediction. J Fam Psychol 1994;8:32–43.

69. Epstein E, McCrady B, Hirsch L. Marital functioning in early versus late-onset alcoholic couples. Alcohol Clin Exp Res 1997;21(3):547–56.

70. Homish G, Leonard K, Kozlowski L, et al. The longitudinal association between multiple substance use discrepancies and marital satisfaction. Addiction 2009; 104(7):1201–9.

71. Addis M, Jacobson N. Reasons for depression and the process and outcome of cognitive-behavioral psychotherapies. J Consult Clin Psychol 1996;64(6): 1417–24.

72. Hooley J, Teasdale J. Predictors of relapse in unipolar depressives: expressed emotion, marital distress, and perceived criticism. J Abnorm Psychol 1989; 98(3):229–35.

73. Zinbarg R, Lee J, Yoon K. Dyadic predictors of outcome in a cognitive-behavioral program for patients with generalized anxiety disorder in committed relationships: a 'spoonful of sugar' and a dose of non-hostile criticism may help. Behav Res Ther 2007;45(4):699–713.

74. Tarrier N, Pilgrim H, Sommerfield C, et al. A randomized trial of cognitive therapy and imaginal exposure in the treatment of chronic posttraumatic stress disorder. J Consult Clin Psychol 1999;67(1):13–8.

75. Chambless D, Steketee G. Expressed emotion and behavior therapy outcome: a prospective study with obsessive-compulsive and agoraphobic outpatients. J Consult Clin Psychol 1999;67(5):658–65.

76. Jacobson N, Dobson K, Fruzzetti A, et al. Marital therapy as a treatment for depression. J Consult Clin Psychol 1991;59(4):547–57.

77. Beach S, O'Leary K. Treating depression in the context of marital discord: outcome and predictors of response of marital therapy versus cognitive therapy. Behav Ther 1992;23(4):507–28.

78. Emanuels-Zuurveen L, Emmelkamp P. Individual behavioural-cognitive therapy v. marital therapy for depression in maritally distressed couples. Br J Psychiatry 1996;169(2):181–8.

79. Glynn SM, Eth S, Randolph ET, et al. A test of behavioral family therapy to augment exposure for combat-related posttraumatic stress disorder. J Consult Clin Psychol 1999;67:243–51.

80. Bodenmann G, Plancherel B, Beach SR, et al. Effects of coping oriented couples therapy on depression: a randomized clinical trial. J Consult Clin Psychol 2008;76:944–54.

81. Powers MB, Vedel E, Emmelkamp PM. Behavioral couples therapy (BCT) for alcohol and drug use disorders: a meta-analysis. Clin Psychol Rev 2008;28:952–62.

82. Miklowitz D, Axelson D, Birmaher B, et al. Family-focused treatment for adolescents with bipolar disorder: results of a 2-year randomized trial. Arch Gen Psychiatry 2008;65(9):1053–61.

83. Zinbarg R. Comment on "Role of emotion in cognitive-behavior therapy": some quibbles, a call for greater attention to patient motivation for change, and implications of adopting a hierarchical model of emotion. Clin Psychol Sci Pract 2000;7:394–9.

84. Miller WR, Rollnick S. Motivational interviewing: preparing people to change addictive behavior. 2nd edition. New York: Guilford; 2002.

85. Newman CF. Understanding client resistance: methods for enhancing motivation to change. Cognit Behav Pract 1994;1:47–69.

86. Arkowitz H, Burke BL. Motivational interviewing as an integrative framework for the treatment of depression. In: Arkowitz H, Westra HA, Miller WR, et al, editors. Motivational interviewing in the treatment of psychological problems. New York: Guilford; 2008. p. 145–72.

87. Arkowitz H, Westra HA. Integrating motivational interviewing and cognitive behavioral therapy in the treatment of depression and anxiety. J Cognit Psychother 2004;18:337–50.

88. Maltby N, Tolin DF. A brief motivational intervention for treatment-refusing OCD patients. Cognit Behav Ther 2005;34:176–84.

89. Murphy RT. Enhancing combat veterans' motivation to change posttraumatic stress disorder symptoms and other problem behaviors. In: Arkowitz H, Westra HA, Miller WR, et al, editors. Motivational interviewing in the treatment of psychological problems. New York: Guilford; 2008. p. 57–84.

90. Simpson HB, Zuckoff A, Page JR, et al. Adding motivational interviewing to exposure and ritual prevention for obsessive-compulsive disorder: an open pilot trial. Cognit Behav Ther 2008;37(1):38–49.

91. Steketee G, Frost RO. Compulsive hoarding and acquiring: therapist guide. New York: Oxford University Press; 2007.

92. Tolin DF, Maltby N. Motivating treatment-refusing patients with obsessive-compulsive disorder. In: Arkowitz H, Westra HA, Miller WR, et al, editors. Motivational interviewing in the treatment of psychological problems. New York: Guilford; 2008. p. 85–108.

93. Treasure J, Schmidt U. Motivational interviewing in the management of eating disorders. In: Arkowitz H, Westra HA, Miller WR, et al, editors. Motivational interviewing in the treatment of psychological problems. New York: Guilford; 2008. p. 194–224.

94. Westra HA. Managing resistance in cognitive behavioural therapy: the application of motivational interviewing in mixed anxiety and depression. Cognit Behav Ther 2004;33:161–75.

95. Westra HA, Arkowitz H, Dozois DJ. Adding a motivational interviewing pretreatment to cognitive behavioral therapy for generalized anxiety disorder: a preliminary randomized controlled trial. J Anxiety Disord 2009;23:1106–17.

96. Westra HA, Dozois DJ. Preparing clients for cognitive behavioral therapy: a randomized pilot study of motivational interviewing for anxiety. Cognit Ther Res 2006;30:481–98.
97. Westra HA, Dozois DJ. Integrating motivational interviewing into the treatment of anxiety. In: Arkowitz H, Westra HA, Miller WR, et al, editors. Motivational interviewing in the treatment of psychological problems. New York: Guilford; 2008. p. 26–56.
98. Zuckoff A, Swartz HA, Grote NK. Motivational interviewing as a prelude to psychotherapy for depression. In: Arkowitz H, Westra HA, Miller WR, et al, editors. Motivational interviewing in the treatment of psychological problems. New York: Guilford; 2008. p. 109–44.
99. Burns DD, Spangler DL. Does psychotherapy homework lead to improvements in depression in cognitive-behavioral therapy or does improvement lead to increased homework compliance? J Consult Clin Psychol 2000;68:46–56.
100. Schmidt NB, Woolaway-Bickel K. The effects of treatment compliance on outcome in cognitive-behavioral therapy for panic disorder: quality versus quantity. J Consult Clin Psychol 2000;68:13–8.
101. Cheavens JS, Feldman DB, Woodward JT, et al. Hope in cognitive psychotherapies: on working with client strengths. J Cognit Psychother 2006;20: 135–45.
102. Hayes AM, Harris MS. The development of an integrative therapy for depression. In: Johnson SL, Hayes AM, Field TM, et al, editors. Stress, coping and depression. Mahwah (NJ): Erlbaum; 2000. p. 291–306.
103. Wingate L, Van Orden KA, Joiner TE, et al. Comparison of compensation and capitalization models when treating suicidality in young adults. J Consult Clin Psychol 2005;73:756–62.
104. Grawe K. Research-informed psychotherapy. Psychother Res 1997;7:1–19.
105. Grawe K. Psychological psychotherapy. Göttingen (Germany): Hogrefe; 2004. (Original work published in German 1998).
106. Grawe K. Neuropsychotherapy. New York: Erlbaum; 2006. (Original work published in German 2004).
107. Flückiger C, Wüsten G, Zinbarg R, et al. Activation of resources—manual. Seattle (WA): Hogrefe; 2010. (Original work published in Gernan in 2008).
108. Arnkoff DB, Glass CR, Constantino MJ. Expectations and preferences. In: Norcross JC, editor. Psychotherapy relationships that work. New York: Oxford University Press; 2002. p. 335–56.
109. Greenberg RP, Constantino MJ, Bruce N. Are patient expectations still relevant for psychotherapy process and outcome? Clin Psychol Rev 2006;26:657–78.
110. Howard KI, Lueger RJ, Maling MS, et al. A phase model of psychotherapy outcome: causal mediation of change. J Consult Clin Psychol 1993;61(4): 678–85.
111. Stulz N, Lutz W. Multidimensional patterns of change in outpatient psychotherapy: the phase model revisited. J Clin Psychol 2007;63:817–33.
112. Wampold BE. The great psychotherapy debate. Mahwah (NJ): Lawrence Erlbaum; 2001.
113. Flückiger C, Caspar F, Grosse Holtforth M, et al. Working with the patient's strengths—a microprocess approach. Psychother Res 2009;19: 213–23.
114. Gassmann D, Grawe K. General change mechanisms. The relation between problem activation and resource activation in successful and unsuccessful therapeutic interactions. J Clin Psychol 2006;13(1):1–11.

115. Stangier U, Von Cronbruch K, Schramm E, et al. Common factors of cognitive therapy and interpersonal psychotherapy in the treatment of social phobia. Anxiety Stress Coping 2009. DOI: 10.1080/10615800903180239.

116. Znoj HJ, Messerli-Burgy N, Tschopp S, et al. Psychotherapeutic process of cognitive-behavioral intervention in HIV-infected persons: results from a controlled, randomized prospective clinical trial. Psychother Res 2009. DOI: 10.1080/10503300903246663.

117. Flückiger C, Grosse Holtforth M. Focusing the therapist's attention on the patient's strengths—a preliminary study to foster a mechanism of change in outpatient psychotherapy. J Clin Psychol 2008;64:1–14.

118. Weisensee L, Rümenapf A, Stein C. et al. Fostering therapist's attention on patient's strengths—a controlled trial [unpublished master thesis]. University of Bamberg, Germany; 2009.

119. Haug S, Gabriel C, Flückiger C, et al. [Activation of resources – Effectiveness of a minimal-intervention in internet chat groups]. Ressourcenaktivierung beim Patienten -Wirksamkeit einer Minimalintervention in Internet-Chatgruppen. Psychotherapeut 2009 [in German]. DOI:10.1007/s00278-009-0657-7.

120. Willutzki U, Neumann B, Haas H, et al. [Psychotherapy for social phobia: Cognitive behavioral therapy in comparison to a combined resource-oriented approach. A randomized controlled trial]. Psychotherapie sozialer Ängste: kognitive Verhaltenstherapie im Vergleich zu einem kombiniert ressourcenorientierten Vorgehen. Z Klin Psychol Psychiatr Psychother 2004;33:42–50 [in German].

121. Caspar F. Plan analysis. In: Eells T, editor. Handbook of psychotherapeutic case formulations. 2nd edition. New York: Guilford; 2007. p. 251–89.

122. Duncan BL, Miller SD, Wampold BE, et al. The heart and soul of change: delivering what works. 2nd edition. Washington, DC: American Psychological Association; 2010.

123. Borkovec TD, Whisman MA. Psychosocial treatment for generalized anxiety disorder. In: Mavissakalian MR, Prien RF, editors. Long-term treatments of anxiety disorders. Washington, DC: American Psychiatric Association; 1996. p. 171–99.

124. Brown TA, Barlow DH. Long-term outcome in cognitive-behavioral treatment of panic disorder: clinical predictors and alternative strategies for assessment. J Consult Clin Psychol 1995;63:754–65.

125. Craske MG, Brown TA, Barlow DH. Behavioral treatment of panic disorder: a two-year follow-up. Behav Ther 1991;22:289–304.

126. Ogles BM, Lambert MJ, Sawyer JD. Clinical significance of the National Institute of mental health treatment of depression collaborative research program data. J Consult Clin Psychol 1995;63:321–6.

127. Burns DD, Nolen-Hoeksema S. Therapeutic empathy and recovery from depression in cognitive-behavior therapy: a structural equation model. J Consult Clin Psychol 1992;60:441–9.

128. Castonguay LG, Goldfried MR, Wiser S, et al. Predicting the effect of cognitive therapy for depression: a study of unique and common factors. J Consult Clin Psychol 1996;64:497–504.

129. Klein DN, Schwartz JE, Santiago NJ, et al. Therapeutic alliance in depression treatment: controlling for prior change and patient characteristics. J Consult Clin Psychol 2003;71:997–1006.

130. Parloff MB. Placebo controls in psychotherapy research: a sine qua non or a placebo for research problems? J Consult Clin Psychol 1986;54:79–87.

131. Tang TZ, DeRubeis RJ. Sudden gains and critical sessions in cognitive-behavioral therapy for depression. J Consult Clin Psychol 1999;67:894–904.
132. Tang TZ, DeRubeis RJ, Beberman R, et al. Cognitive changes, critical sessions, and sudden gains in cognitive-behavioral therapy for depression. J Consult Clin Psychol 2005;73:168–72.
133. Wampold BE, Serlin RC. The consequences of ignoring a nested factor on measures of effect size in analysis of variance. Psychol Methods 2000;5:425–33.

Index

Note: Page numbers of article titles are in **boldface** type.

Psychiatr Clin N Am 33 (2010) 729–740
doi:10.1016/S0193-953X(10)00065-1
0193-953X/10/$ – see front matter © 2010 Elsevier Inc. All rights reserved.

psych.theclinics.com

Printed and bound by CPI Group (UK) Ltd, Croydon, CR0 4YY

03/10/2024

01040447-0007